Liver Cancer: Diagnosis, Prevention and Treatment

Liver Cancer: Diagnosis, Prevention and Treatment

Edited by Arthur Saunders

STATES
ACADEMIC PRESS
www.statesacademicpress.com

States Academic Press,
109 South 5th Street,
Brooklyn, NY 11249, USA

Visit us on the World Wide Web at:
www.statesacademicpress.com

ISBN: 978-1-63989-333-1

Cataloging-in-Publication Data

Liver cancer : diagnosis, prevention and treatment / edited by Arthur Saunders.
p. cm.
Includes bibliographical references and index.
ISBN 978-1-63989-333-1
1. Liver--Cancer. 2. Liver--Cancer--Diagnosis. 3. Cancer--Prevention.
4. Liver--Cancer--Treatment. I. Saunders, Arthur.
RC280.L5 L58 2022
616.994 36--dc23

Table of Contents

Preface

The cancer that begins in the cells of the liver is known as liver cancer. Many types of cancer can form in the liver among which hepatocellular carcinoma is the most common. Other types of liver cancer are hepatoblastoma and intrahepatic cholangiocarcinoma. The cancer that develops in other parts of the body and spreads to the liver is known as metastatic cancer and not liver cancer. There are no signs and symptoms of liver cancer in most people in the primary stages. But when they appear, they include loss of appetite, unintentional weight loss, abdominal swelling, white and chalky stools, general weakness and fatigue, nausea and vomiting, upper abdominal pain and jaundice. This book contains some path-breaking studies in the field of liver cancer. It presents this complex subject in the most comprehensible and easy to understand language. This book will provide comprehensive knowledge to the readers.

The researches compiled throughout the book are authentic and of high quality, combining several disciplines and from very diverse regions from around the world. Drawing on the contributions of many researchers from diverse countries, the book's objective is to provide the readers with the latest achievements in the area of research. This book will surely be a source of knowledge to all interested and researching the field.

In the end, I would like to express my deep sense of gratitude to all the authors for meeting the set deadlines in completing and submitting their research chapters. I would also like to thank the publisher for the support offered to us throughout the course of the book. Finally, I extend my sincere thanks to my family for being a constant source of inspiration and encouragement.

Editor

1

Molecular Mechanisms of Hepatocellular Carcinoma Related to Aflatoxins

Xi-Dai Long, Yan Deng, Xiao-Ying Huang, Jin-Guang Yao, Qun-Ying Su, Xue-Min Wu, Juan Wang, Qun-Qing Xu, Xiao-Ying Zhu, Chao Wang, Bing-Chen Huang and Qiang Xia

Abstract

Hepatocellular carcinoma (hepatocarcinoma) is a major type of primary liver cancer and one of the most frequent human malignant neoplasms. Aflatoxins are I-type chemical carcinogen for hepatocarcinoma. Increasing evidence has shown that hepatocarcinoma induced by aflatoxins is the result of interaction between aflatoxins and hereditary factor. Aflatoxins can induce DNA damage including DNA strand break, adducts formation, oxidative DNA damage, and gene mutation and determine which susceptible individuals feature cancer. Inheritance such as alterations may result in the activation of proto-oncogenes and the inactivation of tumor suppressor genes and determine individual susceptibility to cancer. Interaction between aflatoxins and genetic susceptible factors commonly involve in almost all pathologic sequence of hepatocarcinoma: chronic liver injury, cirrhosis, atypical hyperplastic nodules, and hepatocarcinoma of early stages. In this review, we discuss the biogenesis, toxification, and epidemiology of aflatoxins and signal pathways of aflatoxin-induced hepatocarcinoma. We also discuss the roles of some important genes related to cell apoptosis, DNA repair, drug metabolism, and tumor metastasis in hepatocarcinogenesis related to aflatoxins.

Keywords: hepatocellular carcinoma, molecular mechanism, aflatoxin

1. Introduction

Hepatocellular carcinoma (also called hepatocarcinoma or liver carcinoma) is a major type of primary liver cancer and one of the most frequent human malignant neoplasms. This malignancy has been proved to correlate with aflatoxins, especially aflatoxin B1 (AFB1) [1–3].

Increasing evidence has exhibited that several mechanisms, including the toxic production from metabolism, the accumulation of DNA damage and genic mutation–induced aflatoxins, the decreasing DNA repair capacity, and dysregulation of signal pathways may play a central role in the tumorigenesis of aflatoxin-induced hepatocarcinoma [4–6]. In this review, we discuss the biogenesis, metabolism, and genic toxification of aflatoxins. We also discuss the molecular mechanisms of aflatoxin-induced hepatocarcinoma, involving in aflatoxin toxification, abnormal change of tumor relative genes, the interaction of aflatoxins and genetic factors, and signal pathway for tumorigenesis. The roles of some important genes related to cell apoptosis, DNA repair, drug metabolism, and tumor metastasis in hepatocarcinogenesis related to aflatoxins are further emphasized.

2. Aflatoxin biosynthesis, metabolism, and toxification

2.1. Aflatoxin biosynthesis

The biosynthesis of aflatoxins has been fully summarized in several previous reviews [7, 8]. In brief, aflatoxins are an important type of mycotoxins, which were the most early identified in the *Aspergillus flavus* (*A. flavus*) and regarded as causative agents of "turkey X" disease in the late 1950s and early 1960s. Thus, these toxins were named as "aflatoxins (namely *A. flavus* toxins)" according to their origin fungus [9]. Until now, 17 related aflatoxin isoforms and aflatoxin metabolites have been identified, and 4 of them often contaminated a number of agricultural commodities [10]. According to the amounts and fluorescent reactions, four aflatoxins primarily identified in foodstuffs are named as AFB1, aflatoxin B2 (AFB2), aflatoxin G1 (AFG1), and aflatoxin G2 (AFG2). Among these four known aflatoxins, AFB1 and AFB2 are named as B-type aflatoxins because they are attached to a pentanone and can produce blue-color fluorescent under UV light, whereas AFG1 and AFG2 are termed as G-type aflatoxins because of their attachment to a 6-membered lactone and producing green fluorescent color feature. These aflatoxins are mainly produced by *A. flavus*, *Aspergillus parasiticus* (*A. parasiticus*), *Aspergillus nidulans* (*A. nidulans*), *Aspergillus pseudotamarii* (*A. pseudotamarii*), and *Aspergillus bombycis* (*A. bombycis*) [7, 8].

Toxigenic strains of *A. flavus* produce only B-type aflatoxins, but do not synthesize G-type aflatoxins due to the deletion of an unstable microsome enzyme and a-220 kDa cytosolic protein. The other aflatoxigenic species including *A. parasiticus*, *A. nidulans*, *A. pseudotamarii*, and *A. bombycis* can produce all four aflatoxins [8].

Numeral synthetical genes, such as aflatoxin regulatory protein gene (aflR), are required for aflatoxin biosynthesis and act as a huge neighbor gene cluster consisting of about 60–70 kb in original fungi (**Figure 1**) [8–10]. All corresponding gene-encoding enzymes and transcription factors produce aflatoxin production and regulate biosynthesis. Increasing evidence has proved that aflatoxin biosynthesis involves in at least 3 stages and 18 enzyme steps (**Figures 2–4**). The first stage, including the first (R01) to eighth reaction (R08) of biosynthesis, refers from acetyl CoA to hydroxyversicolorone. The primary product hydroxyversicolorone will be formed and regulated by transcription factors aflR and aflJ (**Figure 2**) [8, 10]. The second (biosynthesis

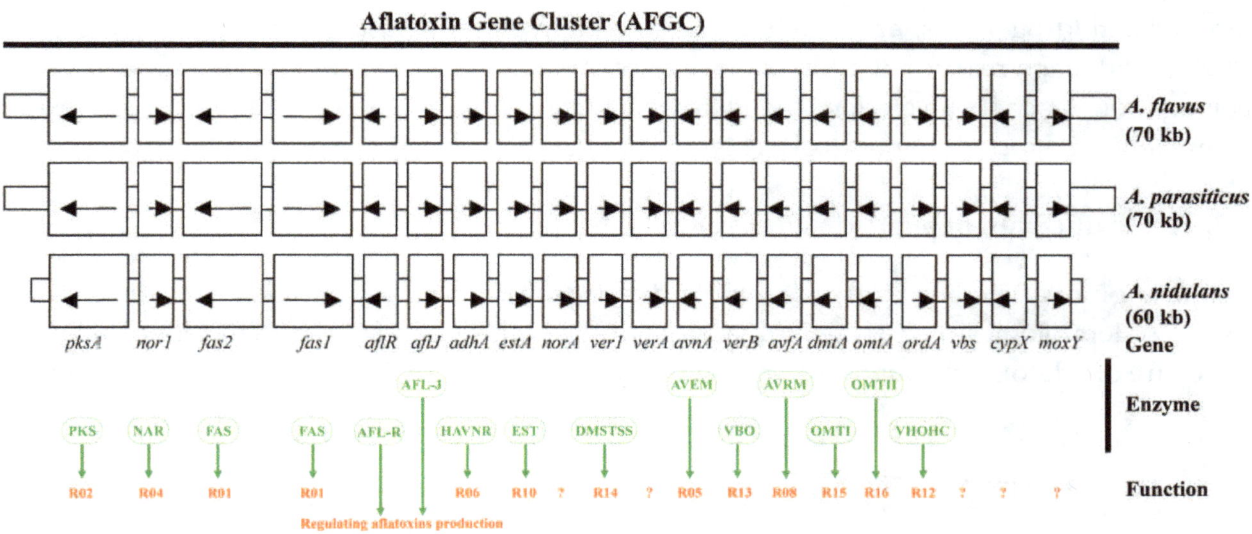

Figure 1. The aflatoxin gene cluster and their expression productions and functions. In the fungus-producing aflatoxins including *A. nidulans, A. parasiticus,* and *A. flavus,* genes encoding the enzymes and the transcription factors involving in aflatoxin biosynthesis commonly locate within a huge gene cluster of about 60–70 kb in the genomes. These genes, except for aflR and aflJ, involve in the 18 enzyme reaction steps (R01–R18) of aflatoxin biosynthesis, whereas aflR and aflJ expressing proteins are two important transcription factors and can regulate enzyme-related gene expression. "?" shows that the function of the corresponding gene is unknown (Note: adapted from Yabe and Nakajima [7]). *Abbreviations.* MCA, malonyl CoA; HAS, hexanoate synthase (also termed fatty acid synthase); PKS, polyketide synthase; NAS, Norsolorinic acid (NA) synthase; NAR, norsolorinic acid (NA) reductase; AVN, averantin; AVNM, averantin (AVN) monooxygenase; HAVN, 5′-hydroxyaverantin; HAVNR, 5′-hydroxyaverantin reductase; OVENC, 5′-oxoaverantin (OAVN) cyclase; AVRM, averufin (AVR) monooxygenase; VHAS, versiconal hemiacetal acetate (VHA) synthase; VHOHC, versiconal (VHOH) cyclase (also called versicolorin B synthase); VHAR, versiconal hemiacetal acetate (VHA) reductase; VBD, versicolorin B (VB) desaturase; DMSTSS, demethylsterigmatocystin (DMST) synthase system; OMTI, *O*-methyltransferase I; OMTII, *O*-methyltransferase II; OAE, OrdA enzyme.

reaction: R09–R12) (**Figure 3**) and third stages (biosynthesis reaction: R13–R18) (**Figure 4**) refer from hydroxyversicolorone to versicolorin B and from versicolorin B (VB) to the formation of ultimate products, respectively. These two stages involve in the formation of hydroxy- and non–hydroxy-versicolorone, and toxins. During the aflatoxin synthesis, more than 10 nicotinamide-adenine dinucleotide phosphate reduced form (NAPDH), one nicotinamide-adenine dinucleotide (NAD), and 2*S*-adenosylmethionine (SAM) are required. These cofactors may play a critical role in the control of aflatoxin biosynthesis [7–10].

2.2. The metabolism of aflatoxins in liver

Aflatoxins synthesized in the mycelia are finally excreted into such mediums as cereals (maize, wheat, sorghum, rice, and millet), nuts (peanuts, pistachios, walnuts, Brazil nut, and coconut), spices (chili, turmeric, paprika, black pepper, and ginger), and seeds. Epidemiological studies have exhibited that AFB1 is the most common in contaminated human foods [8, 10]. Once this aflatoxin in the mediums is taken into body, it is metabolized via two-stage reactions in the liver. The first-stage metabolisms include reduction reaction (ketoreduction to aflatoxicol), oxidative reaction (O-dealkylation to aflatoxin P1), and hydrolytic reactions (hydroxylation to aflatoxin M1, aflatoxin Q1, and aflatoxin B2). This stage reaction involves numerous enzymes such as cytochromes P450 (CYP450), monooxygenases, amino-oxidases, alcohol dehydrogenases, epoxide-hydrolases, aldehyde-reductases, and ketone-reductases. The second-stage reaction mainly comprises covalent binding reaction (toxic produces) and conjugation reaction (excretion and detoxification). Through these metabolites, aflatoxins ultimately transform into nontoxic secretions and toxic products [10, 11].

2.3. The toxification of aflatoxins in liver

Toxification of aflatoxins in liver is mainly divided into acute and chronic toxic effects. Data from epidemiological, experimental, and clinical studies have shown that above 6000 mg exposure of aflatoxin through digestion will cause acute severe liver damage and subsequent

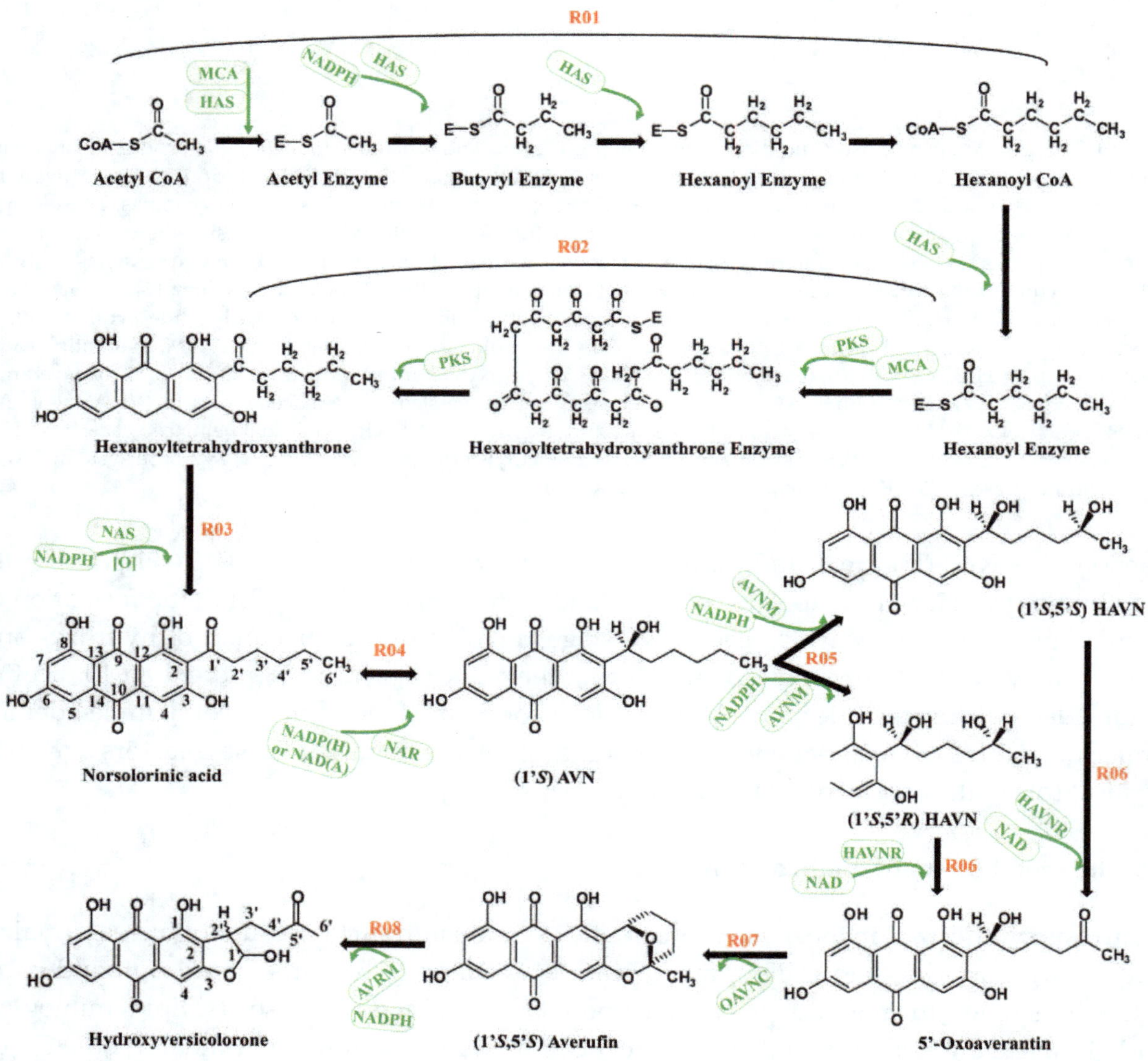

Figure 2. The first stage of aflatoxin biosynthesis. The first stage of aflatoxin biosynthesis, including the first (R01) to eighth reaction (R08) of biosynthesis, refers from acetyl CoA to hydroxyversicolorone. *Abbreviations.* MCA, malonyl CoA; HAS, hexanoate synthase (also termed fatty acid synthase); PKS, polyketide synthase; NAS, norsolorinic acid (NA) synthase; NAR, norsolorinic acid (NA) reductase; AVN, averantin; AVNM, averantin (AVN) monooxygenase; HAVN, 5′-hydroxyaverantin; HAVNR, 5′-hydroxyaverantin reductase; OVENC, 5′-oxoaverantin (OAVN) cyclase; AVRM, averufin (AVR) monooxygenase; NADP, nicotinamide adenine dinucleotide phosphate; NADPH, nicotinamide-adenine dinucleotide phosphate (reduced form); CoA, coenzyme A. *Noted:* adapted from Yabe and Nakajima [7].

illness or death. This kind of acute effect is mainly associated with malfunction of the liver induced by toxic metabolic products. For chronic toxic effects, chronic exposure of aflatoxins can induce DNA damage and produce genotoxicity and carcinogenicity. In the past decades, increasing evidence has proved that AFB1 as aflatoxins often induce genic mutations such as TP53 and are among the most carcinogenic substances known and the major cancerous hepatocarcinoma risk factor.

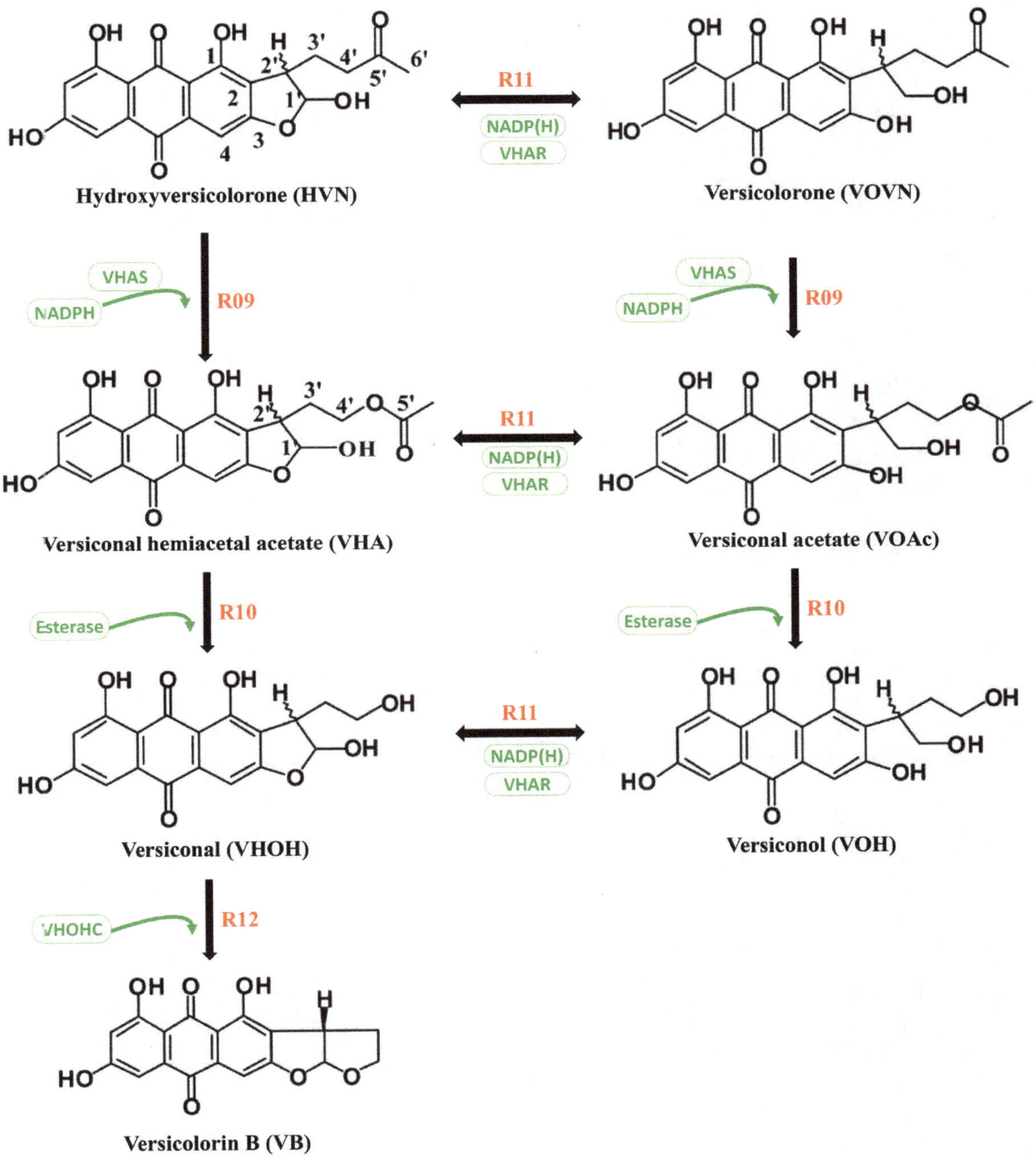

Figure 3. The second stage of aflatoxin biosynthesis. The second stage of aflatoxin biosynthesis, including the ninth (R09) to twelfth reaction (R12) of biosynthesis, refers from hydroxyversicolorone to versicolorin B (VB). *Abbreviations.* VHAS, versiconal hemiacetal acetate (VHA) synthase; VHOHC, versiconal (VHOH) cyclase (also called versicolorin B synthase); VHAR, versiconal hemiacetal acetate (VHA) reductase; NADP, nicotinamide adenine dinucleotide phosphate; NADPH, nicotinamide-adenine dinucleotide phosphate (reduced form). *Noted:* adapted from Yabe and Nakajima [7].

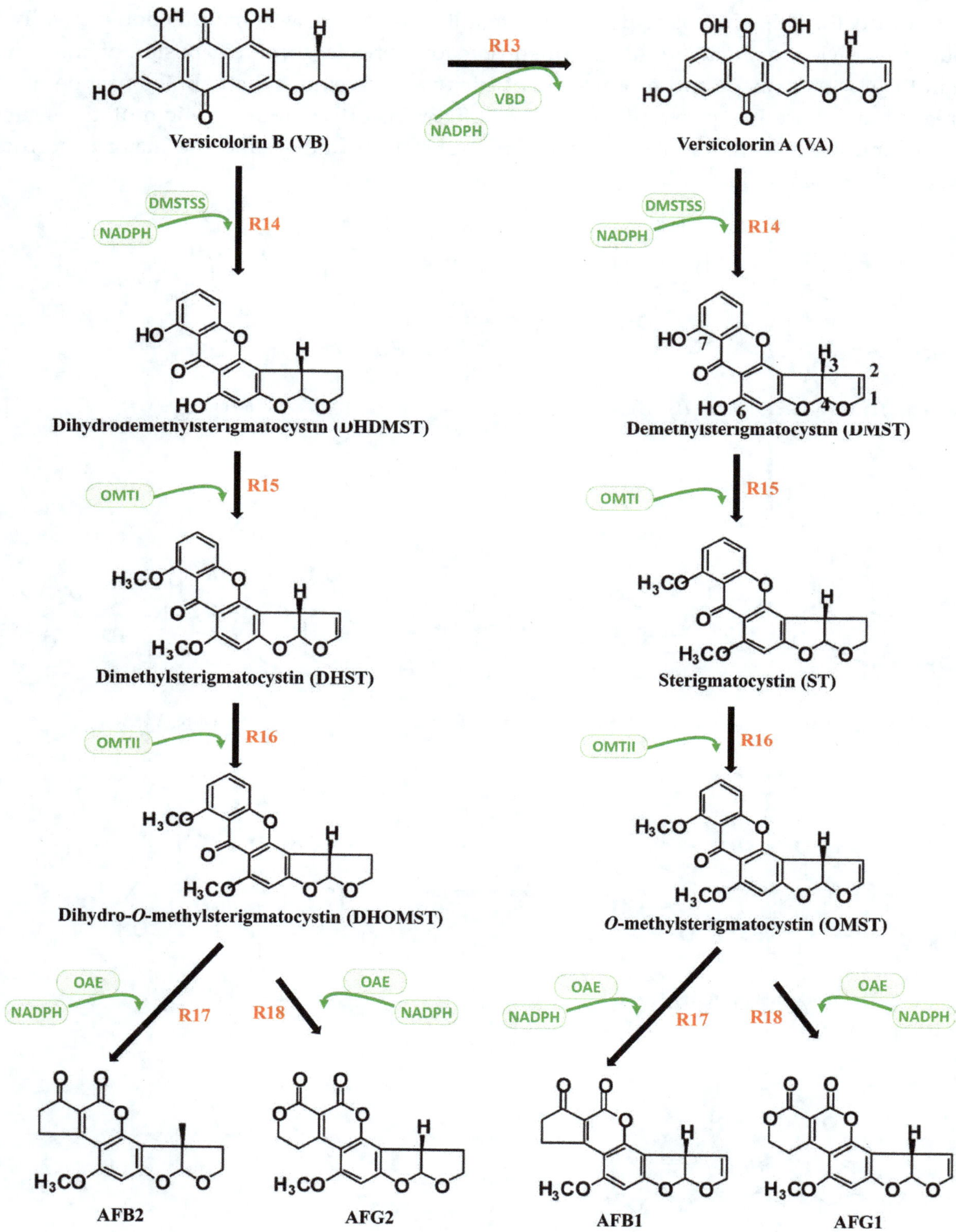

Figure 4. The third stage of aflatoxin biosynthesis. The third stage of aflatoxin biosynthesis, including the 13th (R13) to 18th reaction (R18) of biosynthesis, refers from versicolorin B (VB) to the formation of aflatoxin B1 (AFB1), aflatoxin B2 (AFB2), aflatoxin G1 (AFG1), and aflatoxin G2 (AFG2). *Abbreviations.* VBD, versicolorin B (VB) desaturase; DMSTSS, demethylsterigmatocystin (DMST) synthase system; OMTI, *O*-methyltransferase I; OMTII, *O*-methyltransferase II; OAE, OrdA enzyme; NADP, nicotinamide adenine dinucleotide phosphate; NADPH, nicotinamide-adenine dinucleotide phosphate (reduced form). *Noted:* adapted from Yabe and Nakajima [7].

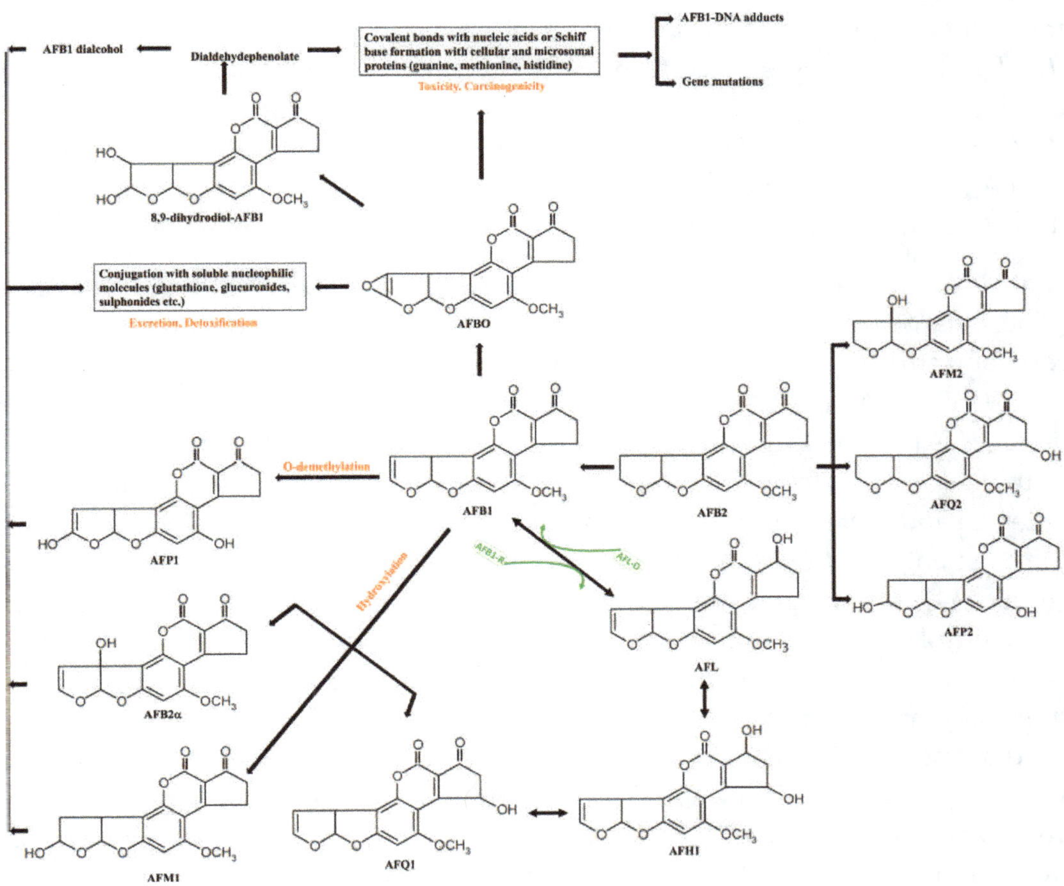

Figure 5. The metabolite of aflatoxins in the liver. Aflatoxins are metabolized via four metabolic pathways: O-dealkylation to aflatoxin P1 (AFP1), ketoreduction to aflatoxicol (AFL), epoxidation to AFB1-8,9-epoxide (AFBO, highly toxic, mutagenic, and carcinogenic), and hydroxylation to aflatoxin M1 (AFM1, highly toxic), AFP1, aflatoxin Q1 (AFQ1), or aflatoxin B2a (AFB2a). *Abbreviations.* AFM2, aflatoxin M2; AFP2, aflatoxin P2; AFQ2, aflatoxin Q2; AFL-D, aflatoxicol dehydrogenase; AFB1-R, aflatoxin B1 reductase. *Noted:* adapted from Wu and Jezkova [10].

3. The molecular mechanisms of aflatoxin-induced hepatocarcinoma

As described earlier, the main chronic toxification of aflatoxins is chronic liver damage and induced tumorigenesis of hepatocarcinoma. AFB1 has been proved as an I-type chemical carcinogen. Mechanisms of AFB1-induced hepatocarcinoma mainly involve in DNA damage and repair, the inactivation of tumor suppressor genes and the activation of oncogenes from genic mutations, abnormal immunoreaction, and inheritance alterations.

3.1. Aflatoxin-induced DNA damage

Increasing evidence has shown that the carcinogenicity of aflatoxins results from aflatoxin-induced DNA damage, including the formation of DNA adducts, DNA single strand breaks (SSBs) or double strand breaks (DSBs), chromosomal aberration damage (CAD), unscheduled DNA synthesis (USDS), abnormal chromatid exchange (ACE), the formation of micronuclei and macronuclei, and oxidation DNA damage. Of these DNA damages, AFB1-DNA adducts are the most common damage types and consist of 8,9-dihydro-8-(N^7-guanyl)-9-hydroxy–AFB1 adduct (AFB1-GA) and ring-opened formamidopyrimidine AFB1 adduct (AFB1-FAPYA). The formation of AFB1-GA begins from AFB1 covalent binding to DNA and its product 8,9-epoxide-AFB1 (AFBE) by CYP450 [12, 13]. This adduct can automatically not only give rise to AFB1-FAYPA, which is accumulated using a time-dependence and nonenzyme pathway, but also be transferred into AFP1, AFM1, AFQ1, and other products by metabolic enzymes.

Additionally, AFB1 also induces oxidation DNA damage such as 8-oxodeoxyguanosine (8-_{oxyG}). These damages induced by aflatoxins, if not timely repaired, can cause subsequent repair-resistant adducts and depurination or lead to error-prone DNA repair resulting in DSBs, SSBs, USDs, CAD, ACE, and frame shift mutations. Interestingly, the accumulation of DNA damages is positively associated with the time and the levels of aflatoxin exposure and modifies the risk of hepatocarcinoma through regulating the expression of some genes such as a disintegrin and metalloproteinase with thrombospondin motifs 5 (ADAMTS5) [14], X-ray repair complementing 4 (XRCC4) [15], microRNA-4651 [16], and so on (**Table 1**). For example, Huang et al. [14] investigated the association between AFB1-DNA adducts via a hospital-based case control study and found increasing AFB1-DNA adducts negatively correlated with ADAMTS5 expression. It is known that ADAMTS5 may act as a tumor suppressor gene via decreasing vascular endothelial growth factor (VEGF) expression and inhibiting tumor angiogenesis and metastasis [17]. The downregulation of XRCC4 by increasing AFB1-DNA adducts decreases repair capacity for SSBs and DSBs and increases risk of tumor suppressor gene TP53 mutation and tumors [15, 18–22]. These genes progress the tumorigenesis and progression of hepatocarcinoma via regulating DNA repair capacity and angiogenesis. Although AFB1-DNA adducts are mainly produced in liver cells, they are also found in the immune cells and may regulate the immune function. Thus, DNA damage may be an important molecular event and may play a crucial role in the carcinogenesis of hepatocarcinoma caused by aflatoxins.

3.2. The mutagenesis of aflatoxins

Aflatoxin-induced DNA adducts can produce depurination, DSBs, the substitution of DNA bases, and frame shift mutations. In the past decades, the *in vivo* and *in vitro* studies have shown that the mutagenesis of aflatoxins can induce the mutation from GC to TA. As previously shown, mispairing of the aflatoxin-DNA adducts can cause both transition and transversion mutations [25–27]. In an *in vitro* non-sense analysis, Foster et al. found that the action form of AFB1 (namely AFBE) can induce more than 90% of GC to TA mutation [28]. This

Gene	Expression change	Role of change in the hepatocarcinoma carcinogenesis	Ref
ADAMTS5	Down	Angiogenesis, metastasis, prognosis	[14]
XRCC4	Down	Low DNA repair capacity, gene mutation	[15]
MicroRNA-4651	Up	Angiogenesis, metastasis, prognosis	[16]
MicroRNA-24	Up	Angiogenesis, metastasis, prognosis	[23]
MicroRNA-429	Up	Angiogenesis, metastasis, prognosis	[24]

Table 1. The change of gene expression related to DNA damage induced by aflatoxins.

mutation was further proved to locate in the GC-rich regions via the plasmid system identifying mutational target enzyme and named as hot-spot regions for aflatoxin-induced mutations [29–31]. Results from quantitative analyses based on the *in vitro* cell model, which was transfected by pS189 (a shuttle vector having mutative targets), also showed that more than 90% of mutative spectra caused by aflatoxins was GC to TA (about 50% of mutations) and GG to TC transversion (about 30% of mutations) [32]. It has been proved that the accumulation of these transversions will result in the mutations of some important genes such as TP53 and Ras and promote hepatocarcinogenesis [31, 33].

3.3. The abnormality of tumor suppressor genes induced by aflatoxins

Studies *in vivo* and *in vitro* have examined the abnormality of tumor suppressor genes by aflatoxin exposure (**Table 2**). Among these known genes, the abnormality of TP53 induced by aflatoxins has been proved to be an important molecule change [34, 35]. In high aflatoxin-exposure areas, the mutations of TP53 gene, especially hot-spot mutation at codon 249, are present among more than 40% of patients with AFB1-related hepatocarcinoma, whereas this kind of mutation is very rare among cases with null or low AFB1 exposure [14, 36, 37]. Therefore, the mutation at codon 249 of TP53 gene has been defined as a molecular symbol for hepatocarcinoma caused by AFB1 exposure. Results from clinical sample and experimental studies further display that consistent exposure of aflatoxins may result in the accumulation of TP53 mutant protein and abnormal DNA damage repair, apoptosis, and immunoreaction [38]. Other genes such as bcl2, p27, p16, and p21 are found to produce different expression or abnormal structural change under the conditions of aflatoxin expression (**Table 2**). Taken together, inactivation of tumor suppressor genes from mutation and increasing mutant expression may be a crucial step of malignant transformation for liver cells.

3.4. The abnormality of oncogenes induced by aflatoxins

In the past decades, the abnormality of oncogenes induced by aflatoxins has mainly been focused on c-myc and ras genes, involving in the activation, expression, and mutation of proto-oncogenes (**Table 3**). For example, Tashiro et al. investigated the effects of AFB1 exposure on oncogenes based on rat model with AFB1-induced hepatomas and found that the expression of both c-myc and c-Ha-ras was upregulated in all the tumors [65]. They also observed c-Ha-ras amplification and rearrangement [65]. In Fischer rat models with AFB1- and AFG1-induced liver tumors, Sinha et al. observed that aflatoxins can induce activation of N-ras and spot mutation of G to A at codon 12 of Ki-ras [66]. This type of activation and mutation will increase in the tissues with liver cancer than those with noncancers [66–69]. Results from *in vitro* studies have further proved that aflatoxins can induce gene mutations of oncogenes [70]. Together, these data suggest that aflatoxins may activate proto-oncogenes by inducing gene mutations and promote the carcinogenesis of hepatocarcinoma.

3.5. The interaction of aflatoxins and hepatitis B virus promoting hepatocarcinogenesis

The interaction of aflatoxins and hepatitis B virus (HBV) has been proved in the carcinogenesis of hepatocarcinoma by molecular epidemiological and clinicopathological studies and sys-

Gene	Study design	Change	Significance	Ref
TP53	Mice model with HNP	Expression ↑	DNA damage ↑	[39]
bcl2	Mice model with HNP	Expression ↓	DNA damage ↑	[39]
p27	Hepatocytes *in vitro*	Expression ↓	DNA damage ↑	[40]
p21	Hepatocytes *in vitro*	Expression ↓	DNA damage ↑	[40]
TP53	HCCs (n = 223)	Expression ↑, multiplot mutation	Carcinogenesis	[41]
TP53	HCCs (n = 124)	Mutation at codon 249: 60%	Carcinogenesis	[42]
H2AX	HCC cells *in vitro*	Phosphorylation	Carcinogenesis	[43]
BP1	HCC cells *in vitro*	Phosphorylation	Carcinogenesis	[43]
TP53	HCCs (n = 52)	Mutation at codon 249: 50%	Carcinogenesis	[44]
p16	HCCs (n = 40)	Methylation	Carcinogenesis	[45]
p53	HCCs (n = 40)	Multiplot mutation	Carcinogenesis	[45]
p53	AFB1-induced mutation *in vitro*	Multiplot mutation at CpG	Carcinogenesis	[46]
TP53	HCCs (n = 64) plus a meta-analysis	Mutation at codon 249: 36%, protein accumulation: 50%	Carcinogenesis	[47]
TP53	Mice model with HNP	Multiplot mutation	Carcinogenesis	[48]
TP53	HCC cells *in vitro*	AFB1-induced mutation at codon 249 promoting IGF-II expression	Carcinogenesis	[49]
TP53	Atcc-Ccl13 *in vitro*	Mutation at codon 249	Carcinogenesis	[50]
TP53	HCCs (n = 36)	Mutation at codon 249	Carcinogenesis	[51]
TP53	Mice model	Mutation at codon 249 and 346, mutant protein increasing	Carcinogenesis	[52–57]
TP53	HCCs (n = 60)	Mutation at codon 249: 69%	Carcinogenesis	[58, 59]
TP53	Hepatocytes *in vitro*	Multiplot mutation	Carcinogenesis	[60]
TP53	HCCs (n = 110)	Mutation at codon 249: 69%	DNA damage, carcinogenesis	[61]
TP53	HCCs (n = 15)	Mutation at codon 249 and 254	Carcinogenesis	[62]
TP53	HCC cells *in vitro*	AFB1-induced Mutation at codon 249	Carcinogenesis	[63]
TP53	HCCs (n = 18)	Mutation at codon 249: 53%	Carcinogenesis	[64]

Abbreviations. HNP, hepatic neoplasms; HCC, hepatocarcinoma.

Table 2. The change information of tumor suppressor genes induced by aflatoxins in hepatic cells and hepatocarcinoma cells.

Gene	Study design	Change	Significance	Ref
N-ras	HCCs (n = 36)	Mutation at codon 61	Carcinogenesis	[51]
c-myc	Mice model with HNP	Expression ↑, amplification, rearrangement	Carcinogenesis	[65]
c-Ha-ras	Mice model with HNP	Expression ↑, amplification, rearrangement	Carcinogenesis	[65]
Ki-ras	Mice model with HNP	Activation	Carcinogenesis	[69]
N-ras	Mice model with HNP	Activation	Carcinogenesis	[66]
Ki-ras	Mice model with HNP	Mutation at codon 12	Carcinogenesis	[66]
N-ras	Mice model with HCC	Activation	Carcinogenesis	[67]
Ki-ras	Mice model with HCC	Activation	Carcinogenesis	[67]
c-Ha-ras	Mice model with HNP	Mutation at codon 61: 40–60%	Carcinogenesis	[71, 72]

Abbreviations. HNP, hepatic neoplasms; HCC, hepatocarcinoma.

Table 3. The change information of oncogenes induced by aflatoxins.

tematically reviewed by several studies [73–75]. In brief, the first clinicopathological evidence of aflatoxins interacting with HBV was provided by Yeh et al. [76]. Through a case-control study design conducted in Guangxi Area, they found that these HBV-positive individuals with high AFB1 exposure consumption featured 10-times the mortality rate compared with those with low exposure consumption. Results from multivariable interactive analyses have further convinced that AFB1 multiplicatively interacted with HBV status for promoting hepatocarcinoma risk [77–80]. For example, Williams et al. reported that the risk of developing hepatocarcinoma was 6.37 for aflatoxin exposure, 11.3 for HBV infection, and 73.0 for the combination of aflatoxin and HBV [77]. The following several molecular epidemiological studies with large-size samples from areas with high aflatoxin exposure and high HBV infection in China showed remarkably multiplicative effect for hepatocarcinoma risk (multiplicative interaction: $63.2_{\text{(both positive)}} > 1.9_{\text{(AFB1 positive)}} \times 9.5_{\text{(HBV positive)}}$ [78–80].

This interaction of two hepatocarcinogenic causes has been proved in the transgenic mice models with overexpressing HBV large envelope polypeptide [81]. Results from this study exhibited that animals will produce more rapid and extensive hepatic dysplasia and hepatocarcinoma under the conditions with aflatoxin consumption [81]. Similar findings have also shown in the studies based on woodchuck and duck models [82–84].

The aflatoxins interacting with HBV infection promoting hepatocarcinoma development mechanically involve in the following aspects. First, HBV infection directly or indirectly increases the sensitivity of hepatocytes on the toxification of aflatoxins. Evidence from observation studies have displayed that HBV-positive carriers have more amount of aflatoxin adducts than those with negative HBV status, although they are from the same high aflatoxin exposure area [85, 86]. The active product of aflatoxin AFBE is found to significantly increase the risk of viral DNA integrating into damaged DNA strand [87]. This promotes malignant transformation of damaged hepatocytes by aflatoxins. Second, HBV infection increases the mutation frequency at codon 249 of TP53 gene and coordinates with aflatoxins for abrogating the normal functions of TP53 (such as the control of cell cycle, DNA damage repair, and cell apoptosis), which contributes to multisteps of hepatic carcinogenesis [64, 88]. Third, the HBV X gene–expressing protein inhibits base excision repair potential and results in an increasing accumulation of aflatoxin-DNA adducts [89]. Finally, HBV infections can cause hepatocytic necrosis, inflammatory proliferation, and oxygen/nitrogen active products, which may increase the likelihood of aflatoxin-induced mutations and the cellular clonal expansion containing mutations [90–92].

3.6. The interaction of aflatoxins and inheritance alterations promoting hepatocarcinogenesis

Increasing evidence has exhibited that the genetic alterations in DNA repair genes increase the amount of AFB1-DNA adducts and the frequency of hot-spot mutation at codon 249 of TP53 gene and may promote hepatic toxification of aflatoxins [1, 19, 20, 22, 37, 93–98]. Joint analyses based on meta-analyses further showed this kind of toxic effects (**Table 4**) [1, 22]. The genetic variants in other genes, such as CYP450, glutathione *S*-transferase T1 (GSTT1), glutathione *S*-transferase M1 (GSTM1), and microsomal epoxide hydrolase (HEHY), also display similar modificative effects on aflatoxin-induced hepatocarcinoma [98–101]. Interestingly, the multiplicatively interactive effects between aflatoxins and genetic alterations in these genes have been identified in the risk elucidation of hepatocarcinoma related to aflatoxins [22]. Taken together, genetic deficiency in the DNA repair and detoxification capacity may play a vital role in the carcinogenetic process of aflatoxin-induced hepatocarcinoma.

3.7. The aflatoxin-caused immunosuppression promoting hepatocarcinogenesis

Increasing evidence from *in vitro* and *in vivo* studies has proved that the immunosuppression induced by aflatoxins plays an important role in the carcinogenesis of hepatocarcinoma. Several known mechanisms may involve in this progression step. First, aflatoxins can significantly suppress the functions of macrophages via affecting the expression and secretions of cytokines such as tumor necrosis factor (TNF)-α, interleukin (IL)-1, IL-2, IL-3, IL-6, and reactive intermediates (including nitric oxide, hydrogen peroxide, and superoxide anion) [102, 103]. The suppression of macrophages by aflatoxins may be also correlated with the arrest in the G1/G0 phase [104] and altered expression of CD14 (a cell surface protein functionally regulating immunoreaction) [105]. This suppression may result in the dysregulation of the immune response and homeostasis, which contributes to the accumulation of abnormal cells with DNA damage and altered genome induced by aflatoxins, and ultimately progresses tumorigenesis. Second, aflatoxin exposure can decrease the secretion of antibody such as IgA [106]. For example, Turner et al. investigated effects of aflatoxin exposure on antibody production based on a large molecular epidemiological study [106]. In their study, they tested the levels of saliva secretory IgA (sIgA) in Gambian children (n = 472) with different degree exposure of aflatoxins and found that these individuals with high aflatoxin exposure featured lower level of sIgA in their saliva compared to those without high exposure (50.4 vs. 70.2 μg/mg protein). Finally, aflatoxins may alter T-cell functions (including decreased T-cell populations and suppressed CD4+ T-cell function) and increase individuals' susceptibility to other carcinogens [77, 107].

Gene	RS#	Genotype	TP53M			DNA adducts	
			%	Risk	*P*	Mean	*P*
XRCC1	rs25487	CC	46.51	Reference		3.276	
		CT	45.25	2.419	3.371×10^{-11}	3.264	0.899
		TT	8.24	5.028	6.651×10^{-6}	3.640	0.026
XRCC3	rs861539	GG	32.17	Reference		2.990	
		GA	43.55	1.380	0.018	3.216	0.025
		AA	24.28	1.524	0.011	3.897	4.962×10^{-14}
XRCC7	rs7003908	AA	21.24	Reference		2.879	
		AC	46.06	1.883	1.372×10^{-5}	3.347	1.663×10^{-5}
		CC	32.71	2.089	4.368×10^{-6}	3.550	1.751×10^{-8}
XRCC4	rs28383151	GG	67.03	Reference		3.308	
		GA	21.68	1.688	0.001	3.405	0.069
		AA	11.29	3.829	7.387×10^{-6}	3.721	2.867×10^{-4}
XRCC4	rs3734091	GG	72.31	Reference		3.229	
		GT	17.56	2.799	9.191×10^{-7}	3.439	0.095
		TT	10.13	5.104	3.826×10^{-6}	3.654	0.005
XPD	rs13181	TT	34.41	Reference		2.926	
		TG	41.85	1.458	0.005	3.253	0.011
		GG	23.75	1.744	0.001	4.062	4.265×10^{-6}
XPC	rs2228001	TT	34.05	Reference		3.083	
		TG	48.30	1.500	0.002	3.332	0.001
		GG	17.65	1.818	0.001	3.666	3.404×10^{-22}

Noted: Adapted from Refs. [13] and [84]. *Abbreviations.* TP53M, hot-spot mutation at codon 249 of TP53 gene; RS#, the number of polymorphism.

Table 4. Polymorphisms in DNA repair genes and HCC risk.

Altogether, the data available to date make it clear that aflatoxins can exert an immunosuppressive effect via different pathways. However, more detailed mechanisms by which this effect is mediated remain unknown.

4. Limitation and further direction

In the past decades, the advance in pathological mechanisms of aflatoxin-related hepatocarcinoma held great promise. However, we are still far from a comprehensive view of this kind of potentials. First, the detailed metabolic step and corresponding enzymes, especially the first-stage reaction and toxicity mechanisms, have not been elucidated. Second, although the activation of aflatoxins is found to act as a crucial step, it is unclear how the tumorigenesis of hepatocarcinoma is triggered by aflatoxins. Third, the vast literature for aflatoxin-induced hepatocarcinoma mainly focuses on the studies on AFB1, and some important information may have been lost. Fourth, in spite of some evidence of AFB1 inducing abnormal immunoreaction and interacting with hepatitis virus and genetic factors, they are at the primary stage and still far from elucidation. Therefore, the detailed toxicity mechanisms of aflatoxins and corresponding carcinogenesis mechanism will greatly benefit our understanding of aflatoxin-related hepatocarcinoma.

5. Summary

It has been shown that increasing exposure of aflatoxins may promote the carcinogenesis of hepatocarcinoma. Molecular mechanisms of aflatoxin-induced hepatocarcinoma involve in DNA damage, gene mutations, the inactivation of such tumor suppressor gene as TP53, the activation of proto-oncogenes, abnormal immunoreaction, and the interaction between aflatoxins and other carcinogens such as HBV. However, an understanding of aflatoxin-induced hepatocarcinoma is far from complete, and further research in this field is looked forward to elucidating more detailed mechanisms responsible for hepatocarcinoma related to aflatoxins in the future.

Conflicts of interest and source of funding

The authors declare no competing financial interests. This study was supported in part by the National Natural Science Foundation of China (Nos. 81760502, 81572353, 81372639, 81472243, 81660495, and 81460423), the Innovation Program of Guangxi Municipal Education Department (Nos. 201204LX674 and 201204LX324), Innovation Program of Guangxi Health Department (No. Z2013781), the Natural Science Foundation of Guangxi (Nos. 2017GXNSFGA198002, 2017JJF10001, 2017GXNSFAA198002, 2016GXNSFDA380003, 2015GXNSFAA139223, 2013GXNSFAA019251, 2014GXNSFDA118021, and 2014GXNSFAA118144), Research Program of Guangxi "Zhouyue Scholar" (No. 2017-38), Research Program of Guangxi Specially-invited Expert (No. 2017-6th), Research Program of Guangxi Clinic Research Center of Hepatobiliary Diseases (No. AD17129025), and Open Research Program from Molecular Immunity Study Room Involving in Acute & Severe Diseases in Guangxi Colleges and Universities (Nos. kfkt20160062 and kfkt20160063).

Abbreviations

AFB1	aflatoxin B1
AFB2	aflatoxin B2
AFG1	aflatoxin G1

AFG2	aflatoxin G2
AFP	α-fetoprotein
A. flavus	*Aspergillus flavus*
A. parasiticus	*Aspergillus parasiticus*
A. nidulans	*Aspergillus nidulans*
A. pseudotamarii	*Aspergillus pseudotamarii*
A. bombycis	*Aspergillus bombycis*
HBV	hepatitis virus B
HCV	hepatitis virus C
Hepatocarcinoma	hepatocellular carcinoma
NAPDH	nicotinamide-adenine dinucleotide phosphate reduced form
NAD	one nicotinamide-adenine dinucleotide
SAM	*S*-adenosylmethionine
CYP450	cytochromes P450

Author details

Xi-Dai Long[1,2,3*†], Yan Deng[4†], Xiao-Ying Huang[1†], Jin-Guang Yao[1†], Qun-Ying Su[1†], Xue-Min Wu[1†], Juan Wang[1†], Qun-Qing Xu[3], Xiao-Ying Zhu[3], Chao Wang[5], Bing-Chen Huang[1] and Qiang Xia[2]

*Address all correspondence to: sjtulongxd@263.net

1 Department of Pathology, the Affiliated Hospital of Youjiang Medical University for Nationalities, Baise, China

2 Department of Liver Surgery, Ren Ji Hospital, School of Medicine, Shanghai Jiao Tong University, Shanghai, China

3 Guangxi Clinic Research Center of Hepatobiliary Diseases, Baise, China

4 Department of Epidemiology, Youjiang Medical University for Nationalities, Baise, China

5 Department of Medicine, the Affiliated Hospital of Youjiang Medical University for Nationalities, Baise, China

† These authors contributed equally to this work.

References

[1] Long XD, Yao JD, Yang Q, Huang CH, Liao P, Nong LG, Tang YJ, Huang XY, Wang C, Wu XM, Huang BC, Ban FZ, Zeng LX, Ma Y, Zhai B, Zhang JQ, Xue F, Lu CX, Xia Q. Polymorphisms of DNA repair genes and toxicological effects of aflatoxin B1 exposure. In: Faulkner AG, editor. Aflatoxins: Food Sources, Occurrence and Toxicological Effects. 1st ed. New York: Nova Science Publishers; 2014. pp. 107-124. DOI: 978-1-63117-298-4

[2] Siegel RL, Miller KD, Jemal A. Cancer statistics, 2017. CA: A Cancer Journal for Clinicians. 2017;**67**:7-30. DOI: 10.3322/caac.21387

[3] Chen W, Zheng R, Baade PD, Zhang S, Zeng H, Bray F, Jemal A, Yu XQ, He J. Cancer statistics in China, 2015. CA: A Cancer Journal for Clinicians. 2016;**66**:115-132. DOI: 10.3322/caac.21338

[4] Umesha S, Manukumar HM, Chandrasekhar B, Shivakumara P, Shiva Kumar J, Raghava S, Avinash P, Shirin M, Bharathi TR, Rajini SB, Nandhini M, Vinaya Rani GG, Shobha M, Prakash HS. Aflatoxins and food pathogens: Impact of biologically active aflatoxins and their control strategies. Journal of the Science of Food and Agriculture. 2017;**97**:1698-1707. DOI: 10.1002/jsfa.8144

[5] Sarma UP, Bhetaria PJ, Devi P, Varma A. Aflatoxins: Implications on health. Indian Journal of Clinical Biochemistry. 2017;**32**:124-133. DOI: 10.1007/s12291-017-0649-2

[6] Kowalska A, Walkiewicz K, Koziel P, Muc-Wierzgon M. Aflatoxins: characteristics and impact on human health. Postepy Higieny i Medycyny Doświadczalnej (Online). 2017;**71**:315-327. DOI: 10.5604/01.3001.0010.3816

[7] Yabe K, Nakajima H. Enzyme reactions and genes in aflatoxin biosynthesis. Applied Microbiology and Biotechnology. 2004;**64**:745-755. DOI: 10.1007/s00253-004-1566-x

[8] Abrar M, Anjum FM, Butt MS, Pasha I, Randhawa MA, Saeed F, Waqas K. Aflatoxins: Biosynthesis, occurrence, toxicity, and remedies. Critical Reviews in Food Science and Nutrition. 2013;**53**:862-874. DOI: 10.1080/10408398.2011.563154

[9] Kensler TW, Roebuck BD, Wogan GN, Groopman JD. Aflatoxin: A 50-year odyssey of mechanistic and translational toxicology. Toxicological Sciences. 2011;**120**(Suppl 1):S28-S48. DOI: 10.1093/toxsci/kfq283

[10] Wu Q, Jezkova A, Yuan Z, Pavlikova L, Dohnal V, Kuca K. Biological degradation of aflatoxins. Drug Metabolism Reviews. 2009;**41**:1-7. DOI: 10.1080/03602530802563850

[11] Woloshuk CP, Shim WB. Aflatoxins, fumonisins, and trichothecenes: A convergence of knowledge. FEMS Microbiology Reviews. 2013;**37**:94-109. DOI: 10.1111/1574-6976.12009

[12] Essigmann JM, Croy RG, Nadzan AM, Busby WF Jr, Reinhold VN, Buchi G, Wogan GN. Structural identification of the major DNA adduct formed by aflatoxin B1 in vitro. Proceedings of the National Academy of Sciences of the United States of America. 1977;**74**:1870-1874. DOI: 10.1073/pnas.PMC431033

[13] Croy RG, Essigmann JM, Reinhold VN, Wogan GN. Identification of the principal aflatoxin B1-DNA adduct formed in vivo in rat liver. Proceedings of the National Academy of Sciences of the United States of America. 1978;**75**:1745-1749. DOI: 10.1073/pnas.PMC392416

[14] Huang XY, Yao JG, Huang BC, Ma Y, Xia Q, Long XD. Polymorphisms of a disintegrin and metalloproteinase with thrombospondin motifs 5 and aflatoxin B1-related hepatocellular carcinoma. Cancer Epidemiology, Biomarkers & Prevention. 2016;**25**:334-343. DOI: 10.1158/1055-9965.EPI-15-0774

[15] Lu J, Wang XZ, Zhang TQ, Huang XY, Yao JG, Wang C, Wei ZH, Ma Y, Wu XM, Luo CY, Xia Q, Long XD. Prognostic significance of XRCC4 expression in hepatocellular carcinoma. Oncotarget. 2017;**8**:87955-87970. DOI: 10.18632/oncotarget.21360

[16] Wu XM, Xi ZF, Liao P, Huang HD, Huang XY, Wang C, Ma Y, Xia Q, Yao JG, Long XD. Diagnostic and prognostic potential of serum microRNA-4651 for patients with hepatocellular carcinoma related to aflatoxin B1. Oncotarget. 2017;**8**:81235-81249. DOI: 10.18632/oncotarget.16027

[17] Li C, Xiong Y, Yang X, Wang L, Zhang S, Dai N, Li M, Ren T, Yang Y, Zhou SF, Gan L, Wang D. Lost expression of ADAMTS5 protein associates with progression and poor prognosis of hepatocellular carcinoma. Drug Design, Development and Therapy. 2015;**9**:1773-1783. DOI: 10.2147/DDDT.S77069

[18] Long XD, Ma Y, Huang YZ, Yi Y, Liang QX, Ma AM, Zeng LP, Fu GH. Genetic polymorphisms in DNA repair genes XPC, XPD, and XRCC4, and susceptibility to helicobacter pylori infection-related gastric antrum adenocarcinoma in Guangxi population. China Molecular Carcinogenesis. 2010;**49**:611-618. DOI: 10.1002/mc.20630

[19] Long XD, Yao JG, Zeng Z, Ma Y, Huang XY, Wei ZH, Liu M, Zhang JJ, Xue F, Zhai B, Xia Q. Polymorphisms in the coding region of X-ray repair complementing group 4 and aflatoxin B1-related hepatocellular carcinoma. Hepatology. 2013;**58**:171-181. DOI: 10.1002/hep.26311

[20] Long XD, Zhao D, Wang C, Huang XY, Yao JG, Ma Y, Wei ZH, Liu M, Zeng LX, Mo XQ, Zhang JJ, Xue F, Zhai B, Xia Q. Genetic polymorphisms in DNA repair genes XRCC4 and XRCC5 and aflatoxin B1-related hepatocellular carcinoma. Epidemiology. 2013;**24**:671-681. DOI: 10.1097/EDE.0b013e31829d2744

[21] Lin ZH, Chen JC, Wang YS, Huang TJ, Wang J, Long XD. DNA repair gene XRCC4 codon 247 polymorphism modified diffusely infiltrating astrocytoma risk and prognosis. International Journal of Molecular Sciences. 2014;**15**:250-260. DOI: 10.3390/ijms15010250

[22] Yao JG, Huang XY, Long XD. Interaction of DNA repair gene polymorphisms and aflatoxin B1 in the risk of hepatocellular carcinoma. International Journal of Clinical and Experimental Pathology. 2014;**7**:6231-6244. DOI: 10.2016/1936-2625.25337275

[23] Liu YX, Long XD, Xi ZF, Ma Y, Huang XY, Yao JG, Wang C, Xing TY, Xia Q. MicroRNA-24 modulates aflatoxin B1-related hepatocellular carcinoma prognosis and tumorigenesis. BioMed Research International. 2014;**2014**:482926. DOI: 10.1155/2014/482926

[24] Huang XY, Yao JG, Huang HD, Wang C, Ma Y, Xia Q, Long XD. MicroRNA-429 modulates hepatocellular carcinoma prognosis and tumorigenesis. Gastroenterology Research and Practice. 2013;**2013**:804128. DOI: 10.1155/2013/804128

[25] Hagiwara N, Mechanic LE, Trivers GE, Cawley HL, Taga M, Bowman ED, Kumamoto K, He P, Bernard M, Doja S, Miyashita M, Tajiri T, Sasajima K, Nomura T, Makino H, Takahashi K, Hussain SP, Harris CC. Quantitative detection of p53 mutations in plasma DNA from tobacco smokers. Cancer Research. 2006;**66**:8309-8317. DOI: 10.1158/0008-5472. CAN-06-0991

[26] Harris LC, Remack JS, Houghton PJ, Brent TP. Wild-type p53 suppresses transcription of the human O6-methylguanine-DNA methyltransferase gene. Cancer Research. 1996; **56**:2029-2032

[27] Harris CC. Tumour suppressor genes, multistage carcinogenesis and molecular epidemiology. IARC Scientific Publications. 1992:67-85 DOI: PMID1428103

[28] Foster PL, Eisenstadt E, Miller JH. Base substitution mutations induced by metabolically activated aflatoxin B1. Proceedings of the National Academy of Sciences of the U S A. 1983;**80**:2695-2698. DOI: PMC393894

[29] Qi LN, Bai T, Chen ZS, Wu FX, Chen YY, De Xiang B, Peng T, Han ZG, Li LQ. The p53 mutation spectrum in hepatocellular carcinoma from Guangxi, China: Role of chronic hepatitis B virus infection and aflatoxin B1 exposure. Liver International. 2014. DOI: 10.1111/liv.12460

[30] Golli-Bennour EE, Kouidhi B, Bouslimi A, Abid-Essefi S, Hassen W, Bacha H. Cytotoxicity and genotoxicity induced by aflatoxin B1, ochratoxin A, and their combination in cultured Vero cells. Journal of Biochemical and Molecular Toxicology. 2010;**24**:42-50. DOI: 10.1002/jbt.20310

[31] Paget V, Sichel F, Garon D, Lechevrel M. Aflatoxin B1-induced TP53 mutational pattern in normal human cells using the FASAY (functional analysis of separated alleles in yeast). Mutation Research. 2008;**656**:55-61. DOI: 10.1016/j.mrgentox.2008.07.009

[32] Levy DD, Groopman JD, Lim SE, Seidman MM, Kraemer KH. Sequence specificity of aflatoxin B1-induced mutations in a plasmid replicated in xeroderma pigmentosum and DNA repair proficient human cells. Cancer Research 1992;**52**:5668-5673. DOI: 10.1158/0008-5472. CAN-Published-October-1992

[33] Wang JS, Groopman JD. DNA damage by mycotoxins. Mutation Research. 1999;**424**:167-181. DOI: 10.1016/S0027-5107(99)00017-2

[34] Long XD, Yao JG, Zeng Z, Huang CH, Huang ZS, Huang YZ, Ban FZ, Huang XY, Yao LM, Fan LD, Fu GH. DNA repair capacity-related to genetic polymorphisms of DNA repair genes and aflatoxin B1-related hepatocellular carcinoma among Chinese population. In: Kruman I, editor. DNA Repair. Rijeka: InTech; 2011. pp. 505-524. DOI: 10.5772/20792

[35] Xia Q, Huang XY, Xue F, Zhang JJ, Zhai B, Kong DC, Wang C, Huang ZQ, Long XD. Genetic polymorphisms of DNA repair genes and DNA repair capacity related to aflatoxin

b1 (AFB1)-induced DNA damages. In: Chen C, editor. New Research Directions in DNA Repair. 1st ed. Rijeka: InTech; 2013. pp. 377-412. DOI: 10.5772/53967

[36] Chen BP, Long XD, Fu GH. Meta-analysis of XRCC1 codon 399 polymorphism and susceptibility of hepatocellular carcinoma. Journal of Shanghai Jiao Tong University (Medical Science). 2011;**31**:1588-1602. DOI: 10.3969/j.issn.1674-8115.2011.11.018

[37] Long XD, Huang HD, Huang XY, Yao JG, Xia Q. XPC codon 939 polymorphism is associated with susceptibility to DNA damage induced by aflatoxin B1 exposure. International Journal of Clinical and Experimental Medicine. 2015;**8**:1197-1204. DOI: PMC4358568

[38] Shen HM, Ong CN. Mutations of the p53 tumor suppressor gene and ras oncogenes in aflatoxin hepatocarcinogenesis. Mutation Research. 1996;**366**:23-44. DOI: 10.1016/S0165-1110(96)90005-6

[39] Alm-Eldeen AA, Basyony MA, Elfiky NK, Ghalwash MM. Effect of the Egyptian propolis on the hepatic antioxidant defense and pro-apoptotic p53 and anti-apoptotic bcl2 expressions in aflatoxin B1 treated male mice. Biomedicine & Pharmacotherapy. 2017;**87**:247-255. DOI: 10.1016/j.biopha.2016.12.084

[40] Ranchal I, Gonzalez R, Bello RI, Ferrin G, Hidalgo AB, Linares CI, Aguilar-Melero P, Gonzalez-Rubio S, Barrera P, Marchal T, Nakayama KI, de la Mata M, Muntane J. The reduction of cell death and proliferation by p27(Kip1) minimizes DNA damage in an experimental model of genotoxicity. International Journal of Cancer. 2009;**125**:2270-2280. DOI: 10.1002/ijc.24621

[41] Qi LN, Bai T, Chen ZS, Wu FX, Chen YY, De Xiang B, Peng T, Han ZG, Li LQ. The p53 mutation spectrum in hepatocellular carcinoma from Guangxi, China: Role of chronic hepatitis B virus infection and aflatoxin B1 exposure. Liver International. 2015;**35**:999-1009. DOI: 10.1111/liv.12460

[42] Chittmittrapap S, Chieochansin T, Chaiteerakij R, Treeprasertsuk S, Klaikaew N, Tangkijvanich P, Komolmit P, Poovorawan Y. Prevalence of aflatoxin induced p53 mutation at codon 249 (R249s) in hepatocellular carcinoma patients with and without hepatitis B surface antigen (HBsAg). Asian Pacific Journal of Cancer Prevention. 2013;**14**:7675-7679. DOI: PMID24460352

[43] Gursoy-Yuzugullu O, Yuzugullu H, Yilmaz M, Ozturk M. Aflatoxin genotoxicity is associated with a defective DNA damage response bypassing p53 activation. Liver International. 2011;**31**:561-571. DOI: 10.1111/j.1478-3231.2011.02474.x

[44] Pineau P, Marchio A, Battiston C, Cordina E, Russo A, Terris B, Qin LX, Turlin B, Tang ZY, Mazzaferro V, Dejean A. Chromosome instability in human hepatocellular carcinoma depends on p53 status and aflatoxin exposure. Mutation Research. 2008;**653**:6-13. DOI: 10.1016/j.mrgentox.2008.01.012

[45] Zhang YJ, Rossner P Jr, Chen Y, Agrawal M, Wang Q, Wang L, Ahsan H, Yu MW, Lee PH, Santella RM. Aflatoxin B1 and polycyclic aromatic hydrocarbon adducts, p53 mutations and p16 methylation in liver tissue and plasma of hepatocellular carcinoma patients. International Journal of Cancer. 2006;**119**:985-991. DOI: 10.1002/ijc.21699

[46] Chan KT, Hsieh DP, Lung ML. In vitro aflatoxin B1-induced p53 mutations. Cancer Letters. 2003;**199**:1-7. DOI: 10.1016/S0304-3835(03)00337-9

[47] Stern MC, Umbach DM, Yu MC, London SJ, Zhang ZQ, Taylor JA. Hepatitis B, aflatoxin B(1), and p53 codon 249 mutation in hepatocellular carcinomas from Guangxi, People's Republic of China, and a meta-analysis of existing studies. Cancer Epidemiology Biomarkers & Prevention. 2001;**10**:617-625. DOI: PMID11401911

[48] Park US, Su JJ, Ban KC, Qin L, Lee EH, Lee YI. Mutations in the p53 tumor suppressor gene in tree shrew hepatocellular carcinoma associated with hepatitis B virus infection and intake of aflatoxin B1. Gene. 2000;**251**:73-80. DOI: 10.1016/S0378-1119(00)00183-9

[49] Lee YI, Lee S, Das GC, Park US, Park SM, Lee YI. Activation of the insulin-like growth factor II transcription by aflatoxin B1 induced p53 mutant 249 is caused by activation of transcription complexes; implications for a gain-of-function during the formation of hepatocellular carcinoma. Oncogene. 2000;**19**:3717-3726. DOI: 10.1038/sj.onc.1203694

[50] Uwaifo O. P53 gene of chang-liver cells (Atcc-Ccl13) exposed to aflatoxin B1 (Afb): The effect of lysine on mutation at codon 249 of exon 7. African Journal of Medicine and Medical Sciences. 1999;**28**:71-75. DOI: PMID12953991

[51] Chao HK, Tsai TF, Lin CS, Su TS. Evidence that mutational activation of the ras genes may not be involved in aflatoxin B(1)-induced human hepatocarcinogenesis, based on sequence analysis of the ras and p53 genes. Molecular Carcinogenesis. 1999;**26**:69-73. DOI: 10.1002/(SICI)1098-2744(199910)26:2<69::AID-MC1>3.0.CO;2-A

[52] Ghebranious N, Sell S. The mouse equivalent of the human p53ser249 mutation p53ser246 enhances aflatoxin hepatocarcinogenesis in hepatitis B surface antigen transgenic and p53 heterozygous null mice. Hepatology. 1998;**27**:967-973. DOI: 10.1002/hep.510270411

[53] Ghebranious N, Sell S. Hepatitis B injury, male gender, aflatoxin, and p53 expression each contribute to hepatocarcinogenesis in transgenic mice. Hepatology. 1998;**27**:383-391. DOI: 10.1002/hep.510270211

[54] Liu YP, Lin Y, Ng ML. Immunochemical and genetic analysis of the p53 gene in liver preneoplastic nodules from aflatoxin-induced rats in one year. Annals of the Academy of Medicine of Singapore. 1996;**25**:31-36

[55] Hulla JE, Chen ZY, Eaton DL. Aflatoxin B1-induced rat hepatic hyperplastic nodules do not exhibit a site-specific mutation within the p53 gene. Cancer Research. 1993;**53**:9-11. DOI: PMID8380129

[56] Lilleberg SL, Cabonce MA, Raju NR, Wagner LM, Kier LD. Alterations in the structural gene and the expression of p53 in rat liver tumors induced by aflatoxin B1. Molecular Carcinogenesis. 1992;**6**:159-172. DOI: 10.1002/mc.2940060211

[57] Lilleberg SL, Cabonce MA, Raju NR, Wagner LM, Kier LD. Alterations in the p53 tumor suppressor gene in rat liver tumors induced by aflatoxin B1. Progress in Clinical and Biological Research. 1992;**376**:203-222

[58] Deng ZL, Ma Y. Aflatoxin sufferer and p53 gene mutation in hepatocellular carcinoma. World Journal of Gastroenterology. 1998;**4**:28-29. DOI: 10.3748/wjg.v4.i1.28

[59] Deng Z, Pan L, Ma Y. Sequence alterations in p53 gene of hepatocellular carcinoma from high aflatoxin risk area in Guangxi. Zhonghua Zhong Liu Za Zhi. 1997;**19**:18-21. DOI: PMID10743047

[60] Mace K, Aguilar F, Wang JS, Vautravers P, Gomez-Lechon M, Gonzalez FJ, Groopman J, Harris CC, Pfeifer AM. Aflatoxin B1-induced DNA adduct formation and p53 mutations in CYP450-expressing human liver cell lines. Carcinogenesis. 1997;**18**:1291-1297. DOI: PMID9230270

[61] Lunn RM, Zhang YJ, Wang LY, Chen CJ, Lee PH, Lee CS, Tsai WY, Santella RM. p53 mutations, chronic hepatitis B virus infection, and aflatoxin exposure in hepatocellular carcinoma in Taiwan. Cancer Reserch. 1997;**57**:3471-3477. DOI: PMID9270015

[62] Hollstein MC, Wild CP, Bleicher F, Chutimataewin S, Harris CC, Srivatanakul P, Montesano R. p53 mutations and aflatoxin B1 exposure in hepatocellular carcinoma patients from Thailand. International Journal of Cancer. 1993;**53**:51-55. DOI: 10.1002/ijc.2910530111

[63] Aguilar F, Hussain SP, Cerutti P. Aflatoxin B1 induces the transversion of G-->T in codon 249 of the p53 tumor suppressor gene in human hepatocytes. Proceedings of the National Academy of Sciences U S A. 1993;**90**:8586-8590. DOI: PMC47402

[64] Ozturk M. p53 mutation in hepatocellular carcinoma after aflatoxin exposure. Lancet. 1991;**338**:1356-1359. DOI: 10.1016/0140-6736(91)92236-U

[65] Tashiro F, Morimura S, Hayashi K, Makino R, Kawamura H, Horikoshi N, Nemoto K, Ohtsubo K, Sugimura T, Ueno Y. Expression of the c-Ha-ras and c-myc genes in aflatoxin B1-induced hepatocellular carcinomas. Biochemical and Biophysical Research Communications. 1986;**138**:858-864. DOI: 10.1016/S0006-291X(86)80575-7

[66] Sinha S, Webber C, Marshall CJ, Knowles MA, Proctor A, Barrass NC, Neal GE. Activation of ras oncogene in aflatoxin-induced rat liver carcinogenesis. Proceedings of the National Academy of Sciences U S A. 1988;**85**:3673-3677. DOI: PMC280280

[67] Soman NR, Wogan GN. Activation of the c-Ki-ras oncogene in aflatoxin B1-induced hepatocellular carcinoma and adenoma in the rat: Detection by denaturing gradient gel electrophoresis. Proceedings of the National Academy of Sciences U S A. 1993;**90**:2045-2049. DOI: PMC46017

[68] McMahon G, Hanson L, Lee JJ, Wogan GN. Identification of an activated c-Ki-ras oncogene in rat liver tumors induced by aflatoxin B1. Proceedings of the National Academy of Sciences U S A. 1986;**83**:9418-9422. DOI: PMC387149

[69] McMahon G, Davis EF, Huber LJ, Kim Y, Wogan GN. Characterization of c-Ki-ras and N-ras oncogenes in aflatoxin B1-induced rat liver tumors. Proceedings of the National Academy of Sciences U S A. 1990;**87**:1104-1108. DOI: PMC53419

[70] Riley J, Mandel HG, Sinha S, Judah DJ, Neal GE. In vitro activation of the human Harvey-ras proto-oncogene by aflatoxin B1. Carcinogenesis. 1997;**18**:905-910. DOI: PMID9163674

[71] Bauer-Hofmann R, Buchmann A, Wright AS, Schwarz M. Mutations in the Ha-ras proto-oncogene in spontaneous and chemically induced liver tumours of the CF1 mouse. Carcinogenesis. 1990;**11**:1875-1877. DOI: PMID2119910

[72] Wiseman RW, Stowers SJ, Miller EC, Anderson MW, Miller JA. Activating mutations of the c-Ha-ras protooncogene in chemically induced hepatomas of the male B6C3 F1 mouse. Proceedings of the National Academy of Sciences U S A. 1986;**83**:5825-5829. DOI: PMC386388

[73] Kew MC. Synergistic interaction between aflatoxin B1 and hepatitis B virus in hepatocarcinogenesis. Liver International. 2003;**23**:405-409. DOI: 10.1111/j.1478-3231.2003.00869.x

[74] Kew MC. Aflatoxins as a cause of hepatocellular carcinoma. Journal of Gastrointestinal and Liver Diseases. 2013;**22**:305-310. DOI: PMID24078988

[75] Moudgil V, Redhu D, Dhanda S, Singh JA. Review of molecular mechanisms in the development of hepatocellular carcinoma by aflatoxin and hepatitis B and C viruses. Journal of Environmental Pathology, Toxicology and Oncology. 2013;**32**:165-175. DOI: 10.1615/JEnvironPatholToxicolOncol.2013007166

[76] Yeh FS, Mo CC, Yen RC. Risk factors for hepatocellular carcinoma in Guangxi, People's Republic of China. National Cancer Institute Monograph. 1985;**69**:47-48. DOI: PMID3010122

[77] Williams JH, Phillips TD, Jolly PE, Stiles JK, Jolly CM, Aggarwal D. Human aflatoxicosis in developing countries: A review of toxicology, exposure, potential health consequences, and interventions. The American Journal of Clinical Nutrition. 2004;**80**:1106-1122. DOI: PMID15531656

[78] Qian GS, Ross RK, Yu MC, Yuan JM, Gao YT, Henderson BE, Wogan GN, Groopman JD. A follow-up study of urinary markers of aflatoxin exposure and liver cancer risk in Shanghai, People's Republic of China. Cancer Epidemiology, Biomarkers & Prevention. 1994;**3**:3-10. DOI: PMID8118382

[79] Wang JS, Qian GS, Zarba A, He X, Zhu YR, Zhang BC, Jacobson L, Gange SJ, Munoz A, Kensler TW, et al. Temporal patterns of aflatoxin-albumin adducts in hepatitis B surface antigen-positive and antigen-negative residents of Daxin, Qidong County, People's Republic of China. Cancer Epidemiology, Biomarkers & Prevention: A publication of the American Association for Cancer Research, Cosponsored by the American Society of Preventive Oncology. 1996;**5**:253-261. DOI: PMID8722216

[80] Ross RK, Yuan JM, MC Y, Wogan GN, Qian GS, JT T, Groopman JD, Gao YT, Henderson BE. Urinary aflatoxin biomarkers and risk of hepatocellular carcinoma. Lancet. 1992;**339**:943-946. DOI: 10.1016/0140-6736(92)91528-G

[81] Sell S, Hunt JM, Dunsford HA, Chisari FV. Synergy between hepatitis B virus expression and chemical hepatocarcinogens in transgenic mice. Cancer Reserch. 1991;**51**:1278-1285. DOI: PMID1847661

[82] Bannasch P, Khoshkhou NI, Hacker HJ, Radaeva S, Mrozek M, Zillmann U, Kopp-Schneider A, Haberkorn U, Elgas M, Tolle T, et al. Synergistic hepatocarcinogenic effect of hepadnaviral infection and dietary aflatoxin B1 in woodchucks. Cancer Reserch. 1995;**55**:3318-3330. DOI: PMID7614467

[83] Li Y, Su JJ, Qin LL, Yang C, Ban KC, Yan RQ. Synergistic effect of hepatitis B virus and aflatoxin B1 in hepatocarcinogenesis in tree shrews. Annals of the Academy of Medicine Singapore. 1999;**28**:67-71. DOI: PMID10374028

[84] Cova L, Wild CP, Mehrotra R, Turusov V, Shirai T, Lambert V, Jacquet C, Tomatis L, Trepo C, Montesano R. Contribution of aflatoxin B1 and hepatitis B virus infection in the induction of liver tumors in ducks. Cancer Reserch. 1990;**50**:2156-2163. DOI: PMID2107970

[85] Allen SJ, Wild CP, Wheeler JG, Riley EM, Montesano R, Bennett S, Whittle HC, Hall AJ, Greenwood BM. Aflatoxin exposure, malaria and hepatitis B infection in rural Gambian children. Transactions of the Royal Society of Tropical Medicine and Hygiene. 1992;**86**: 426-430. DOI: PMID1440826

[86] Turner PC, Mendy M, Whittle H, Fortuin M, Hall AJ, Wild CP, Hepatitis B. Infection and aflatoxin biomarker levels in Gambian children. Tropical Medicine & International Health. 2000;**5**:837-841. DOI: 10.1046/j.1365-3156.2000.00664.x

[87] Groopman JD, Wang JS, Scholl P. Molecular biomarkers for aflatoxins: From adducts to gene mutations to human liver cancer. Canadian Journal of Physiology and Pharmacology. 1996;**74**:203-209. DOI: PMID8723033

[88] Coursaget P, Depril N, Chabaud M, Nandi R, Mayelo V, LeCann P, Yvonnet B. High prevalence of mutations at codon 249 of the p53 gene in hepatocellular carcinomas from Senegal. British Journal of Cancer. 1993;**67**:1395-1397. DOI: PMC1968506

[89] Kew MC, Hepatitis B. Virus x protein in the pathogenesis of hepatitis B virus-induced hepatocellular carcinoma. Journal of Gastroenterology and Hepatology. 2011;**26**(Suppl 1): 144-152. DOI: 10.1111/j.1440-1746.2010.06546.x

[90] Gomez-Moreno A, Garaigorta U, Hepatitis B. Virus and DNA damage response: Interactions and consequences for the infection. Virus. 2017;**9**. DOI: 10.3390/v9100304

[91] Castelli G, Pelosi E, Testa U. Liver cancer: Molecular characterization, clonal evolution and cancer stem cells. Cancers (Basel). 2017;**9**. DOI: 10.3390/cancers9090127

[92] Ghouri YA, Mian I, Rowe JH. Review of hepatocellular carcinoma: Epidemiology, etiology, and carcinogenesis. Journal of Carcinogenesis. 2017;**16**:1. DOI: 10.4103/jcar.JCar_9_16

[93] Long XD, Huang HD, Xia Q. The polymorphism of XRCC3 codon 241 and the hotspot mutation in the TP53 gene in hepatocellular carcinoma induced by aflatoxin B1. Journal of Tumor. 2014;**2**:272-277. DOI: 10.6051/j.issn.1819-6187.2014.02.57

[94] Long XD, Yao JG, Huang YZ, Huang XY, Ban FZ, Yao LM, Fan LDDNA. Repair gene XRCC7 polymorphisms (rs#7003908 and rs#10109984) and hepatocellular carcinoma related to AFB1 exposure among Guangxi population, China. Hepatology Research. 2011;**41**:1085-1093. DOI: 10.1111/j.1872-034X.2011.00866.x

[95] Long XD, Ma Y, Zhou YF, Ma AM, Fu GH. Polymorphism in xeroderma pigmentosum complementation group C codon 939 and aflatoxin B1-related hepatocellular carcinoma in the Guangxi population. Hepatology. 2010;**52**:1301-1309. DOI: 10.1002/hep.23807

[96] Long XD, Ma Y, Zhou YF, Yao JG, Ban FZ, Huang YZ, Huang BC. XPD Codon 312 and 751 polymorphisms, and AFB1 exposure, and hepatocellular carcinoma risk. BMC Cancer. 2009;**9**:400. DOI: 10.1186/1471-2407-9-400

[97] Long XD, Ma Y, Huang HD, Yao JG, Qu de Y, Lu YL. Polymorphism of XRCC1 and the frequency of mutation in codon 249 of the p53 gene in hepatocellular carcinoma among Guangxi population, China. Molecular Carcinogenesis 2008;**47**:295-300. doi: 10.1002/mc.20384

[98] Long XD, Ma Y, Wei YP, Deng ZL. The polymorphisms of GSTM1, GSTT1, HYL1*2, and XRCC1, and aflatoxin B1-related hepatocellular carcinoma in Guangxi population, China. Hepatology Research. 2006;**36**:48-55. DOI: 10.1016/j.hepres.2006.06.004

[99] Long XD, Ma Y, Deng ZL. GSTM1 and XRCC3 polymorphisms: Effects on levels of aflatoxin B1-DNA adducts. Chinese Journal of Cancer Research. 2009;**21**:177-184. DOI: 10.1007/s11670-009-0177-6

[100] Long XD, Ma Y, Wei YP, Deng ZL. A study about the association of detoxication gene GSTM1 polymorphism and the susceptibility to aflatoxin B1-related hepatocellular carcinoma. Zhonghua Gan Zang Bing Za Zhi. 2005;**13**:668-670. DOI: PMID16174455

[101] Long XD, Ma Y, Wei YP, Deng ZL. Study on the detoxication gene gstM1-gstT1-null and susceptibility to aflatoxin B1 related hepatocellular carcinoma in Guangxi. Zhonghua Liu Xing Bing Xue Za Zhi. 2005;**26**:777-781. DOI: PMID16536303

[102] Moon EY, Rhee DK, Pyo S. In vitro suppressive effect of aflatoxin B1 on murine peritoneal macrophage functions. Toxicology. 1999;**133**:171-179. DOI: PMID10378483

[103] Moon EY, Rhee DK, Pyo S. Inhibition of various functions in murine peritoneal macrophages by aflatoxin B1 exposure in vivo. International Journal of Immunopharmacology. 1999;**21**:47-58. DOI: 10.1016/S0192-0561(98)00069-1

[104] Bianco G, Russo R, Marzocco S, Velotto S, Autore G, Severino L. Modulation of macrophage activity by aflatoxins B1 and B2 and their metabolites aflatoxins M1 and M2. Toxicon. 2012;**59**:644-650. DOI: 10.1016/j.toxicon.2012.02.010

[105] Bruneau JC, Stack E, O'Kennedy R, Loscher CE. Aflatoxins B(1), B(2) and G(1) modulate cytokine secretion and cell surface marker expression in J774A.1 murine macrophages. Toxicology In Vitro. 2012;**26**:686-693. DOI: 10.1016/j.tiv.2012.03.003

[106] Turner PC, Moore SE, Hall AJ, Prentice AM, Wild CP. Modification of immune function through exposure to dietary aflatoxin in Gambian children. Environmental Health Perspectives. 2003;**111**:217-220. DOI: PMC1241353

[107] Oswald IP, Marin DE, Bouhet S, Pinton P, Taranu I, Accensi F. Immunotoxicological risk of mycotoxins for domestic animals. Food Additives and Contaminants. 2005;**22**:354-360. DOI: 10.1080/02652030500058320

2

Pathogenesis of Hepatitis B Virus Associated Chronic Liver Disease

Mark A. Feitelson

Abstract

Hepatitis B virus (HBV) infection is associated with chronic liver diseases (CLD), which progress from hepatitis to fibrosis, cirrhosis, and finally hepatocellular carcinoma (HCC) over 30–50 years. The pathogenesis of CLD is immune mediated, which is characterized by persistent immune responses against virus infected hepatocytes. During bouts of CLD, the virus gene encoding the hepatitis B x antigen (HBx) is increasingly found integrated at multiple sites within the human genome. Many of these integrated templates express HBx, which is a *trans*-regulatory protein that supports virus gene expression and replication on one hand, but also alters patterns of gene expression in the infected cell. HBx alters gene expression by constitutively activating signal transduction pathways in the cytoplasm and promoting epigenetic mediated changes in the expression of cellular genes. In doing so, HBx contributes to the persistence of virus infected cells and to the pathogenesis of CLD by triggering multiple hallmarks which are characteristic of cancer.

Keywords: hepatitis B virus, chronic liver disease, hepatocellular carcinoma, hepatitis B x, immune mediated liver disease, epigenetics, hallmarks of cancer

1. Introduction

Hepatitis B virus (HBV) is a blood-borne virus that infects the liver. Until the discovery of the virus in the 1960s [1], it was transmitted sexually and by transfusion of contaminated blood and blood fractions. Today, the virus has been virtually eliminated from the blood supply by a simple blood test while infection has been prevented by a highly efficacious vaccine [2, 3]. Prior to establishment of vaccination programs in various countries, infants born to infected mothers replicating virus often acquired the virus at birth by exposure to contaminated maternal blood.

More than 90% of these children became HBV carriers, characterized by the persistence of virus or virus antigens in their blood for years to decades. These children were a high risk for the development of chronic liver disease (CLD), which progressed from hepatitis, to fibrosis, cirrhosis, and hepatocellular carcinoma (HCC) [4]. Fortunately, newborns in many countries receive the HBV vaccine at birth, which helps to prevent mother-to-infant transmission as well as protect from exposure later in life. Among unvaccinated adults engaging in unprotected sex, roughly 5–10% become carriers, and these individuals are also at high risk for the development of CLD and HCC. Although estimates vary, there are ~300–350 million carriers of HBV worldwide [5]. HCC is the sixth most prevalent cancer worldwide, with about 600,000 newly diagnosed cases annually, and the second leading cause of cancer deaths [6]. Interferon, and in more recent years, powerful nucleoside analogs, have successfully treated patients with chronic hepatitis B, but presently there is no cure [7, 8]. HCC is curable by surgical resection, but this is often accompanied by relapse. Dozens of drugs, alone or in combination, have been evaluated in clinical trials for patients with advanced HCC, but only the multi-kinase inhibitors, Sorafenib and regorafenib, and the immune checkpoint inhibitor nivolumab, have been useful in modestly extending the lifespan of such patients [9, 10]. Given that the carrier state and CLD are the major risk factors for HCC [11], there is strong rationale to better understand the host-virus relationship that contributes to the pathogenesis of chronic infection.

2. Variations in pathogenesis

A hallmark in the pathogenesis of HBV infection is its' variability. Among acutely infected adults, up to 65% develop a subclinical infection characterized only by the appearance of one or more viral antibodies in the blood, while another 25% develop acute resolving infection, which may or may not include a bout of hepatitis. The remaining 10% of patients develop chronic infection (i.e., the persistence of virus and virus antigens in the blood for more than 6 months). In chimpanzees [12] and woodchucks [13], acute infections are characterized by the nearly complete clearance of virus from the blood and liver followed by seroconversion from surface antigen to corresponding antibody. In this case, virus is mostly cleared by non-cytolytic cytokines (e.g., interferon gamma [IFNɣ] and tumor necrosis factor alpha [TNFα]) prior to the appearance of T and other inflammatory cells in the liver, suggesting that most virus clearance occurs prior to the development of acute hepatitis. Further work showed that $CD4^+$ and $CD8^+$ T cells, natural killer (NK) cells, Fas, various IFNs and corresponding receptors, and the TNF receptor 1 participate in virus clearance, suggesting redundant pathways inhibit HBV replication in the liver [14]. The subsequent contribution of a T cell response appears to clear virus infected cells by cytolytic mechanisms involving Fas and granzymes. In this context, $CD4^+$ T cells are required to prime $CD8^+$ T cells to facilitate virus elimination in acute infection [14]. When this happens in acute, resolving infection, the T cell response to HBV is vigorous, polyclonal and multi-specific, while among those who go on to develop chronic infection, adaptive immunity is relatively weak and narrowly focused, suggesting that clearance of HBV is T cell dependent. When T cell responses are not adequate, CLD may develop and progress to cirrhosis and HCC. However, CLD may spontaneously resolve at any of these stages. While the origin of this variability is not completely characterized, it is clear that the ability of the host to mount adaptive immune responses is a key element to limiting virus spread.

3. Contributions of hepatitis B surface, core and e antigens to the pathogenesis of chronic infection

3.1. Hepatitis B surface antigen (HBsAg)

HBV is a small virus consisting of only four open reading frames (ORF) [15]. One ORF encodes a family of envelope polypeptides (**Figure 1**). The major envelope polypeptide, HBsAg, triggers neutralizing antibody which is central to virus clearance after acute exposure and is the major component of the HBV vaccine [2]. HBsAg polypeptides are transmembrane proteins and glycoproteins that are on the envelope of virus particles, and are also secreted as small, spherical and variably long filamentous subviral particles that lack the virus nucleocapsid and HBV DNA. It is thought that these subviral particles, which are produced at concentrations several logs above that of infectious virus particles, absorb neutralizing antibody and trigger immunological tolerance, both of which promote virus persistence in the blood. Moreover, in patients with CLD, there does not seem to be any correlation between intrahepatic HBsAg expression patterns and inflammatory infiltrates [16, 17], nor have HBsAg specific T cell clones been isolated from such patients [18]. In addition, T cell sensitization to HBsAg in acute and chronic HBV infection is usually undetectable [19],

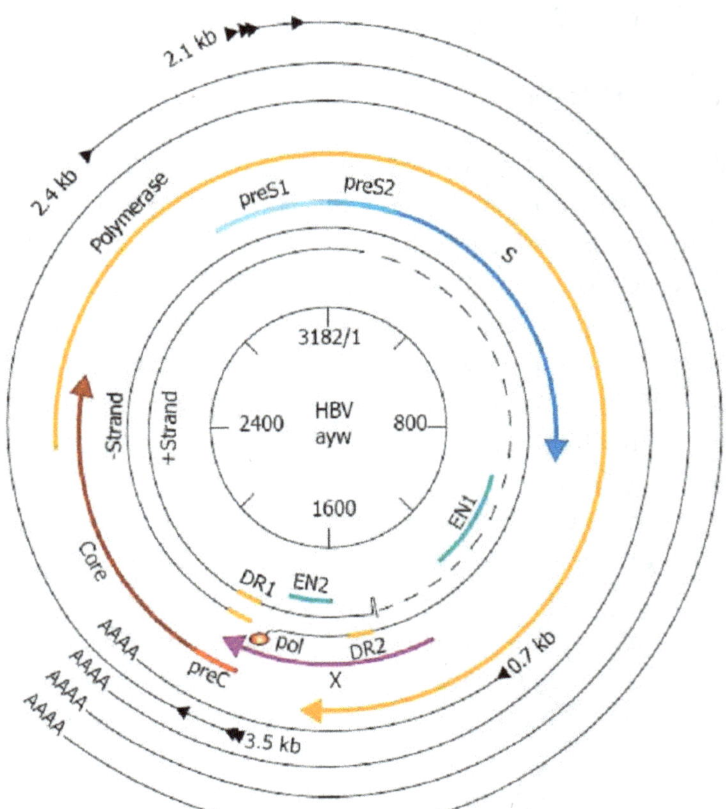

Figure 1. Genetic organization of HBV showing the ORFs (in color). The positions of enhancer 1 (EN1) and 2 (EN2) are also shown. The direct repeat 1 (DR1) and 2 (DR2) sequences at the ends of the long and short DNA strands are also indicted. The pregenomic RNA (3.5 kb) is greater than genome length, while the 2.1 and 2.4 kb subgenomic mRNAs encode surface antigen polypeptides, and the 0.7 kb mRNA encodes the X protein. Reproduced from [20] with permission.

so while HBsAg clearance occurs in acute, resolving infections, it is not clear that it is an immunological target in established infections.

3.2. Hepatitis B core antigen (HBcAg)

The second ORF, or core gene, encodes the hepatitis B core antigen (HBcAg) or nucleocapsid protein that polymerizes as an icosahedron around the virus replication complex, the latter of which consists of the virus nucleic acid and HBV encoded polymerase [20]. The fact that the pregenomic RNA and the reverse transcribed viral DNA product are sequestered within a nucleocapsid means that they are not readily detected by pattern recognition receptors, (e.g., toll-like receptors, retinoic acid inducible gene 1 [RIG-1], and mitochondrial anti-viral signaling [MAVS]) that trigger innate immunity [21]. Moreover, innate immune responses do not develop in the liver of acutely infected chimpanzees [22], suggesting that HBV replication and spread may be conducted in "stealth" mode with virus nucleocapsids upon infection and again during virus replication. If so, then this may explain why up to 70% of acutely infected adults who become carriers do not develop CLD. However, carriers who develop CLD also have intrahepatic core antigen, suggesting that HBcAg may be an important immunological target in CLD [23]. Alternatively, patients with acute, resolving hepatitis show a vigorous peripheral blood mononuclear cell response to HBcAg that is temporally associated with the clearance of HBsAg, while in patients with chronic infection, T cell responsiveness to HBcAg is relatively weak, providing an opportunity for HBV to spread in the liver and establish a chronic infection [19].

3.3. Hepatitis B e antigen (HBeAg)

A proteolytic fragment of HBcAg, known as HBeAg, is secreted into the circulation and serves as a surrogate marker of virus replication. Seroconversion from HBeAg to anti-HBe is usually accompanied by a significant decrease in virus replication in both the liver and blood and resolution of CLD [24]. The detection of HBcAg specific cytotoxic T lymphocytes (CTL) is associated with the clearance of virus replication, often a transient exacerbation of CLD, and seroconversion to anti-HBe during the natural history of infection [24], suggesting that HBcAg is an important virus target in CLD. HBcAg specific T cells have been detected in the peripheral blood and liver [18, 25] of patients with CLD, suggesting that HBcAg is an immunological target in chronic hepatitis B. Interestingly, HBeAg in serum may attenuate immune responses against virus infected liver, because some patients who develop mutations in HBV that no longer express HBeAg, continue to support high levels of virus replication and ongoing, CLD [26, 27]. In fact, HBeAg appears to be a T cell tolerogen that down-regulates immune responses against HBcAg [28]. HBeAg may also stimulate the appearance of regulatory dendritic cells, which would also suppress virus specific immunity and promote virus persistence [29] by up-regulating the expression of suppressor of cytokine signaling 2 (SOCS2), which in turn represses IFN signaling, thereby blunting innate anti-viral responses and promoting virus persistence [30]. Thus, HBeAg polypeptides, like subviral HBsAg particles, promote chronicity by acting as tolerogens.

3.4. Hepatitis B polymerase

The HBV encoded polymerase, encoded by a third ORF, has DNA dependent and RNA dependent DNA polymerase (DNAp) activities, and RNase H activity. Upon infection, the partially

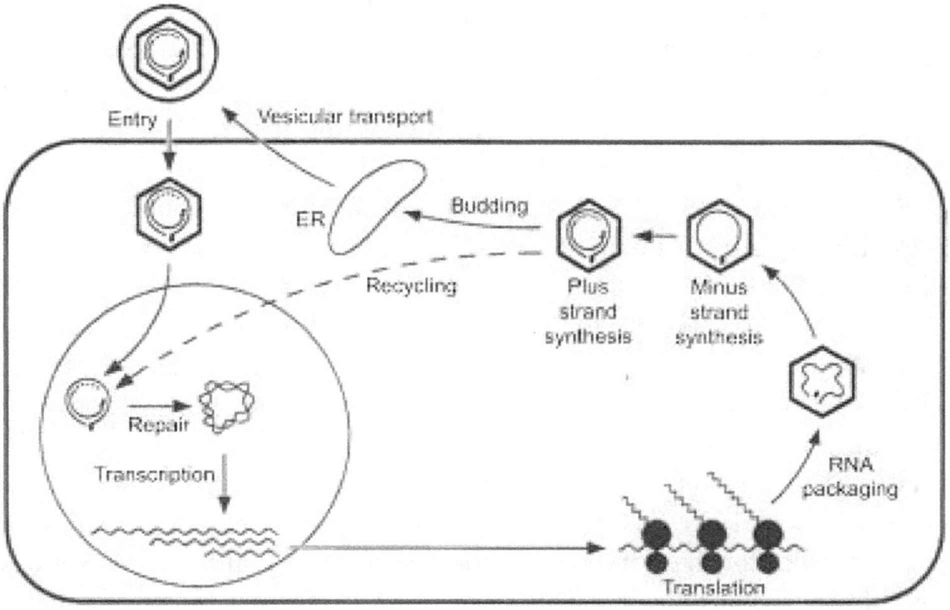

Figure 2. General scheme of HBV replication. See the text for additional details. Reproduced from [20] with permission.

double stranded viral DNA is made fully double stranded by the endogenous DNAp activity [20] (**Figure 2**). The HBV genome then appears as a supercoiled mini-chromosome in the nuclei of infected cells, and this acts as a template for the transcription of subgenomic RNAs and a greater than genome length pre-genomic RNA. The latter then migrates into the cytoplasm, where it is packaged with the virus polymerase into nascent ("immature") core (or nucleocapsid) particles, where the pregenomic RNA is reverse transcribed into minus strand DNA, with the latter then being used as a template for partial plus strand synthesis just prior to the budding and secretion of progeny virus (**Figure 2**). Some immature core particles are recycled into the nucleus to replenish the pool of covalently closed circular (ccc) HBV DNA. Although the HBV polymerase triggers antibody responses [31], there is no evidence that immune responses against the polymerase directly impact pathogenesis or virus persistence. However, HBV polymerase inhibits RIG-1 and nuclear factor kappa B (NF-κB) induction of IFNβ, suggesting that the polymerase could block innate signaling [32, 33], thereby contributing to virus persistence.

4. Relationship between persistent virus replication, integration of HBV DNA, and the risk for the development of HCC

There is evidence to suggest that persistent, high levels of HBV replication correlate with the progression of CLD to HCC [34]. However, independent work showed an elevated risk for HCC among patients with CLD but low virus titers [35, 36]. Other observations have shown no correlation between HBV DNA levels in serum (>10^5 copies/ml) and histological grade or stage of liver disease in carriers [37, 38]. In addition, it is controversial as to whether long term nucleoside analog therapy resulted in a decreased risk for the development of HCC [6, 35]. Given that HBV is not directly cytopathic [39], that carriers with high levels of HBV DNA in serum are often asymptomatic, and that the pathogenesis of CLD is immune mediated [17,

40], a correlation between virus replication and CLD may contribute to, but not by itself, determine disease progression. Moreover, most carriers with CLD who develop cirrhosis and HCC have long since seroconverted from HBeAg (reflecting high levels of virus replication) to anti-HBe (reflecting low or undetectable virus replication), indicating that disease progression may occur at low virus titers [36]. Among patients with sustained high levels of HBV replication and successive bouts of CLD, there is a wave of liver regeneration following each episode of hepatitis to restore full liver function. At these times, fragments of HBV DNA, mostly encoding the HBx ORF (and sometimes the HBx plus preS/S ORFs), become integrated at multiple sites within host DNA [41, 42] (**Figure 3**). Over time, these integration events result in increased intrahepatic expression levels of HBx that alter patterns of host (and support virus) gene expression (**Figure 3**). HBV integrates early after infection, not only in permissive liver cell lines, but also in non-replicating primary human hepatocytes [43]. Many fragments of integrated HBV DNA encode HBx that is capable of *trans*-activation [44]. Although the relatively low levels of HBx made from the virus mini-chromosome support virus gene expression and replication, it is hypothesized that as intrahepatic levels of HBx increase [45] (**Figure 3**), it epigenetically alter the expression patterns of selected host genes [46] that contribute to both virus persistence and to malignant transformation. Thus, the changing intrahepatic levels of HBx promote virus persistence and ultimately, contribute to malignant transformation [47].

4.1. Covalently closed circular HBV (ccc) DNA

Given that the current treatment of chronic hepatitis B with nucleoside analogs is not curative, there has been a major effort to eliminate ccc DNA [47], especially since ccc DNA is the template for all virus transcripts. Since nucleoside analogs do not eliminate integrated HBV templates or the HBV mini-chromosome, continued virus gene expression from these templates will drive pathogenesis toward HCC. Formation of ccc DNA is a complex process that involves a variety of host proteins, including several DNA polymerases [48] that could potentially be therapeutic targets, although this approach may be accompanied by toxicity. As outlined below, HBx regulates the formation, function and intracellular copy number of ccc DNA by several epigenetic mechanisms that involve altered expression of histone methyltransferases and histone deacetylases, by promoting degradation of the anti-viral restriction factor Smc5/6, and by increasing expression of DNA methyltransferases [48]. Anti-viral immune responses in which selected cytokines mediate non-cytolytic degradation of ccc DNA have also been documented *in vitro* [48, 49]. Among these, IFN alpha up-regulated expression of APOBEC3

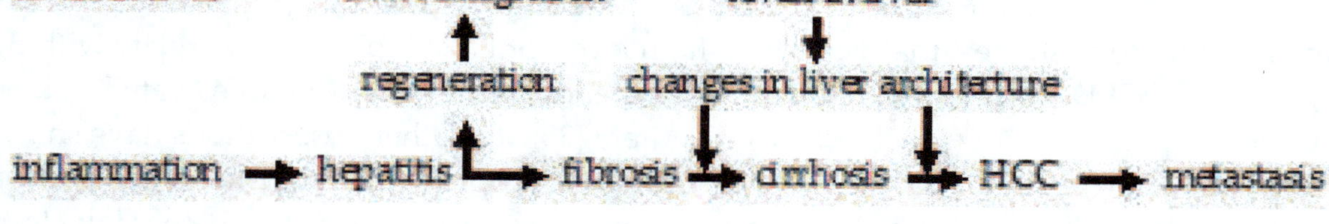

Figure 3. Natural history of chronic hepatitis B featuring the progressive lesions that develop in CLD compared to increased number of integration events, many of which produce functional HBx (modified from [53] with permission).

nuclear deaminase resulted in a modest reduction in ccc DNA copy number via deamination [50]. Gene editing approaches, such as CRISPR/Cas9 have also been demonstrated to work *in vitro* and *in vivo* [51], but off-target effects, ability to access and act on all susceptible cells, and recognition of all HBV genotypes, remain to be addressed. In addition, the recent finding of ccc host DNA in both normal and tumor cells, as a mechanism whereby host cells regulate gene expression [52], implies that targeting ccc DNA may also have toxic effects on the treated cells whether or not they are virally infected. Thus, it is not clear whether this approach in a liver which is already damaged will exacerbate that damage and/or have an anti-tumor effect.

5. Contribution of HBx to pathogenesis of CLD by regulation of HBV replication

HBx, the *trans*-activation protein of HBV, *trans*-activates virus gene expression and replication *in vitro* [54, 55]. The contribution of this regulatory protein to virus persistence in the carrier state was shown in woodchucks experimentally infected with the HBV-like virus, woodchuck hepatitis virus (WHV). Wild type WHV readily establishes a chronic infection, characterized by persistent virus replication and CLD that progresses to HCC [56]. However, experimental infection with a mutant of WHV that does not encode woodchuck hepatitis x (WHx) antigen yielded no carrier state and no CLD [57, 58], suggesting that *trans*-activation of virus gene expression and replication is central to the establishment of the carrier state. Among infected woodchucks, there was co-staining between WHV core antigen (where virus replication takes place) and WHx [59, 60], while in human infection, HBx often co-existed with HBe in serum [61] and replication complexes (i.e., with HBcAg) in the liver [62]. Thus, HBx expression is associated with virus replication.

5.1. Mechanisms regulating HBV replication

At the molecular level, HBx regulates HBV replication by binding to various cellular proteins. For example, HBx binds to jumonji C-domain-containing 5 (JMJD5), a arginyl-hydroxylase, which promotes the expression of transcription factors (e.g., such as hepatocyte nuclear factors 3 gamma and 4 alpha [HNF3G and HNF4A] and CCAAT/enhancer-binding protein alpha) that facilitate hepatocyte differentiation [63]. Given that HBV replicates in differentiated hepatocytes, the binding of HBx to JMJD5 facilitates HBV replication via epigenetic alterations in host gene expression. In addition, HBx promotes the formation of ccc DNA by recruiting the transcriptional scaffold, p300; the cAMP response element binding protein CREB; the CREB transcription factor binding protein, CBP; the histone acetyltransferase p300/CBP-associated factor, as well as the histone deactylases HDAC1, Sirt1 [48] and Sirt2 [12]. Once ccc DNA is formed, HBx up-regulates HBV replication, in part, by binding to cullin4-damage specific DNA binding protein (CUL4-DDB1) ubiquitin ligase [64, 65], suggesting that HBx may function, at least in part, at the level of the proteasome. HBx modulates proteasome activity by direct binding to the 26S proteasomal subunit [66], which is responsible for degradation of HBx and several anti-viral proteins. One of the latter is Smc5/6, which is involved in the structural maintenance of chromosomes (i.e., genome stability) and DNA repair [67]. Smc5/6 and HBx bind to the HBV mini-chromosome [67, 68], resulting in epigenetic changes of virus gene expression. HBx binding to CUL4-DDB1 triggers altered enzymatic activity of the E3 ligase CRL4, which then stimulates the ubiquitination and subsequent proteasomal degradation of Smc5/6 [68–70], thereby promoting virus replication. Other anti-viral systems, such as IFN induced APOBEC3A [50], may also be similarly degraded. In this context, HBV is not very good in triggering innate immunity, which may underscore why there are hundreds of millions of carriers worldwide [71]. As mentioned above, sequestration and reverse transcription of pregenomic HBV RNA in immature nucleocapsids (**Figure 2**) may block the induction of innate immunity. In addition, although HBV replication is exquisitely sensitive to inhibition by IFNs, HBx appears to block IFN expression and signaling [72–74], suggesting that both innate and adaptive immunity could be compromised, thereby permitting virus persistence. Under these circumstances, CLD would continue to damage the liver while being unable to resolve the virus infection. HBx also regulates HBV replication by stimulating the expression of DNA methyl-transferases (DNMTs), which suppresses HBV transcription via DNA methylation [75]. DNMTs also methylate tumor suppressor genes, thereby down-regulating their expression, and permitting the accumulation of mutations and chromosomal instability that contribute importantly to HCC. Thus, HBx regulates the activity of ccc DNA in both positive and negative ways, and in doing so, impacts upon the pathogenesis of CLD. The reason why it is important to regulate the intrahepatic levels of ccc DNA is because when virus antigens are greatly overproduced, they could trigger cytopathic effects (CPE), thereby limiting virus replication. For example, mutations in the preS region of the S gene prevent secretion of surface antigen and complete virus particles, and eventually CPE. Pre-S mutations also promote recycling of viral DNA into the nucleus where it results in increased levels of viral ccc DNA, which potentially promotes virus persistence [76] (**Figure 2**). In transgenic mice overproducing HBsAg, CPE develops and eventually evolves into HCC [77]. Although the latter is not characteristic of HCC pathogenesis among human carriers, it does underscore that selected HBV mutants that may arise during chronic infection potentially contribute to pathogenesis via CPE.

5.2. Oxidative damage and inflammation

Although HBV is not cytopathic, HBx strongly activates NF-κB [78], which promotes the expression of many pro-inflammatory cytokines and chemokines that attenuate virus replication and contribute to the pathogenesis of CLD and HCC. For example, HBx stimulates the expression of IFN inducible proteins, such as the CXC chemokine IP-10 [79] which promotes leukocyte chemotaxis. HBx also stimulates production of interleukin-23 (IL-23) [79], which contributes to the maintenance and expansion of pro-inflammatory Th17 cells. Among others, IL-6 is up-regulated by HBx in a MyD88 manner [80], which indicates that HBx is activating a pro-inflammatory environment via innate immune pathways early on after infection. The repressive effect of IL-6 upon HBV replication is demonstrated by the fact that IL-6 treatment of infected cells results in the loss of HNF1a and HNF4a, both of which bind to ccc DNA. Il-6 also redistributes signal transducers and activators of transcription 3 (STAT3) signaling from ccc DNA to IL-6 target genes [49]. HBx targets up-regulation of IL-18, which up-regulates FasL [81], which in this case blocks the killing of infected cells by CTLs. HBx also up-regulates tumor TNFα [82], which was shown to suppress HBcAg expression [83], thereby inhibiting virus replication. In addition, the pro-inflammatory IL-32 was up-regulated by HBx in a NF-κB dependent manner [84]. This is not an exhaustive list. Many of these molecules are turned on as a result of HBx stimulating multiple signal transduction pathways in the cytoplasm (in addition to NF-κB), but the bigger question is trying to understand how a non-cytopathic virus is mediating these and other related changes in infected cells.

The fact that HBx plays a central role in HBV replication suggests that intracellular conditions that stimulate HBx activity would also promote the carrier state, which would be evolutionally selected for because it would provide a large window of time for virus to be transmitted to other hosts. In this context, the expression and activity of HBx is stimulated in an oxidative environment, since the addition of anti-oxidants to cells expressing HBx strongly diminish HBx *trans*-activation activity [85, 86]. An oxidative environment (accompanied by oxidative stress of cellular organelles) could be created in the infected cell by virtue of the association of HBx with mitochondria [87]. HBx interacts with the voltage dependent anion channel on the outer mitochondrial membrane, altering transmembrane potential [88], resulting in diminished electron transport, increased free radical accumulation, including elevated lipid peroxidation products [89], release of calcium into the cytosol [55], and under specific circumstances, cell death [90]. Release of calcium into the cytosol, resulted in the activation of the protein tyrosine kinase 2 and Src kinase families, leading to stimulation of ras, raf, mitogen activated protein kinase, and Jun, which stimulate HBV transcription and replication [55]. HBx also induces oxidative stress in the endoplasmic reticulum, which activates the unfolded protein response and expression of pro-inflammatory cyclooxygenase-2 through the activating transcription factor 4 pathway [91]. Free radicals are also characteristic of immune responses aimed at damaging and destroying infected cells that are replicating HBV. In addition, mitochondrial associated HBx induces oxidative stress, which activates selected transcription factors, such as NF-κB, STAT3 and activating protein 1 [86]. However, HBx is also known to block mitochondrial triggered cell death, not only by activation of survival [21, 92] and hepato-protective pathways such as NF-κB that over-ride apoptosis signaling, but also by blocking key caspases and promoting autophagy [93] and mitophagy [94]. The maintenance of mitochondrial and cellular homeostasis by mitophagy acts to attenuate virus induced apoptosis, so that on the one hand, autophagy and mitophagy promote cell survival and virus persistence, while simultaneous mitochondrial damage may contribute to CLD [94].

5.3. HBx and inflammation

In this chronic pro-inflammatory environment, one would expect to see a correlation between HBx staining and the intensity of CLD. In fact, WHx staining has been observed around inflammatory foci in chronically infected woodchuck livers [95], and among human carriers, relatively low levels of intrahepatic HBx staining was observed in patient biopsy samples from people with low grade hepatitis, while intense and widespread HBx staining was observed in patient biopsies from those with advanced fibrosis and cirrhosis [45, 96], suggesting a direct correlation between HBx staining and liver damage. Independent work also showed low levels of HBx mRNA in the livers of patients with mild CLD (e.g., mild hepatitis), and much higher levels among patients with severe lesions in the liver (advanced fibrosis and cirrhosis) [97]. The relationship of HBx expression to disease severity is also consistent with the idea that when the liver regenerates following each bout of hepatitis, fragments of HBV

DNA encoding the HBx region (and sometimes part of the preS/S encoding gene as well) increasingly integrate into multiple regions of the host genome during normal host DNA replication, resulting in increasing accumulation of intrahepatic HBx as CLD progresses. In contrast, the copy number of ccc DNA per cell decreases with regeneration.

The relationship between HBx expression and CLD has been recapitulated in HBx transgenic mice, where the presence, frequency and distribution of HBx in the liver increase with age, as does liver pathology, which progressively develops from hepatitis and steatosis, to dysplasia and microscopic nodules of HCC, and finally to multi-nodular macroscopic HCC with age [98]. In this model, HBx is expressed from its own enhancer and promoter, which is not active until after birth when appropriate transcription factors in the liver begin to appear. HBx expression triggers immune responses in the absence of other HBV gene products, so it is likely that the pathogenesis observed is due to the impact of increasing levels of HBx upon host gene expression combined with immune responses directed against virus infected cells. There is no ccc DNA in this system, just as it is difficult to detect HBV replication among patients with advanced stages of CLD (i.e., cirrhosis). Thus, it is possible that early in chronic infection, and immune responses to virus antigens emanating from ccc DNA templates play an important role in triggering and sustaining immune mediated pathogenesis, but following bouts of CLD and liver regeneration, where the levels of virus replication decrease at the same time that integration of virus DNA fragments increase, pathogenesis appears to be increasingly driven by one or more antigens made from integrated HBV DNA. Although *cis*-acting mechanisms have been postulated to contribute importantly to the pathogenesis of HCC in selected cases, the broadly distributed integration events of the HBx ORF into most chromosomes [99], suggests that the HBx proteins encoded by most integration events promote CLD and HCC in *trans* [47]. In this model, integration of HBV sequences would accumulate in areas of euchromatin and fragile sites much more frequently that at or within specific genes [100].

The model above suggests that targeting ccc DNA in HBeAg carriers with CLD may be an important therapeutic goal to bring about a functional (but not sterilizing) cure due to the presence of integrated virus DNA that express one or more virus proteins. Among anti-HBe carriers with advanced CLD, targeting the much lower levels of ccc DNA may not be effective in preventing progression to cirrhosis and HCC, because at this stage, most of the HBx made probably comes from integrated templates. Under these circumstances, ccc DNA may persist in a transcriptionally inactive form, which is consistent with the absence of HBV DNA in the blood, even after treatment with direct acting anti-viral agents or therapy aimed at stimulating immune responses against virus infected cells [101, 102]. In fact, early work already pointed out that seroconversion to anti-HBe is sometimes associated with the progression of CLD [103, 104], even though later work showed that disease progression was associated with continued replication of HBV DNA carrying one or more mutations in the core gene that blocks production of HBeAg [27]. These mutations were probably selected for during the natural history of infection by immune responses targeting HBcAg [105]. Although these findings suggest that CLD progresses in the liver supporting replication of selected virus mutants, it has also recently been suggested that linear HBV DNA, and not ccc DNA, is the template for integration into host DNA [43], from which one or more virus gene products are made, and contribute to pathogenesis. Thus, persistent inflammation in a chronically damaged liver may result in the development of HCC despite low levels or undetectable levels of virus replication.

6. Conclusions

HBV encodes polypeptides from four ORFs that trigger corresponding immune responses during acute and chronic infections. When these responses are rapid, strong and multi-specific, acute, resolving infection can be achieved. When these immune responses are weak and of limited specificity (against few virus epitopes), the carrier state may develop. Although the pathogenesis of HBV is variable in different hosts, the virus encodes proteins that blunt innate immunity, and as a consequence, adaptive immunity is not triggered at all or to a limited extent. The latter causes liver damage over many years without eliminating the virus. Even though available treatments suppress virus replication, none are curative, and the persistence of viral ccc DNA sustains infection. Production of HBx regulates virus gene expression and replication, but over time, increased integration of HBV DNA fragments encoding HBx results in high levels of HBx expression that epigenetically alter the expression of numerous host genes that up- or down-regulate HBV replication and impact disease activity. For example, HBx activation of AKT decreased HBV replication, but this was accompanied by an inhibition of apoptosis, suggesting that HBx balances HBV replication and cell survival by stimulating signaling that enhance hepatocyte survival at the expense of higher levels of HBV replication [106]. The generation of free radicals by immune responses against virus infected cells, combined with HBx mediated alterations in mitochondrial function, promote HBx activity. These events result in the activation of signaling pathways (e.g., AP-1 and NF-κB) that over-ride apoptosis and/or directly block the activation of critical caspases, so that whether HBx stimulates or block apoptosis depends upon whether the liver is experiencing inflammation and oxidative stress. It also depends upon whether HBx is being expressed in normal hepatocytes, where apoptotic pathways could be triggered, or whether HBx is expressed at high levels in cells where apoptotic pathways are compromised. In addition to being pro-inflammatory, activated NF-κB protects infected cells against immune elimination. Thus, the dichotomy of HBx activity may be a reflection of the environment wherein HBx is expressed. Importantly, the epigenetic mechanisms whereby HBx regulates virus replication also have an impact on cell growth and survival, and many of these same alterations in host gene expression are also hallmarks of cancer [107], which may explain why there is such a high risk of HCC among carriers with CLD [11]. The common denominator is that many of the pathways and molecules that support HBV gene expression and replication also protect infected cells from elimination, and contribute centrally to malignant transformation.

Acknowledgements

The author wants to acknowledge Temple University for providing him with the opportunity to work on this project.

Author details

Mark A. Feitelson

Address all correspondence to: feitelso@temple.edu

College of Science and Technology, Temple University, Philadelphia, Pennsylvania, United States

References

[1] Blumberg BS. Australia antigen and the biology of hepatitis B. Science. 1977;**197**:17-25

[2] Szmuness W, Stevens CE, Zang EA, Harley EJ, Kellner A. A controlled clinical trial of the efficacy of the hepatitis B vaccine (Heptavax B): A final report. Hepatology. 1981;**1**:377-385

[3] Senior JR, London WT, Sutnick AI. The Australia antigen and role of the late Philadelphia general hospital in reducing post-transfusion hepatitis and sequelae. Hepatology. 2011;**54**:753-756. DOI: 10.1002/hep.24593

[4] Villeneuve JP. The natural history of chronic hepatitis B virus infection. Journal of Clinical Virology. 2005;**34**(Suppl 1):S139-S142

[5] Nguyen VT, Law MG, Dore GJ. Hepatitis B-related hepatocellular carcinoma: Epidemiological characteristics and disease burden. Journal of Viral Hepatitis. 2009;**16**:453-463. DOI: 10.1111/j.1365-2893.2009.01117.x

[6] Yoo J, Hann HW, Coben R, Conn M, DiMarino AJ. Update treatment for HBV infection and persistent risk for hepatocellular carcinoma: Prospect for an HBV cure. Diseases. 2018;**6**. pii: E27. DOI: 10.3390/diseases6020027

[7] Clark DN, Hu J. Hepatitis B virus reverse transcriptase—Target of current antiviral therapy and future drug development. Antiviral Research. 2015;**123**:132-137. DOI: 10.1016/j.antiviral.2015.09.011

[8] Sun D, Zhu L, Yao D, Chen L, Fu L, Ouyang L. Recent progress in potential anti-hepatitis B virus agents: Structural and pharmacological perspectives. European Journal of Medicinal Chemistry. 2018;**147**:205-217. DOI: 10.1016/j.ejmech.2018.02.001

[9] Ikeda M, Morizane C, Ueno M, Okusaka T, Ishii H, Furuse J. Chemotherapy for hepatocellular carcinoma: Current status and future perspectives. Japanese Journal of Clinical Oncology. 2018;**48**:103-114. DOI: 10.1093/jjco/hyx180

[10] Kudo M. Immune checkpoint inhibition in hepatocellular carcinoma: Basics and ongoing clinical trials. Oncology. 2017;**92**(Suppl 1):50-62. DOI: 10.1159/000451016

[11] Beasley RP, Hwang LY, Lin CC, Chien CS. Hepatocellular carcinoma and hepatitis B virus. A prospective study of 22 707 men in Taiwan. Lancet. 1981;**2**:1129-1133

[12] Guidotti LG, Rochford R, Chung J, Shapiro M, Purcell R, Chisari FV. Viral clearance without destruction of infected cells during acute HBV infection. Science. 1999;**284**:825-829

[13] Wang Y, Jacob JR, Menne S, Bellezza CA, Tennant BC, Gerin JL, Cote PJ. Interferon-gamma-associated responses to woodchuck hepatitis virus infection in neonatal woodchucks and virus-infected hepatocytes. Journal of Viral Hepatitis. 2004;**11**:404-417

[14] Yang PL, Althage A, Chung J, Maier H, Wieland S, Isogawa M, Chisari FV. Immune effectors required for hepatitis B virus clearance. Proceedings of the National Academy of Sciences of the United States of America. 2010;**107**:798-802. DOI: 10.1073/pnas.0913498107

[15] Tiollais P, Pourcel C, Dejean A. The hepatitis B virus. Nature. 1985;**317**:489-495

[16] Kasprzak A, Biczysko W, Zabel M, Wysocki J, Surdyk-Zasada J. Studies on tissue expression of HBV in children with chronic hepatitis type B using Immunomax technique. Polish Journal of Pathology. 1999;**50**:249-258

[17] Feitelson MA. Hepatitis B virus gene products as immunological targets in chronic infection. Molecular Biology & Medicine. 1989;**6**:367-393

[18] Ferrari C, Penna A, Giuberti T, Tong MJ, Ribera E, Fiaccadori F, Chisari FV. Intrahepatic, nucleocapsid antigen-specific T cells in chronic active hepatitis B. Journal of Immunology. 1987;**139**:2050-2058

[19] Ferrari C, Penna A, Bertoletti A, Valli A, Antoni AD, Giuberti T, Cavalli A, Petit MA, Fiaccadori F. Cellular immune response to hepatitis B virus-encoded antigens in acute and chronic hepatitis B virus infection. Journal of Immunology. 1990;**145**:3442-3449

[20] Tong S, Li J, Wands JR, Wen YM. Hepatitis B virus genetic variants: Biological properties and clinical implications. Emerging Microbes and Infections. 2013;**2**:e10. DOI: 10.1038/emi.2013.10

[21] Faure-Dupuy S, Lucifora J, Durantel D. Interplay between the hepatitis B virus and innate immunity: From an understanding to the development of therapeutic concepts. Viruses. 2017;**9**. pii: E95. DOI: 10.3390/v9050095

[22] Wieland S, Thimme R, Purcell RH, Chisari FV. Genomic analysis of the host response to hepatitis B virus infection. Proceedings of the National Academy of Sciences of the United States of America. 2004;**101**:6669-6674. DOI: 10.1073/pnas.0401771101

[23] Kim CW, Yoon SK, Jung ES, Jung CK, Jang JW, Kim MS, Lee SY, Bae SH, Choi JY, Choi SW, Han NI, Lee CD. Correlation of hepatitis B core antigen and beta-catenin expression on hepatocytes in chronic hepatitis B virus infection: Relevance to the severity of liver damage and viral replication. Journal of Gastroenterology and Hepatology. 2007;**22**: 1534-1542. DOI: 10.1111/j.1440-1746.2007.04849.x

[24] Lin CL, Kao JH. Hepatitis B viral factors and clinical outcomes of chronic hepatitis B. Journal of Biomedical Science. 2008;**15**:137-145. DOI: 10.1007/s11373-007-9225-8

[25] Vento S, Hegarty JE, Alberti A, O'Brien CJ, Alexander GJ, Eddleston AL, Williams R. T lymphocyte sensitization to HBcAg and T cell-mediated unresponsiveness to HBsAg in hepatitis B virus-related chronic liver disease. Hepatology. 1985;**5**:192-197

[26] Alexopoulou A, Karayiannis P. HBeAg negative variants and their role in the natural history of chronic hepatitis B virus infection. World Journal of Gastroenterology. 2014;**20**:7644-7652. DOI: 10.3748/wjg.v20.i24.7644

[27] Lin CL, Liao LY, Wang CS, Chen PJ, Lai MY, Chen DS, Kao JH. Basal core-promoter mutant of hepatitis B virus and progression of liver disease in hepatitis B e antigen-negative chronic hepatitis B. Liver International. 2005;**25**:564-570. DOI: 10.1111/j.1478-3231.2005.01041.x

[28] Chen MT, Billaud JN, Sällberg M, Guidotti LG, Chisari FV, Jones J, Hughes J, Milich DR. A function of the hepatitis B virus precore protein is to regulate the immune response to the core antigen. Proceedings of the National Academy of Sciences of the United States of America. 2004;**101**:14913-14918. DOI: 10.1073/pnas.0406282101

[29] Lan S, Wu L, Wang X, Wu J, Lin X, Wu W, Huang Z. Impact of HBeAg on the maturation and function of dendritic cells. International Journal of Infectious Diseases. 2016;**46**: 42-48. DOI: 10.1016/j.ijid.2016.03.024

[30] Yu Y, Wan P, Cao Y, Zhang W, Chen J, Tan L, Wang Y, Sun Z, Zhang Q, Wan Y, Zhu Y, Liu F, Wu K, Liu Y, Wu J. Hepatitis B virus e antigen activates the suppressor of cytokine signaling 2 to repress interferon action. Scientific Reports. 2017;**7**:1729. DOI: 10.1038/s41598-017-01773-6

[31] Feitelson MA, Millman I, Duncan GD, Blumberg BS. Presence of antibodies to the polymerase gene product(s) of hepatitis B and woodchuck hepatitis virus in natural and experimental infections. Journal of Medical Virology. 1988;**24**:121-136

[32] Liu Y, Li J, Chen J, Li Y, Wang W, Du X, Song W, Zhang W, Lin L, Yuan Z. Hepatitis B virus polymerase disrupts K63-linked ubiquitination of STING to block innate cytosolic DNA-sensing pathways. Journal of Virology. 2015;**89**:2287-2300. DOI: 10.1128/JVI.02760-14

[33] Liu D, Wu A, Cui L, Hao R, Wang Y, He J, Guo D. Hepatitis B virus polymerase suppresses NF-κB signaling by inhibiting the activity of IKKs via interaction with Hsp90β. PLoS One. 2014;**9**:e91658. DOI: 10.1371/journal.pone.0091658

[34] Chen CJ, Yang HI. Natural history of chronic hepatitis B REVEALed. Journal of Gastroenterology and Hepatology. 2011;**26**:628-638. DOI: 10.1111/j.1440-1746.2011.06695.x

[35] Sinn DH, Lee J, Goo J, Kim K, Gwak GY, Paik YH, Choi MS, Lee JH, Koh KC, Yoo BC, Paik SW. Hepatocellular carcinoma risk in chronic hepatitis B virus-infected compensated cirrhosis patients with low viral load. Hepatology. 2015;**62**:694-701. DOI: 10.1002/hep.27889

[36] Chen JD, Yang HI, Iloeje UH, You SL, Lu SN, Wang LY, Su J, Sun CA, Liaw YF, Chen CJ. Risk evaluation of viral load elevation and associated liver disease/cancer in HBV (REVEAL-HBV) study group. Carriers of inactive hepatitis B virus are still at risk for hepatocellular carcinoma and liver-related death. Gastroenterology. 2010;**138**:1747-1754. DOI: 10.1053/j.gastro.2010.01.042

[37] Shao J, Wei L, Wang H, Sun Y, Zhang LF, Li J, Dong JQ. Relationship between hepatitis B virus DNA levels and liver histology in patients with chronic hepatitis B. World Journal of Gastroenterology. 2007;**13**:2104-2107. DOI: 10.3748/wjg.v13.i14.2104

[38] Mendy ME, Welzel T, Lesi OA, Hainaut P, Hall AJ, Kuniholm MH, McConkey S, Goedert JJ, Kaye S, Rowland-Jones S, Whittle H, Kirk GD. Hepatitis B viral load and risk for liver cirrhosis and hepatocellular carcinoma in the Gambia, West Africa. Journal of Viral Hepatitis. 2010;**17**:115-122. DOI: 10.1111/j.1365-2893.2009.01168.x

[39] Bertoletti A, Gehring A. Immune response and tolerance during chronic hepatitis B virus infection. Hepatology Research. 2007;**37**(Suppl 3):S331-S338. DOI: 10.1111/j.1872-034X.2007.00221.x

[40] Dudley FJ, Fox RA, Sherlock S. Cellular immunity and hepatitis-associated, Australia antigen liver disease. Lancet. 1972;**1**:723-726

[41] Matsubara K, Tokino T. Integration of hepatitis B virus DNA and its implications for hepatocarcinogenesis. Molecular Biology & Medicine. 1990;**7**:243-260

[42] Feitelson MA, Lee J. Hepatitis B virus integration, fragile sites, and hepatocarcinogenesis. Cancer Letters. 2007;**252**:157-170. DOI: 10.1016/j.canlet.2006.11.010

[43] Tu T, Budzinska MA, Vondran FWR, Shackel NA, Urban S. Hepatitis B virus DNA integration occurs early in the viral life cycle in an *in vitro* infection model via NTCP-dependent uptake of enveloped virus particles. Journal of Virology 2018;**92**:e02007-17. DOI: 10.1128/JVI.02007-17

[44] Wollersheim M, Debelka U, Hofschneider PH. A transactivating function encoded in the hepatitis B virus X gene is conserved in the integrated state. Oncogene. 1988;**3**:545-552

[45] Wang WL, London WT, Lega L, Feitelson MA. HBxAg in the liver from carrier patients with chronic hepatitis and cirrhosis. Hepatology. 1991;**14**:29-37

[46] Tian Y, Yang W, Song J, Wu Y, Ni B. Hepatitis B virus X protein-induced aberrant epigenetic modifications contributing to human hepatocellular carcinoma pathogenesis. Molecular and Cellular Biology. 2013;**33**:2810-2816. DOI: 10.1128/MCB.00205-13

[47] Caselmann WH. Transactivation of cellular gene expression by hepatitis B viral proteins: A possible molecular mechanism of hepatocarcinogenesis. Journal of Hepatology. 1995;**22**(1 Suppl):34-37

[48] Ji M, Hu K. Recent advances in the study of hepatitis B virus covalently closed circular DNA. Virologica Sinica. 2017;**32**:454-464. DOI: 10.1007/s12250-017-4009-4

[49] Palumbo GA, Scisciani C, Pediconi N, Lupacchini L, Alfalate D, Guerrieri F, Calvo L, Salerno D, Di Cocco S, Levrero M, Belloni L. IL6 inhibits HBV transcription by targeting the epigenetic control of the nuclear ccc DNA minichromosome. PLoS One. 2015;**10**:e0142599. DOI: 10.1371/journal.pone.0142599. Erratum in: PLoS One. 2015; **10**(12):e0145555

[50] Lucifora J, Xia Y, Reisinger F, Zhang K, Stadler D, Cheng X, Sprinzl MF, Koppensteiner H, Makowska Z, Volz T, Remouchamps C, Chou WM, Thasler WE, Hüser N, Durantel D, Liang TJ, Münk C, Heim MH, Browning JL, Dejardin E, Dandri M, Schindler M, Heikenwalder M, Protzer U. Specific and nonhepatotoxic degradation of nuclear hepatitis B virus ccc DNA. Science. 2014;**343**:1221-1228. DOI: 10.1126/science.1243462

[51] Lin SR, Yang HC, Kuo YT, Liu CJ, Yang TY, Sung KC, Lin YY, Wang HY, Wang CC, Shen YC, Wu FY, Kao JH, Chen DS, Chen PJ. The CRISPR/Cas9 system facilitates clearance of the intrahepatic HBV templates *in vivo*. Molecular Therapy: Nucleic Acids. 2014;**3**:e186. DOI: 10.1038/mtna.2014.38

[52] Møller HD, Mohiyuddin M, Prada-Luengo I, Sailani MR, Halling JF, Plomgaard P, Maretty L, Hansen AJ, Snyder MP, Pilegaard H, Lam HYK, Regenberg B. Circular DNA elements of chromosomal origin are common in healthy human somatic tissue. Nature Communications. 2018;**9**:1069. DOI: 10.1038/s41467-018-03369-8

[53] Arzumanyan A, Reis HM, Feitelson MA. Pathogenic mechanisms in HBV- and HCV-associated hepatocellular carcinoma. Nature Reviews. Cancer. 2013;**13**:123-135. DOI: 10.1038/nrc3449

[54] Tang H, Oishi N, Kaneko S, Murakami S. Molecular functions and biological roles of hepatitis B virus x protein. Cancer Science. 2006;**97**:977-983. DOI: 10.1111/j.1349-7006.2006.00299.x

[55] Bouchard MJ, Schneider RJ. The enigmatic X gene of hepatitis B virus. Journal of Virology. 2004;**78**:12725-12734. DOI: 10.1128/JVI.78.23.12725-12734.2004

[56] Cote PJ, Toshkov I, Bellezza C, Ascenzi M, Roneker C, Ann Graham L, Baldwin BH, Gaye K, Nakamura I, Korba BE, Tennant BC, Gerin JL. Temporal pathogenesis of experimental neonatal woodchuck hepatitis virus infection: Increased initial viral load and decreased severity of acute hepatitis during the development of chronic viral infection. Hepatology. 2000;**32**(4 Pt 1):807-817. DOI: 10.1053/jhep.2000.17681

[57] Zoulim F, Saputelli J, Seeger C. Woodchuck hepatitis virus X protein is required for viral infection in vivo. Journal of Virology. 1994;**68**:2026-2030

[58] Chen HS, Kaneko S, Girones R, Anderson RW, Hornbuckle WE, Tennant BC, Cote PJ, Gerin JL, Purcell RH, Miller RH. The woodchuck hepatitis virus X gene is important for establishment of virus infection in woodchucks. Journal of Virology. 1993;**67**:1218-1226

[59] Dandri M, Schirmacher P, Rogler CE. Woodchuck hepatitis virus X protein is present in chronically infected woodchuck liver and woodchuck hepatocellular carcinomas which are permissive for viral replication. Journal of Virology. 1996;**70**:5246-5254

[60] Jacob JR, Ascenzi MA, Roneker CA, Toshkov IA, Cote PJ, Gerin JL, Tennant BC. Hepatic expression of the woodchuck hepatitis virus X-antigen during acute and chronic infection and detection of a woodchuck hepatitis virus X-antigen antibody response. Hepatology. 1997;**26**:1607-1615. DOI: 10.1002/hep.510260632

[61] Feitelson MA, Clayton MM. X antigen polypeptides in the sera of hepatitis B virus-infected patients. Virology. 1990;**177**:367-371

[62] Feitelson MA, Clayton MM, Phimister B. Monoclonal antibodies raised to purified woodchuck hepatitis virus core antigen particles demonstrate X antigen reactivity. Virology. 1990;**177**:357-366

[63] Kouwaki T, Okamoto T, Ito A, Sugiyama Y, Yamashita K, Suzuki T, Kusakabe S, Hirano J, Fukuhara T, Yamashita A, Saito K, Okuzaki D, Watashi K, Sugiyama M, Yoshio S, Standley DM, Kanto T, Mizokami M, Moriishi K, Matsuura Y. Hepatocyte factor JMJD5 regulates hepatitis B virus replication through interaction with HBx. Journal of Virology. 2016;**90**:3530-3542. DOI: 10.1128/JVI.02776-15

[64] Guo L, Wang X, Ren L, Zeng M, Wang S, Weng Y, Tang Z, Wang X, Tang Y, Hu H, Li M, Zhang C, Liu C. HBx affects CUL4-DDB1 function in both positive and negative manners. Biochemical and Biophysical Research Communications. 2014;**450**:1492-1497. DOI: 10.1016/j.bbrc.2014.07.019

[65] Leupin O, Bontron S, Schaeffer C, Strubin M. Hepatitis B virus X protein stimulates viral genome replication via a DDB1-dependent pathway distinct from that leading to cell death. Journal of Virology. 2005;**79**:4238-4245. DOI: 10.1128/JVI.79.7.4238-4245.2005

[66] Hu Z, Zhang Z, Doo E, Coux O, Goldberg AL, Liang TJ. Hepatitis B virus X protein is both a substrate and a potential inhibitor of the proteasome complex. Journal of Virology. 1999;**73**:7231-7240

[67] Decorsière A, Mueller H, Van Breugel PC, Abdul F, Gerossier L, Beran RK, Livingston CM, Niu C, Fletcher SP, Hantz O, Strubin M. Hepatitis B virus X protein identifies the Smc5/6 complex as a host restriction factor. Nature. 2016;**531**:386-389. DOI: 10.1038/nature17170

[68] Belloni L, Pollicino T, De Nicola F, Guerrieri F, Raffa G, Fanciulli M, Raimondo G, Levrero M. Nuclear HBx binds the HBV minichromosome and modifies the epigenetic regulation of ccc DNA function. Proceedings of the National Academy of Sciences of the United States of America. 2009;**106**:19975-19979. DOI: 10.1073/pnas.0908365106

[69] Liang TJ. Virology: The X-files of hepatitis B. Nature. 2016;**531**:313-314. DOI: 10.1038/531313a

[70] Murphy CM, Xu Y, Li F, Nio K, Reszka-Blanco N, Li X, Wu Y, Yu Y, Xiong Y, Su L. Hepatitis B virus X protein promotes degradation of SMC5/6 to enhance HBV replication. Cell Reports. 2016;**16**:2846-2854. DOI: 10.1016/j.celrep.2016.08.026

[71] Guidotti LG, Isogawa M, Chisari FV. Host-virus interactions in hepatitis B virus infection. Current Opinion in Immunology. 2015;**36**:61-66. DOI: 10.1016/j.coi.2015.06.016

[72] Tsunematsu S, Suda G, Yamasaki K, Kimura M, Izumi T, Umemura M, Ito J, Sato F, Nakai M, Sho T, Morikawa K, Ogawa K, Tanaka Y, Watashi K, Wakita T, Sakamoto N. Hepatitis B virus X protein impairs α-interferon signaling via up-regulation of

suppressor of cytokine signaling 3 and protein phosphatase 2A. Journal of Medical Virology. 2017;**89**:267-275. DOI: 10.1002/jmv.24643

[73] Cho IR, Oh M, Koh SS, Malilas W, Srisuttee R, Jhun BH, Pellegrini S, Fuchs SY, Chung YH. Hepatitis B virus X protein inhibits extracellular IFN-α-mediated signal transduction by downregulation of type I IFN receptor. International Journal of Molecular Medicine. 2012;**29**:581-586. DOI: 10.3892/ijmm.2012.879

[74] Kumar M, Jung SY, Hodgson AJ, Madden CR, Qin J, Slagle BL. Hepatitis B virus regulatory HBx protein binds to adaptor protein IPS-1 and inhibits the activation of beta interferon. Journal of Virology. 2011;**85**:987-995. DOI: 10.1128/JVI.01825-10

[75] Vivekanandan P, Daniel HD, Kannangai R, Martinez-Murillo F, Torbenson M. Hepatitis B virus replication induces methylation of both host and viral DNA. Journal of Virology. 2010;**84**:4321-4329. DOI: 10.1128/JVI.02280-09

[76] Zhang YY, Hu KQ. Rethinking the pathogenesis of hepatitis B virus (HBV) infection. Journal of Medical Virology. 2015;**87**:1989-1999. DOI: 10.1002/jmv.24270

[77] Chisari FV, Klopchin K, Moriyama T, Pasquinelli C, Dunsford HA, Sell S, Pinkert CA, Brinster RL, Palmiter RD. Molecular pathogenesis of hepatocellular carcinoma in hepatitis B virus transgenic mice. Cell. 1989 Dec 22;**59**(6):1145-1156

[78] Su F, Schneider RJ. Hepatitis B virus HBx protein activates transcription factor NF-kappaB by acting on multiple cytoplasmic inhibitors of rel-related proteins. Journal of Virology. 1996;**70**:4558-4566

[79] Xia L, Tian D, Huang W, Zhu H, Wang J, Zhang Y, Hu H, Nie Y, Fan D, Wu K. Upregulation of IL-23 expression in patients with chronic hepatitis B is mediated by the HBx/ERK/NF-κB pathway. Journal of Immunology. 2012;**188**:753-764. DOI: 10.4049/jimmunol.1101652

[80] Xiang WQ, Feng WF, Ke W, Sun Z, Chen Z, Liu W. Hepatitis B virus X protein stimulates IL-6 expression in hepatocytes via a MyD88-dependent pathway. Journal of Hepatology. 2011;**54**:26-33. DOI: 10.1016/j.jhep.2010.08.006

[81] Lee MO, Choi YH, Shin EC, Kang HJ, Kim YM, Jeong SY, Seong JK, Yu DY, Cho H, Park JH, Kim SJ. Hepatitis B virus X protein induced expression of interleukin 18 (IL-18): A potential mechanism for liver injury caused by hepatitis B virus (HBV) infection. Journal of Hepatology. 2002;**37**:380-386. DOI: 10.1016/S0168-8278(02)00181-2

[82] Lara-Pezzi E, Majano PL, Gómez-Gonzalo M, García-Monzón C, Moreno-Otero R, Levrero M, López-Cabrera M. The hepatitis B virus X protein up-regulates tumor necrosis factor alpha gene expression in hepatocytes. Hepatology. 1998;**28**:1013-1021. DOI: 10.1002/hep.510280416

[83] Romero R, Lavine JE. Cytokine inhibition of the hepatitis B virus core promoter. Hepatology. 1996;**23**:17-23. DOI: 10.1002/hep.510230103

[84] Pan X, Cao H, Lu J, Shu X, Xiong X, Hong X, Xu Q, Zhu H, Li G, Shen G. Interleukin-32 expression induced by hepatitis B virus protein X is mediated through activation of NF-κB. Molecular Immunology. 2011;**48**:1573-1577. DOI: 10.1016/j.molimm.2011.03.012

[85] Meyer M, Caselmann WH, Schlüter V, Schreck R, Hofschneider PH, Baeuerle PA. Hepatitis B virus transactivator MHBst: Activation of NF-kappa B, selective inhibition by antioxidants and integral membrane localization. The EMBO Journal. 1992;**11**:2991-3001

[86] Waris G, Huh KW, Siddiqui A. Mitochondrially associated hepatitis B virus X protein constitutively activates transcription factors STAT-3 and NF-kappa B via oxidative stress. Molecular and Cellular Biology. 2001;**21**:7721-7730

[87] Chen J, Siddiqui A. Hepatitis B virus X protein stimulates the mitochondrial translocation of Raf-1 via oxidative stress. Journal of Virology. 2007;**81**:6757-6760

[88] Rahmani Z, Huh KW, Lasher R, Siddiqui A. Hepatitis B virus X protein co-localizes to mitochondria with a human voltage-dependent anion channel, HVDAC3, and alters its transmembrane potential. Journal of Virology. 2000;**74**:2840-2846

[89] Lee YI, Hwang JM, Im JH, Lee YI, Kim NS, Kim DG, Yu DY, Moon HB, Park SK. Human hepatitis B virus-X protein alters mitochondrial function and physiology in human liver cells. The Journal of Biological Chemistry. 2004;**279**:15460-15471. DOI: 10.1074/jbc.M309280200

[90] Shirakata Y, Koike K. Hepatitis B virus X protein induces cell death by causing loss of mitochondrial membrane potential. The Journal of Biological Chemistry. 2003;**278**:22071-22078. DOI: 10.1074/jbc.M301606200

[91] Cho HK, Cheong KJ, Kim HY, Cheong J. Endoplasmic reticulum stress induced by hepatitis B virus X protein enhances cyclo-oxygenase 2 expression via activating transcription factor 4. The Biochemical Journal. 2011;**435**:431-439. DOI: 10.1042/BJ20102071

[92] Minczuk M, Mroczek S, Pawlak SD, Stepien PP. Human ATP-dependent RNA/DNA helicase hSuv3p interacts with the cofactor of survivin HBXIP. The FEBS Journal. 2005; **272**:5008-5019. DOI: 10.1111/j.1742-4658.2005.04910.x

[93] Mao Y, Da L, Tang H, Yang J, Lei Y, Tiollais P, Li T, Zhao M. Hepatitis B virus X protein reduces starvation-induced cell death through activation of autophagy and inhibition of mitochondrial apoptotic pathway. Biochemical and Biophysical Research Communications. 2011;**415**:68-74. DOI: 10.1016/j.bbrc.2011.10.013

[94] Kim SJ, Khan M, Quan J, Till A, Subramani S, Siddiqui A. Hepatitis B virus disrupts mitochondrial dynamics: Induces fission and mitophagy to attenuate apoptosis. PLoS Pathogens. 2013;**9**:e1003722. DOI: 10.1371/journal.ppat.1003722

[95] Feitelson MA, Lega L, Duan LX, Clayton M. Characteristics of woodchuck hepatitis X-antigen in the livers and sera from infected animals. Journal of Hepatology. 1993; **17**(Suppl 3):S24-S34

[96] Wang WL, London WT, Feitelson MA. Hepatitis B x antigen in hepatitis B virus carrier patients with liver cancer. Cancer Research. 1991;**51**:4971-4977

[97] Diamantis ID, McGandy CE, Chen TJ, Liaw YF, Gudat F, Bianchi L. Hepatitis B X-gene expression in hepatocellular carcinoma. Journal of Hepatology. 1992;**15**:400-403

[98] Yu DY, Moon HB, Son JK, Jeong S, Yu SL, Yoon H, Han YM, Lee CS, Park JS, Lee CH, Hyun BH, Murakami S, Lee KK. Incidence of hepatocellular carcinoma in transgenic mice expressing the hepatitis B virus X-protein. Journal of Hepatology. 1999;**31**:123-132

[99] Furuta M, Tanaka H, Shiraishi Y, Unida T, Imamura M, Fujimoto A, Fujita M, Sasaki-Oku A, Maejima K, Nakano K, Kawakami Y, Arihiro K, Aikata H, Ueno M, Hayami S, Ariizumi SI, Yamamoto M, Gotoh K, Ohdan H, Yamaue H, Miyano S, Chayama K, Nakagawa H. Characterization of HBV integration patterns and timing in liver cancer and HBV-infected livers. Oncotarget. 2018;**9**:25075-25088. DOI: 10.18632/oncotarget.25308

[100] Robinson WS. Molecular events in the pathogenesis of hepadnavirus-associated hepatocellular carcinoma. Annual Review of Medicine. 1994;**45**:297-323. DOI: 10.1146/annurev.med.45.1.297

[101] Lin CL, Kao JH. Review article: Novel therapies for hepatitis B virus cure - advances and perspectives. Alimentary Pharmacology & Therapeutics. 2016;**44**:213-222. DOI: 10.1111/apt.13694

[102] Cao G-W. Cancer Evo-Dev, a novel hypothesis derived from studies on hepatitis B virus-induced carcinogenesis. Hepatoma Research. 2017;**3**:241-259. ISSN: 2454-2520. Available at: http://hrjournal.net/article/view/2267

[103] Sheen IS, Liaw YF, Tai DI, Chu CM. Hepatic decompensation associated with hepatitis B e antigen clearance in chronic type B hepatitis. Gastroenterology. 1985;**89**:732-735

[104] Bonino F, Rosina F, Rizzetto M, Rizzi R, Chiaberge E, Tardanico R, Callea F, Verme G. Chronic hepatitis in HBsAg carriers with serum HBV-DNA and anti-HBe. Gastroenterology. 1986;**90**(5 Pt 1):1268-1273

[105] Lee YI, Hur GM, Suh DJ, Kim SH. Novel pre-C/C gene mutants of hepatitis B virus in chronic active hepatitis: Naturally occurring escape mutants. The Journal of General Virology. 1996;**77**(Pt 6):1129-1138

[106] Rawat S, Bouchard MJ. The hepatitis B virus (HBV) HBx protein activates AKT to simultaneously regulate HBV replication and hepatocyte survival. Journal of Virology. 2015;**89**:999-1012. DOI: 10.1128/JVI.02440-14

[107] Mesri EA, Feitelson MA, Munger K. Human viral oncogenesis: A cancer hallmarks analysis. Cell Host & Microbe. 2014;**15**:266-282. DOI: 10.1016/j.chom.2014.02.011

3

Surgical Resection in HCC

Kevin Labadie, Kevin M. Sullivan and James O. Park

Abstract

Hepatocellular carcinoma (HCC) is a deadly disease. Its incidence is rising worldwide without significant improvement in survival in spite of improving therapies. A wide array of treatment options for HCC exist and include surgery, catheter-based therapies, radiation and systemic therapy. These modalities are often used in combination for optimal management in a multidisciplinary approach. Surgical resection remains one of the only curative therapeutic options for HCC, although it is indicated in select patients with localized disease. Herein, we cover the role of surgical resection in the management of HCC, reviewing the perioperative and operative considerations, in addition to highlighting the advances in minimally invasive surgery and novel navigation technologies.

Keywords: hepatocellular carcinoma, liver cancer, surgery, minimally invasive, multidisciplinary

1. Introduction

Hepatocellular carcinoma (HCC) is the second most lethal malignancy worldwide [1]. Despite the advent of effective antiviral drugs to eradicate hepatitis C infection, the prevalence of HCC is projected to increase secondary to increasing rates of fatty liver disease from diabetes and the obesity epidemic [2]. Unfortunately, there has been little to no change in the survivability of HCC over the last three decades [3] in spite of the increasing array of therapeutic options, leaving much room for improvement. The armamentarium for managing HCC is wide and includes surgical resection, orthotopic liver transplantation (OLT), ablative techniques using ethanol (percutaneous ethanol injection, PEI), microwave (MWA) or radiofrequency (RFA), catheter-directed transarterial chemoembolization (TACE) or radioembolization (TARE), external beam radiation therapy in the form of stereotactic body radiation therapy (SBRT) or proton beam therapy (PBT), systemic targeted small molecule tyrosine kinase inhibitors, check-point inhibitor immunotherapy and investigational agents. These modalities are often used together in a multidisciplinary approach.

Surgical resection, or partial hepatectomy (PH), is a potentially curative surgical treatment option for up to 15–20% of patients with HCC. The primary objective of PH is to remove the HCC with an adequate margin, while preserving as much functional liver parenchyma to avoid post-resection hepatic failure. With improvements in preoperative assessment, patient selection, surgical and anesthetic techniques, intraoperative ultrasound, PH for HCC is now routine and safe. Operative mortality has been reduced to less than 5% with a 5-year overall survival of 60–75%.

2. Preoperative considerations

Several factors are considered in determining the eligibility for PH, including the patient's health status (e.g. age, ECOG PS), tumor-specific factors (e.g. extent and tumor biology), and the reserve of the liver remnant. Determined by the degree of liver dysfunction and the size of the postoperative liver remnant. While there is no strict age limit, one must consider the liver's regenerative capabilities in elderly patients, and the patient's ability to tolerate the physiologic consequences of portal pedicle clamping and acute hemorrhage on their cardiopulmonary system. In addition, patients undergoing a minimally invasive approach must also be able to endure the effects of the pneumoperitoneum and reverse Trendelenburg positioning on their physiology.

Several different clinical staging systems exist to stratify patients according to prognostic variables [4]. One of the most commonly used is the Barcelona Clinic Liver Cancer (BCLC) system which incorporates tumor size, number of nodules and hepatic function as classified by the Child-Pugh score [5]. The system classifies patients into early, intermediate, advanced and terminal stages and proposes recommended treatment strategy. According to this staging system, only stage 0 or early stage patients with small tumors are recommended for surgical resection or liver transplant.

However, many view the BCLC criterion for resection to be restrictive. For patients with large tumors (beyond any down-staging or expanded OLT criteria) who are ineligible for OLT, PH is the only potentially curative treatment. With improvements in perioperative management, preoperative morphological assessment and manipulation of the future liver remnant, PH for large HCC has been safely performed with good oncologic outcome [6, 7]. Therefore, large tumor size alone is not a contraindication to PH, rather factors such as multiple or bilobar tumors, extrahepatic metastasis, involvement of the main bile duct, portal venous or other macroscopic vascular invasion, and portal hypertension are all relative contraindications to PH. When clinically not evident, portal hypertension can be evaluated by measuring the transjugular intrahepatic portosystemic gradient (PSG). PSG values greater than 10 mmHg are indicative of significant portal hypertension and these patients must be approached with caution.

85–90% of patients with HCC have concomitant liver dysfunction. It is critical to account for the degree of liver dysfunction in addition to the patient's overall functional and nutritional status. Patients with liver disease are often malnourished with diminished performance status and comorbid conditions. To help stratify clinical liver dysfunction, patients are classified by the Child-Turcotte-Pugh (CTP) score and the Model for End-Stage Liver Disease (MELD) system. These two systems classify patients based on physical exam and laboratory data, with increasing scores associated with higher overall surgical risk. In general, patients with CTP score up to B7, MELD score <9 without significant portal hypertension can be considered for PH. Patients with more severe liver dysfunction and HCC can be considered for OLT if they meet specific criteria [8, 9].

Assessment of the hepatic function and future liver remnant (FLR) is important for patient selection prior to surgical resection [10]. The volume of the FLR and the regenerative capacity are key predictors of postoperative morbidity. Several laboratory tests have been used to evaluate hepatic reserve in cirrhotic patients including assessment of clearance of indocyanine green, sorbitol and 99mTc-galactosyl serum albumin scintigraphy [11]. Preoperative volumetric analysis can be performed with 3D computerized tomography volumetry [12]. To minimize the chance of post-hepatectomy liver failure, data suggest a liver remnant to be at minimum >20% of preoperative liver volume in a normal functioning liver, >30% for patients who have undergone >3 months systemic chemotherapy and >40% in those with advanced liver disease [13, 14].

Several techniques for preoperative optimization of the FLR exist including portal vein embolization (PVE) and the associated liver partition with portal vein ligation for staged hepatectomy (ALPPS) [15]. Initially developed in 1986, PVE results in atrophy of the embolized segments and compensatory hypertrophy of the perfused segments [16], within approximately 4–6 weeks, with at least >10% growth of the FLR predicting adequate regeneration post-PH. PVE has been shown to reduce the rate of postoperative complications in select patients with chronic liver disease [17], and can also be used safely in patients undergoing concurrent chemotherapy for colorectal metastases. One study demonstrated improved prognosis after PH in patients with impaired hepatic function [18].

ALPPS was developed in 2007 to induce liver hypertrophy in patients planned for extended liver resections with marginal FLR. A two-step operation, the initial data demonstrated it to be quite effective with rapid hypertrophy [15], however, it has not gained wide acceptance secondary to significant morbidity and mortality and the need for larger scale studies [19–21]. However, there are more recent reports of "mini-ALPPS" where the procedure is performed minimally invasively and with limited peripheral division of the parenchyma.

3. Surgical considerations

3.1. Surgical anatomy

The surgical anatomy of the liver is based on Claude Couinaud's classification system and further refined in the Brisbane 2000 Terminology of Liver Anatomy and Resections (**Figure 1**)

[22]. In this classification, the liver is divided into first, second and third order divisions based on internal anatomy rather than surface landmarks. First order division splits the liver into a right and left hemiliver along Cantlie's line, a plane extending from the middle of the gall-bladder fossa to the center of the inferior vena cava. Second order divisions split the hemilivers into two respective sections or sectors, the medial and lateral sections/sectors on the left and anterior and posterior sections/sectors on the right. The third order division divides each section/sector into two segments, constituting the 9 individual hepatic segments defined by Couinaud. In general, each segment has a unique vascular inflow, outflow and biliary duct enabling segments to be removed without damage to other segments.

The proper hepatic artery and portal vein bifurcate prior to the hilum of the liver and form the right and left hepatic artery and portal vein which supply the right and left hemiliver. Joined by the biliary duct, the portal triad generally runs centrally within hepatic segments. The right hepatic artery enters the parenchyma soon after branching while the left has a longer extrahepatic course. In contrast, the three hepatic veins run between section/sectors in three portal scissurae. The right hepatic vein drains directly into the inferior vena cava (IVC) while the middle and left hepatic veins often form a common trunk prior to entering the IVC.

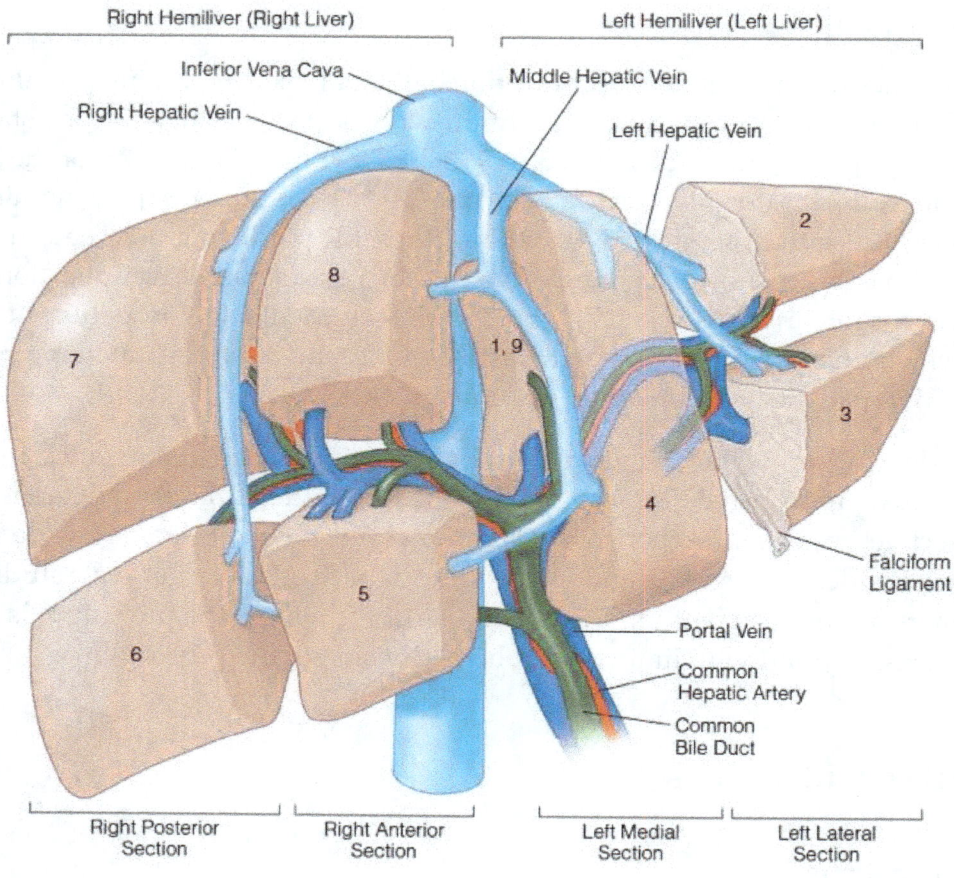

Figure 1. Schematic of liver anatomy separating the parenchyma into 9 anatomic segments. Each segment has unique blood supply and biliary drainage. Source: Cho, Fong. Hepatic Resection. In: Ashley SW, editor. Scientific American Surgery. Hamilton: Decker. 7th ed; 2014. pp. 1094–1114.

The liver is encapsulated by a fibrous capsule, known as Glisson's capsule. The capsule envelops the portal triads as they enter the liver parenchyma which makes it identifiable on intraoperative ultrasound. Furthermore, the dense capsule allows for control of the portal triad during dissection and enables pedicle ligation.

3.2. Anesthetic considerations

Some important perioperative anesthetic considerations should be accounted for to increase the safety of hepatectomy. To minimize the possibility of major intraoperative hemorrhage, the central venous pressure should be maintained at less than 5 mmHg to reduce the intrahepatic venous pressure. This is achieved using various anesthetic maneuvers and agents such as IVF restriction, and administration of isoflurane, fentanyl, mannitol, and cisatricurium. For open hepatectomy, the patient can be placed in slight reverse Trendelenburg position if pressures allow and switched to Trendelenburg position if there is significant hemorrhage with hemodynamic derangement to increase cardiac output and maintain end-organ perfusion. For laparoscopic/robotic hepatectomy, the patient is placed in reverse Trendelenburg position for a caudal approach which improves visualization of the vasculature, and the pneumoperitoneum creates a tamponade effect on the hepatic veins, which aids in limiting hemorrhage. Adequate vascular access should be obtained using large bore IVs, with appropriate invasive hemodynamic monitoring using A-line. Blood products should be readily available and resuscitation of operative blood loss should be with an appropriate combination of crystalloid, albumin and blood product as necessary. End-tidal CO_2 is measured to monitor for CO_2 embolism in the laparoscopic/robotic approach.

4. Operative technique

Resections are either "anatomic" or "non-anatomic". Anatomic resection defines a resection that obeys Brisbane divisions and is preferred for malignant disease because it has been found to lower rate of positive margins, decrease regional recurrences and improve surgical outcome. Non-anatomic resection refers to parenchymal transection that does not respect segmental planes and is typically used for debulking procedures, benign tumors or when trying to preserve remnant parenchyma. Achieving a microscopic margin negative (R0) resection is paramount to reducing local recurrence. 1 cm surgical margins have historically been considered standard, but narrower margins have been safely demonstrated [23].

There are six standard, anatomic hepatic resections as defined by the Brisbane classification (**Figure 2**). Right hemi-hepatectomy consists of surgical resection of segments V-VIII and left hepatectomy includes segments II-IV and occasionally segment I. In an extended right hepatectomy or a right trisectionectomy/trisectorectomy, segments IV-VIII, and in an extended left hepatectomy or a left trisectionectomy, segments II-IV, V and VIII are resected. A left lateral sectorectomy involves resection of segments II-III and a right posterior sectionectomy includes segments VI-VII. Segmentectomies denote resection of any individual segment.

The common principle of anatomic hepatectomies involves parenchymal transection after both vascular inflow and outflow have been controlled. Given that each hepatic segment has

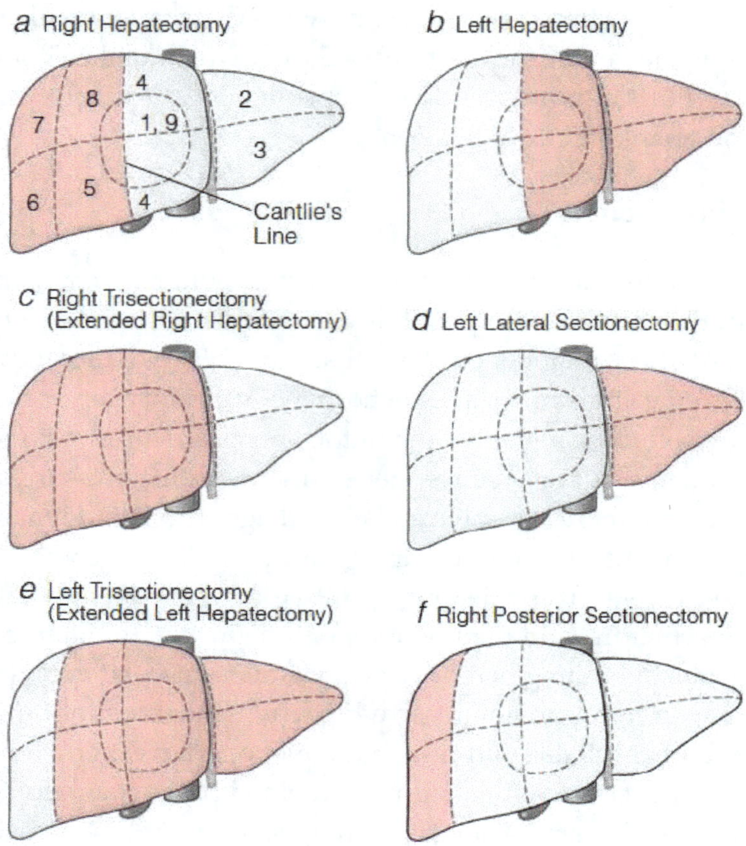

Figure 2. Schematic illustrations of the standard hepatic resections as labeled. Source: Cho, Fong. Hepatic Resection. In: Ashley SW, editor. Scientific American Surgery. Hamilton: Decker. 7th ed; 2014. pp. 1094–1114.

their unique vascular inflow and outflow, each segment can be safely excised without damage to surrounding hepatic segments. Intraoperative ultrasonography is used routinely for identification of the vascular structures, evaluation of tumor location, extent and relationship to the surrounding vasculature.

After initial laparoscopic inspection excludes unresectable disease (in selected cases), the incision is made. In an open conventional approach, appropriate incision and exposure is critical to safe hepatectomy. There are several incisions used including the bilateral subcostal (Chevron), right/left subcostal, J-type or the inverted Y (Mercedes) incision.

Once the liver is mobilized by dividing ligamentous attachments, careful inspection, palpation and ultrasound examination are performed to evaluate for any missed tumors. Arterial aberrancies are identified and portal triad inflow is controlled with sutures and clips or staple ligation. The corresponding hepatic vein is isolated and ligated. Parenchymal transection is performed along the line of devascularization. Different techniques for parenchymal transection exist, varying from clamp-crushing, waterjet, monopolar/bipolar cautery, radiofrequency ablative devices, bipolar vessel sealing devices, ultrasonic dissection devices to staplers. The clamp-crush technique is rapid and has been associated with lower rates of blood loss compared to other methods [24]. Once the resected segment is removed, hemostasis is obtained with sutures, clips, argon beam coagulator and application of various hemostatic agents. Biliary leaks are controlled with clipping and suture ligation. Prior to abdominal closure, drains are placed if there is an infected operative field or if a biliary reconstruction is performed [25].

5. Minimally invasive hepatectomy

5.1. Laparoscopic-assisted partial hepatectomy

Although established as a safe and beneficial approach for numerous intra-abdominal operations, laparoscopic techniques were slow to be adopted for liver surgery for several reasons [26]. Concerns over technical feasibility of vascular dissection and control, organ mobilization, parenchymal dissection and management of intraoperative complications were prohibitive. Furthermore, it was unknown if port-site seeding, inadequate margins and poor oncologic outcomes would be more common in the minimally invasive approach.

The benefits of laparoscopic liver surgery are numerous. In addition to the generalized benefits of laparoscopic surgery including a more rapid functional recovery, smaller incisions which reduce the incidence of surgical site infections and postoperative pulmonary complications, there are additional advantages specific to laparoscopic liver surgery. Steep Trendelenburg positioning reduces intrahepatic venous pressure and the pneumoperitoneum exerts tamponade effect on vasculature leading to reduced intraoperative blood loss. Laparoscopy creates a caudal-cranial surgical view which affords improved visualization of major vascular structures compared to the ventral-dorsal angle of visualization of an open hepatectomy. For cirrhotic patients, small laparoscopic incisions avoid disruption of abdominal wall collaterals and the constraint on fluid shifts in a laparoscopic partial hepatectomy can decrease the incidence of liver-related complications. Minimally invasive hepatectomy also results in less adhesion formation which facilitates additional surgery in the future.

There have been numerous studies to date demonstrating the safety and efficacy of laparoscopic liver surgery. In 2009, a worldwide experience of 127 series including 2804 cases of laparoscopic partial hepatectomy demonstrated comparable 5-year overall survival and disease free survival compared to open hepatectomy [27]. Half of these cases were done for malignant disease with greater than 80% of resections boasting negative surgical margins. In 2015, a randomized control trial was published demonstrating safety and feasibility of laparoscopic liver resection with reduction in length of stay and intraoperative blood loss compared to open hepatectomy [28]. Numerous systematic analyses have substantiated these data, demonstrating that the laparoscopic partial hepatectomy is associated with decreased intraoperative blood loss, shorter length of hospital stay, and decreased number of positive resection margins. Overall, there were consistently fewer complications found in the laparoscopic group in these reviews [29]. A case–control propensity matched studies also found no difference in 1-, 3-, and 5-year overall survival and disease-free survival [30]. The National Surgical Quality Improvement Program database was evaluated to compare short-term outcomes among patients undergoing minimally invasive partial hepatectomy. Over 3000 patients were include in the study and it demonstrated lower postoperative morbidity and shorter length of stay compared with patients undergoing open liver resection [31].

Specific to the treatment of HCC, the safety and efficacy of the laparoscopic approach has been evaluated in several meta-analyses and propensity score analyses. These studies demonstrated the equivalent or superior perioperative outcomes of laparoscopic compared to open resection [32, 33]. In a propensity score analysis, the overall and disease-free survival were similar and for the secondary outcomes, the laparoscopic group had shorter hospital stay, lower morbidity, with fewer transient liver failure and wound complications, and a larger tumor margin [34].

Multiple meta-analyses and case control series were reviewed and analyzed at the second international conference for laparoscopic liver resection in Morioka in 2014. Minor resections were validated as standard practice in the assessment stage, while major or complex resections were considered to be in the exploration stage, with incompletely defined risks. The Jury at Morioka made strong recommendations for higher quality studies including registries to define the role and benefits of laparoscopic major hepatectomy.

Patient selection is critical to ensuring safe laparoscopic partial hepatectomy. Although is technically feasible, resection of lesions in right posterior sections or the hepatic dome can be challenging and should be approached with caution. The patient is placed in the supine position and securely fastened to the table to allow for safe intraoperative repositioning. Generally, five ports are required for laparoscopic resection including two 12 mm and three 5 mm ports. Port placement is dependent upon laterality of the lesion as shown in **Figure 3**. Some surgeons advocate using a hand access port to assist with intraoperative manipulation, intra-corporeal suturing as well as serve as the specimen removal site.

5.2. Robotic-assisted partial hepatectomy

Further advances in surgical technology has created new opportunities in minimally invasive liver surgery. Robotic surgical systems offer unique advantages to the liver surgeon that enhances the minimally invasive approach. There are several key improvements on the robotic surgical system including a camera with optics providing a 3-dimensional stereotactic visual field. In addition, the instruments allow for seven degrees of freedom in their motion, providing easier suturing for hemorrhage control. There is no fulcrum effect on the body wall of the patient as in laparoscopic surgery, and it has been associated with reduction in surgeon fatigue compared to the laparoscopic approach.

Similar to laparoscopic partial hepatectomy, the patient is placed in the supine position and in steep reverse Trendelenburg position. The table is tilted with right side up approximately 25 degrees for right-sided resections. Five ports are placed including four robot-controlled ports and one assistant port (**Figure 4**). The ports are placed based on the laterality of the resection. In general, for a right-sided hepatectomy, the camera port is placed to the right-side of midline. Once the ports have been placed, the robot is docked from the cephalad position (**Figure 5**). Intraoperative ultrasound is critical to establishing vascular anatomy and defining oncologic planes of resection. After vascular control and establishing the line of transection, parenchymal transection is performed using one of many published techniques [35].

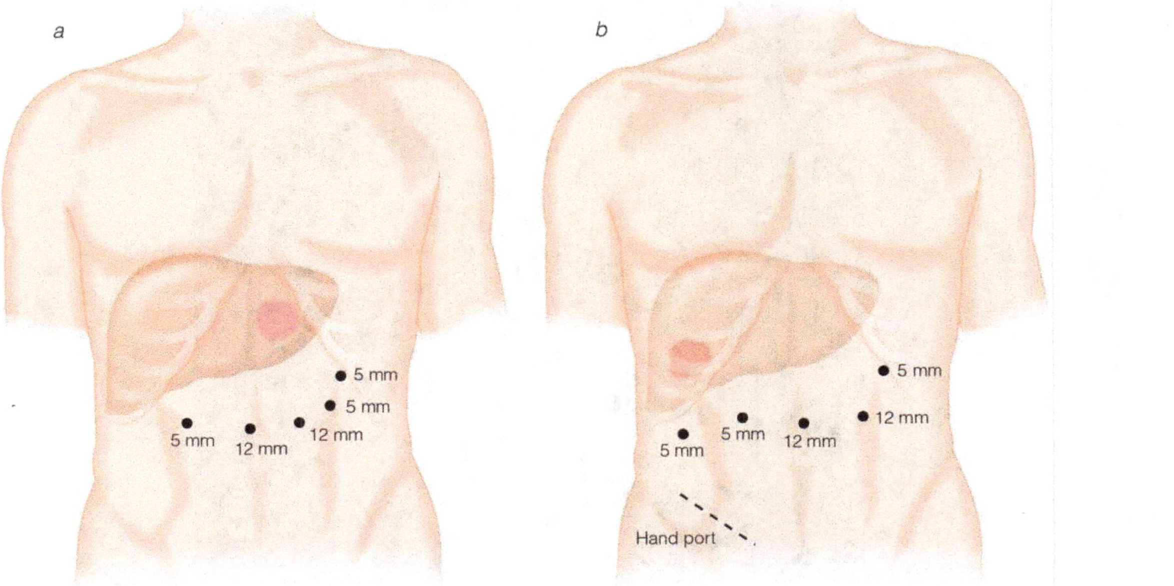

Figure 3. Suggested port placements for laparoscopic left lateral sectionectomy (a) and hand-assisted laparoscopic right hepatectomy (b). Source: Cho, Fong. Hepatic Resection. In: Ashley SW, editor. Scientific American Surgery. Hamilton: Decker. 7th ed; 2014. pp. 1094–1114.

Several large case series have been published demonstrating the success of robotic liver resection [36, 37]. The first large case series of 70 patients included 38.5% major liver resections without any mortalities [36]. An early systematic review of the literature demonstrated safety and feasibility of the robotic technique, with conversion to open rate of 4.6% and complication rate of 20.3% [38]. In 2018, an international, multicenter retrospective review of robotic liver surgery was published specifically evaluating long-term oncologic outcomes in patients with primary hepatobiliary malignancies after a median follow up of 75 months [39]. This study demonstrated comparable outcomes between robotic, open and laparoscopic liver surgery with 3-year overall survival of 90% for HCC. The majority of the cases were non-anatomic resections with an R0 resection achieved in 95% of HCC resections, 68% in cholangiocarcinoma and 82% in gallbladder cancer.

Minimally invasive approach to liver surgery, both laparoscopic and robotic-assisted, have their share of limitations. An important potential complication associated with the establishment of pneumoperitoneum and laparoscopic liver surgery is carbon dioxide gas embolism. Reports have demonstrated that this event rate is low, particularly if the pneumoperitoneal pressure is maintained below 12 mmHg [40]. Studies have published and event rate of as low as at 0.5~1.5% [41]. There is a learning curve with gaining proficiency in the laparoscopic technique of liver resection with expert centers estimating the learning curve for laparoscopic liver resection at approximately 45~70 cases with senior partner proctoring [42]. Other limitations include the need for a skilled bedside assistant, and the diminished tactile sense when dealing with friable tissue such as steatotic liver parenchyma or thin venules within a cirrhotic liver can make the case challenging. And in the rare event when massive venous bleeding ensues, it can be difficult to control.

Cost is one major barrier to the wide adoption of the robotic approach. There is a significant initial capital investment in addition to maintenance fees and costs of staff training. However, one

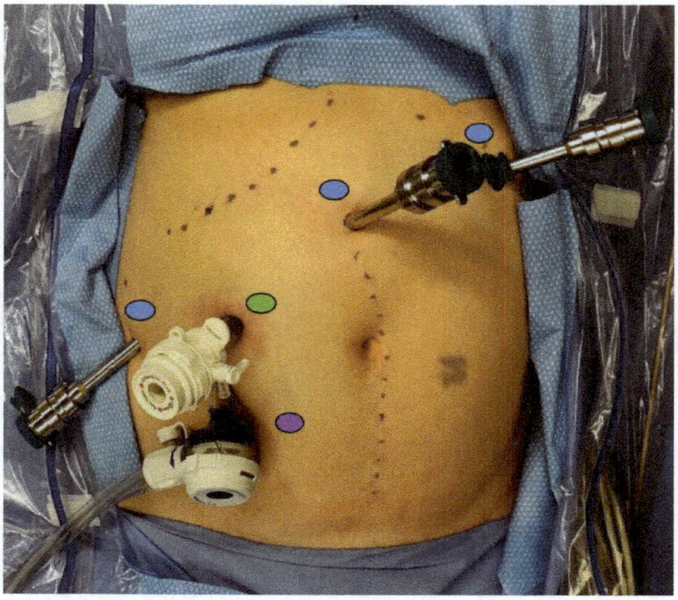

Figure 4. Image of port placement for a robot-assisted surgeries left lateral sectionectomy. Blue dots denote da Vinci 8-mm reusable cannulas (3). Green dot denotes 12-mm camera port. Purple dot denotes AirSeal® assistant port. Costal margin and midline marked in dotted pen.

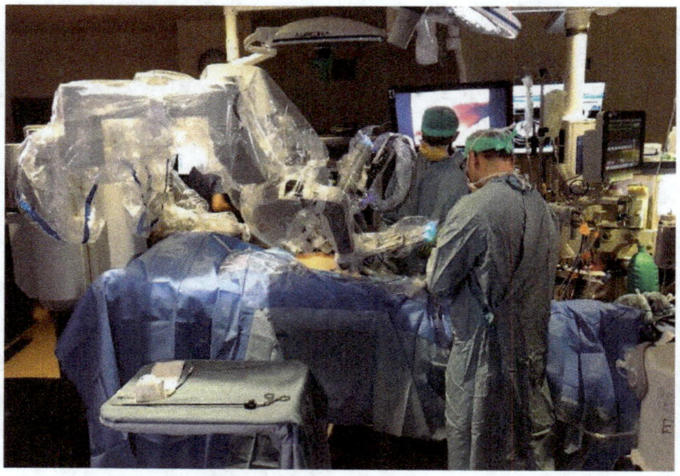

Figure 5. Standard operating room set up for robotic-assisted liver surgery. Head of bed is on left side of image, anesthesia equipment and personnel on right side of image.

study demonstrated that while perioperative costs are higher with the robot, the overall total direct hospital costs are lower at least in part due to the decrease length of stay with robotic minimally invasive resection [43]. There are several generations of the robot with older generation units best suited for an operation in a single work field, with cumbersome redocking steps to perform multi-quadrant operations. The majority of studies indicate a longer operating time secondary to robot set up and draping. Technically speaking, the robot does not provide haptic feedback challenging the surgeon to "feel with their eyes" and occasionally resulting in excessive tissue damage in inexperienced hands. Further studies are needed to examine the comparative effectiveness of robotic versus laparoscopic minimally invasive hepatectomy.

6. Postoperative complications

The main postoperative complications include postoperative hemorrhage, liver dysfunction, biliary leak and fluid collections. Postoperative hemorrhage is uncommon after liver resection if meticulous attention is given to confirmation of hemostasis at the conclusion of the case. Bleeding may occasionally occur from retroperitoneal structures, such as the adrenal gland, or diaphragmatic musculature. Argon beam coagulator and a variety of topical hemostatic applications are utilized to reduce liver surface related bleeding.

Post hepatectomy liver failure (PHLF) is a major postoperative complication with mortality of approximately 30%. The definition of post-hepatectomy liver is the impaired ability of the liver to maintain its synthetic, excretory and detoxifying functions, characterized by an increase in international normalized ratio and bilirubin on or after postoperative day 5 [44]. The most effective treatment of PHLF is liver transplantation but that is reserved for the most severe cases. Initial care is supportive and often includes mechanical ventilation, hemodynamic support and hemodialysis. Administration of colloid products and nutritional supplementation is also advocated.

The best way to treat post-hepatectomy liver failure is to prevent it. Preoperative weight loss, nutritional supplementation, careful preoperative selection and risk stratification are important to minimize the risk of PHLF [10]. Intra-operatively, minimizing blood loss and blood transfusion, close attention to hemostasis and minimizing skeletonization of the hepatoduodenal ligament will lower risk of PHLF. In the postoperative period, recognizing and aggressively treating postoperative hemorrhage, biliary obstructions or leaks and intra-abdominal infections will reduce the hepatic stress and likelihood of developing hepatic failure.

Postoperative fluid collections collect in the resected liver bed. These collections are varied in etiology but can include hematoma, seroma or biloma. They often to not result in symptoms, but occasionally they can cause pain or fullness requiring drainage. These collections also are at risk for infection and abscess formation. Biliary leakage from the raw surface of the resected liver can occur in up to 8% of patients after liver resection [45].

7. Emerging technologies

7.1. Near-infrared fluorescent imaging in hepatic surgery

New technologies continue to be developed to enhance minimally invasive liver surgery. One example is intra-operative near-infrared fluorescence (NIF) imaging. NIF imaging has become commonplace in many laparoscopic and robotic camera systems enabling the identification of various dyes, such as indocyanine green, injected preoperatively. Indocyanine green is a green dye that is preferentially metabolized by hepatocytes and excreted in the biliary tree. It lights up the biliary tree and has been utilized for robotic and laparoscopic assisted cholecystectomy. It has been more recently utilized to guide parenchymal dissection after vascular control by identifying perfused from poorly perfused hepatic parenchyma.

7.2. Intelligent imaging in robotic-assisted surgery

Future directions within the realm of robotic liver surgery include the application of preoperative planning with virtual reality (VR) models and real-time augmented reality (AR) intraoperative endoscopic overlays to aid with surgical navigation on *da Vinci* ® surgical systems. The current practice standard for operative planning involves preoperative cross-sectional imaging using contrast-enhanced, multiphase liver protocol computed tomography (CT) or magnetic resonance imaging (MRI) scans to evaluate the tumor's extent (size and number) and location with respect to critical structures including the major vasculature and biliary architecture. Surgeons rely on years of training to develop the ability to mentally reconstruct 2D images into a mental 3D model in order to preoperatively plan for a surgery while referencing the 2D images intraoperatively.

Computer-based three-dimensional (3D) reconstructions of liver tumors have been shown to increase accuracy of tumor localization and precision of operative planning for liver surgery [46]. While useful for operative planning, intraoperative review of 2D images on a traditional PACS system requires diversion of attention away from the operative field. Intraoperative ultrasound is routinely used for real-time localization of liver tumors and

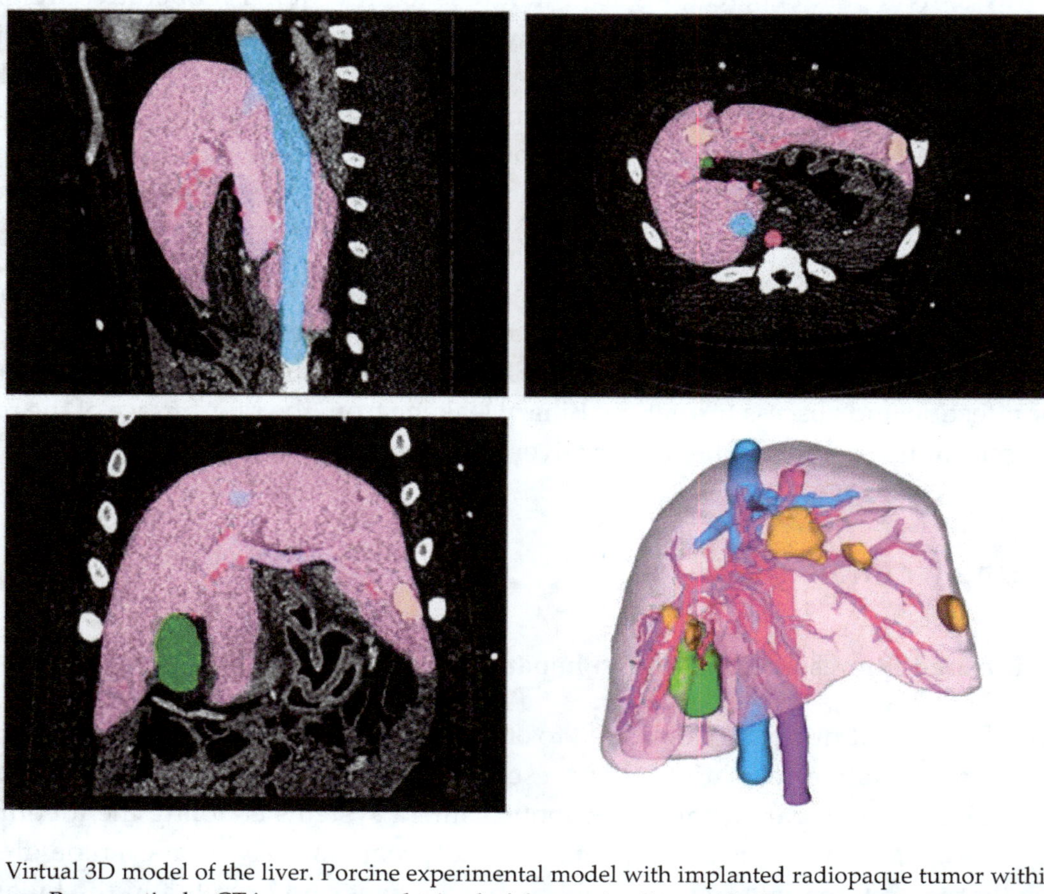

Figure 6. Virtual 3D model of the liver. Porcine experimental model with implanted radiopaque tumor within the liver parenchyma. Preoperatively, CT images were obtained of the porcine liver with 3D segmented reconstructions created from the DICOM images. The 3D reconstructions can be viewed for preoperative planning with intuitive Surgical's *da Vinci*® Surgical System.

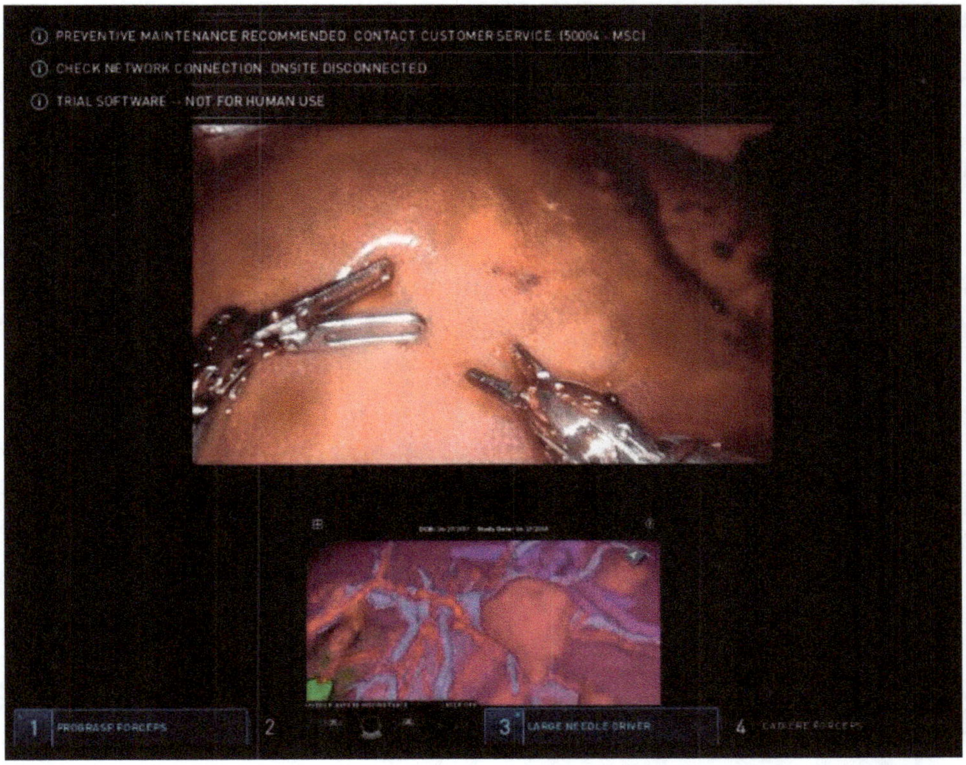

Figure 7. Real-time endoscopic overlay of 3D reconstruction over the surgical field on the *da Vinci* ® Xi Surgical System. The relationship between the tumor (light pink) and adjacent vasculature including the hepatic veins (light blue), hepatic arteries (red) and portal veins (blue) is present on the overlay. After initial registration, the overlay is mapped onto the patient-specific anatomy changing in real-time with camera movement.

identification of vessels and biliary structures. However, its use is limited in minimally invasive liver surgery due to the need for an additional port site and the need to interpret the 2D ultrasound images and mentally reconstruct the 3D anatomy being projected based on the orientation of the ultrasound probe. Preoperative planning with a VR model (**Figure 6**) and the application of AR endoscopic overlay (**Figure 7**) of patient-specific anatomy into the robotic surgical system could potentially improve surgical efficiency in real-time with intelligent surgical navigation.

AR may be developed to overlay accurate 3D reconstruction data onto the operative field itself, thereby eliminating the need to divert the attention from the operative field and to translate the 2D images into a 3D construct. These advancements with planning and guidance can potentially reduce the cognitive load burden on the surgeon. Augmented reality for spatial recognition has been shown to improve localization accuracy in an experimental model of uterine myomectomy [47],and our recent experience has shown promise and feasibility in an experimental porcine liver model (**Figures 1** and **2**). Next steps in the application of VR and AR to hepatobiliary surgery include overcoming technical obstacles of continuous co-registration to a mobile liver with tissue deformation while continuing to define the utility of the technology with patient education, tumor board evaluations, preoperative planning and intraoperative navigation.

8. Conclusion

Hepatocellular carcinoma (HCC) is a deadly disease that represents major challenges for patients and healthcare providers alike. Numerous therapeutic options exist for the treatment of HCC that are often used in combination for local and regional control. Surgical resection remains an important intervention that can be curative. Minimally invasive surgical technologies continue to improve increasing its safety and applicability for oncologic liver surgery.

Acknowledgements

We would like to acknowledge Drs. Kyle Miller and Jonathan Sorger of Intuitive Surgical Inc. for their collaboration on the emerging robotic surgical technologies.

Author details

Kevin Labadie, Kevin M. Sullivan and James O. Park*

*Address all correspondence to: jopark@uw.edu

University of Washington, Seattle, WA, USA

References

[1] Ferlay J, Soerjomataram I, Dikshit R, et al. Cancer incidence and mortality worldwide: Sources, methods and major patterns in GLOBOCAN 2012. International Journal of Cancer. 2015;**136**(5):E359-E386. DOI: 10.1002/ijc.29210

[2] Starley BQ, Calcagno CJ, Harrison SA. Nonalcoholic fatty liver disease and hepatocellular carcinoma: A weighty connection. Hepatology. 2010;**51**(5):1820-1832. DOI: 10.1002/hep.23594

[3] Altekruse SF, McGlynn KA, Reichman ME. Hepatocellular carcinoma incidence, mortality, and survival trends in the United States from 1975 to 2005. Journal of Clinical Oncology. 2009;**27**(9):1485-1491. DOI: 10.1200/JCO.2008.20.7753

[4] Pons F, Varela M, Llovet JM. Staging systems in hepatocellular carcinoma. HPB: The Official Journal of the International Hepato Pancreato Biliary Association. 2005;**7**(1):35-41. DOI: 10.1080/13651820410024058

[5] Llovet J, Brú C, Bruix J. Prognosis of hepatocellular carcinoma: The BCLC staging classification. Seminars in Liver Disease. 1999;**19**(03):329-338. DOI: 10.1055/s-2007-1007122

[6] Ng KK, Vauthey J-N, Pawlik TM, et al. Is hepatic resection for large or multinodular hepatocellular carcinoma justified? Results from a multi-institutional database. Annals of Surgical Oncology. 2005;**12**(5):364-373. DOI: 10.1245/ASO.2005.06.004

[7] Régimbeau JM, Farges O, Shen BY, Sauvanet A, Belghiti J. Is surgery for large hepatocellular carcinoma justified? Journal of Hepatology. 1999;**31**(6):1062-1068

[8] Mazzaferro V, Regalia E, Doci R, et al. Liver transplantation for the treatment of small hepatocellular carcinomas in patients with cirrhosis. The New England Journal of Medicine. 1996;**334**(11):693-700. DOI: 10.1056/NEJM199603143341104

[9] Iwatsuki S, Starzl TE, Sheahan DG, Yokoyama I, Demetris AJ, Todo S, et al. Hepatic resection versus transplantation for hepatocellular carcinoma. Annals of Surgery. 1991; **214**(Table 1):221-228

[10] Kauffmann R, Fong Y. Post-hepatectomy liver failure. Hepatobiliary Surgery and Nutrition. 2014;**3**(5):238-246. DOI: 10.3978/j.issn.2304-3881.2014.09.01

[11] Ge P-L, Du S-D, Mao Y-L. Advances in preoperative assessment of liver function. Hepatobiliary & Pancreatic Diseases International. 2014;**13**(4):361-370

[12] Okamoto E, Kyo A, Yamanaka N, Tanaka N, Kuwata K. Prediction of the safe limits of hepatectomy by combined volumetric and functional measurements in patients with impaired hepatic function. Surgery. 1984;**95**(5):586-592

[13] Kishi Y, Abdalla EK, Chun YS, et al. Three hundred and one consecutive extended right Hepatectomies. Transactions of the Meeting of the American Surgical Association. 2009;**127**(4):171-179. DOI: 10.1097/SLA.0b013e3181b674df

[14] Shindoh J, Tzeng C-WD, Aloia TA, et al. Optimal future liver remnant in patients treated with extensive preoperative chemotherapy for colorectal liver metastases. Annals of Surgical Oncology. 2013;**20**(8):2493-2500. DOI: 10.1245/s10434-012-2864-7

[15] Schnitzbauer AA, Lang SA, Goessmann H, et al. Right portal vein ligation combined with In situ splitting induces rapid left lateral liver lobe hypertrophy enabling 2-staged extended right hepatic resection in small-for-size settings. Annals of Surgery. 2012;**255**(3):405-414. DOI: 10.1097/SLA.0b013e31824856f5

[16] Kinoshita H, Sakai K, Hirohashi K, Igawa S, Yamasaki O, Kubo S. Preoperative portal vein embolization for hepatocellular carcinoma. World Journal of Surgery. 1986;**10**(5):803-808

[17] Farges O, Belghiti J, Kianmanesh R, et al. Portal vein embolization before right hepatectomy. Annals of Surgery. 2003;**237**(2):208-217. DOI: 10.1097/01.SLA.0000048447.16651.7B

[18] Tanaka H, Hirohashi K, Kubo S, Shuto T, Higaki I, Kinoshita H. Preoperative portal vein embolization improves prognosis after right hepatectomy for hepatocellular carcinoma in patients with impaired hepatic function. The British Journal of Surgery. 2000;**87**(7): 879-882. DOI: 10.1046/j.1365-2168.2000.01438.x

[19] Torres OJM, Fernandes ESM, Herman P. ALPPS: Past, present and future. Arquivos Brasileiros de Cirurgia Digestiva. 2015;**28**(3):155-156. DOI: 10.1590/S0102-67202015000300001

[20] Torres OJM, Fernandes E de SM, Oliveira CVC, et al. Associating liver partition and portal vein ligation for staged hepatectomy (ALPPS): The Brazilian experience. Arquivos Brasileiros de Cirurgia Digestiva;**26**(1):40-43

[21] Zhang G-Q, Zhang Z-W, Lau W-Y, Chen X-P. Associating liver partition and portal vein ligation for staged hepatectomy (ALPPS): A new strategy to increase resectability in liver surgery. International Journal of Surgery. 2014;**12**(5):437-441. DOI: 10.1016/j.ijsu.2014.03.009

[22] Strasberg S, Belghiti J, Clavien P, et al. The Brisbane 2000 terminology of liver anatomy and resections. HPB: The Official Journal of the International Hepato Pancreato Biliary Association. 2000;**2**:333-339. DOI: 10.1016/S1365-182X(17)30755-4

[23] Shi M, Guo R-P, Lin X-J, et al. Partial hepatectomy with wide versus narrow resection margin for solitary hepatocellular carcinoma. Annals of Surgery. 2007;**245**(1):36-43. DOI: 10.1097/01.sla.0000231758.07868.71

[24] Pamecha V, Gurusamy KS, Sharma D, Davidson BR. Techniques for liver parenchymal transection: A meta-analysis of randomized controlled trials. HPB: The Official Journal of the International Hepato Pancreato Biliary Association. 2009;**11**(4):275-281. DOI: 10.1111/j.1477-2574.2009.00057.x

[25] Cho, Park, Fong. Hepatic resection. In: Ashley SW, editor. Scientific American Surgery. 7th ed. Decker, Hamilton; 2014. pp. 1094-1114

[26] Coelho FF, Kruger JAP, Fonseca GM, et al. Laparoscopic liver resection: Experience based guidelines. World Journal of Gastrointestinal Surgery. 2016;**8**(1):5-26. DOI: 10.4240/wjgs.v8.i1.5

[27] Nguyen KT, Gamblin TC, Geller DA. World review of laparoscopic liver resection—2,804 patients. Annals of Surgery. 2009;**250**(5):831-841. DOI: 10.1097/SLA.0b013e3181b0c4df

[28] Ding G, Cai W, Qin M. Pure laparoscopic versus open liver resection in treatment of Hepatolithiasis within the left lobes. Surgical Laparoscopy, Endoscopy & Percutaneous Techniques. 2015;**25**(5):392-394. DOI: 10.1097/SLE.0000000000000120

[29] Viganò L, Tayar C, Laurent A, Cherqui D. Laparoscopic liver resection: A systematic review. Journal of Hepato-Biliary-Pancreatic Surgery. 2009;**16**(4):410-421. DOI: 10.1007/s00534-009-0120-8

[30] Han H-S, Shehta A, Ahn S, Yoon Y-S, Cho JY, Choi Y. Laparoscopic versus open liver resection for hepatocellular carcinoma: Case-matched study with propensity score matching. Journal of Hepatology. 2015;**63**(3):643-650. DOI: 10.1016/j.jhep.2015.04.005

[31] Bagante F, Spolverato G, Strasberg SM, et al. Minimally invasive vs. open hepatectomy: A comparative analysis of the National Surgical Quality Improvement Program Database. Journal of Gastrointestinal Surgery. 2016;**20**(9):1608-1617. DOI: 10.1007/s11605-016-3202-3

[32] Jiang B, Yan X-F, Zhang J-H. Meta-analysis of laparoscopic versus open liver resection for hepatocellular carcinoma. Hepatology Research. 2018;**48**(8):635-663. DOI: 10.1111/hepr.13061

[33] Chen K, Pan Y, Zhang B, Liu X-L, Maher H, Zheng X-Y. Laparoscopic versus open surgery for hepatocellular carcinoma: A meta-analysis of high-quality case-matched studies. Canadian Journal of Gastroenterology and Hepatology. 2018;**2018**:1746895. DOI: 10.1155/2018/1746895

[34] Sposito C, Battiston C, Facciorusso A, et al. Propensity score analysis of outcomes following laparoscopic or open liver resection for hepatocellular carcinoma. The British Journal of Surgery. 2016;**103**(7):871-880. DOI: 10.1002/bjs.10137

[35] Nota CL, Rinkes IHB, Hagendoorn J. Setting up a robotic hepatectomy program: A Western-European experience and perspective. Hepatobiliary Surgery and Nutrition. 2017;**6**(4):239-245. DOI: 10.21037/hbsn.2016.12.05

[36] Giulianotti PC, Coratti A, Sbrana F, et al. Robotic liver surgery: Results for 70 resections. Surgery. 2011;**149**(1):29-39. DOI: 10.1016/j.surg.2010.04.002

[37] Goh B, Lee S, Chan C, et al. Early experience with robot-assisted laparoscopic hepatobiliary and pancreatic surgery in Singapore: Single-institution experience with 20 consecutive patients. Singapore Medical Journal. 2018;**59**(3):133-138. DOI: 10.11622/smedj.2017092

[38] Ho C-M, Wakabayashi G, Nitta H, Ito N, Hasegawa Y, Takahara T. Systematic review of robotic liver resection. Surgical Endoscopy. 2013;**27**(3):732-739. DOI: 10.1007/s00464-012-2547-2

[39] Khan S, Beard RE, Kingham PT, et al. Long-term oncologic outcomes following robotic liver resections for primary Hepatobiliary malignancies: A multicenter study. Annals of Surgical Oncology. July 2018. DOI: 10.1245/s10434-018-6629-9

[40] Otsuka Y, Katagiri T, Ishii J, et al. Gas embolism in laparoscopic hepatectomy: What is the optimal pneumoperitoneal pressure for laparoscopic major hepatectomy? Journal of Hepato-Biliary-Pancreatic Sciences. 2013;**20**(2):137-140. DOI: 10.1007/s00534-012-0556-0

[41] Qiu J, Chen S, Chengyou D. A systematic review of robotic-assisted liver resection and meta-analysis of robotic versus laparoscopic hepatectomy for hepatic neoplasms. Surgical Endoscopy. 2016;**30**(3):862-875. DOI: 10.1007/s00464-015-4306-7

[42] Komatsu S, Scatton O, Goumard C, et al. Development Process and Technical Aspects of Laparoscopic Hepatectomy: Learning Curve Based on 15 Years of Experience. Journal of the American College of Surgeons. 2017;**224**(5):841-850

[43] Sham JG, Richards MK, Seo YD, Pillarisetty VG, Yeung RS, Park JO. Efficacy and cost of robotic hepatectomy: Is the robot cost-prohibitive? Journal of Robotic Surgery. 2016;**10**(4):307-313. DOI: 10.1007/s11701-016-0598-4

[44] Rahbari NN, Garden OJ, Padbury R, et al. Posthepatectomy liver failure: A definition and grading by the International Study Group of Liver Surgery (ISGLS). Surgery. 2011;**149**(5):713-724. DOI: 10.1016/j.surg.2010.10.001

[45] Zimmitti G, Roses RE, Andreou A, et al. Greater complexity of liver surgery is not associated with an increased incidence of liver-related complications except for bile leak: An experience with 2,628 consecutive resections. Journal of Gastrointestinal Surgery. 2013;**17**(1):57-65. DOI: 10.1007/s11605-012-2000-9

[46] Lamadé W, Glombitza G, Fischer L, et al. The impact of 3-dimensional reconstructions on operation planning in liver surgery. Archives of Surgery. 2000;**135**(11):1256-1261

[47] Bourdel N, Collins T, Pizarro D, et al. Augmented reality in gynecologic surgery: Evaluation of potential benefits for myomectomy in an experimental uterine model. Surgical Endoscopy. 2017;**31**(1):456-461. DOI: 10.1007/s00464-016-4932-8

4

Biologic and Immunotherapy Developments in Advanced Hepatocellular Carcinoma

Mohammad Telfah, Mohammed Al-Jumayli and Anwaar Saeed

Abstract

Hepatocellular carcinoma (HCC) is the most common primary cancer of the liver, and the second leading cause of cancer-related mortality worldwide with a very poor 5-year survival. Treatment for HCC includes surgery, liver-directed therapies and systemic therapies. Until 2008, no effective systemic therapy was available for advanced HCC. Sorafenib is the first drug to show improvement in overall survival among patients with advanced HCC in comparison to placebo, and it is approved by U.S. Food and Drug Administration (FDA) as a first-line treatment of advanced HCC. After sorafenib approval, several targeted and immune therapies were tested and showed efficacy in advanced HCC. Lenvatinib has been shown to be non-inferior to sorafenib as first-line treatment. Both nivolumab and regorafenib showed improvement in overall survival among patients with advanced HCC as a second line treatment after progression on sorafenib, and both are FDA approved for this indication. There is a limited role for cytotoxic agents in the treatment of advanced HCC.

Keywords: hepatocellular, carcinoma, HCC, kinase, inhibitors, TKI, VEGFR, sorafenib, lenvatinib, regorafenib, immunotherapy, PD-L1, nivolumab

1. Introduction

Hepatocellular carcinoma (HCC) is the most common primary cancer of the liver. HCC is the second leading cause of cancer-related mortality worldwide with a very poor 5-year survival. The incidence of HCC has been increasing over the past decades [1]. Risk factors for HCC include hepatitis B and C infection, alcohol use, non-alcoholic steatohepatitis, and aflatoxin.

Treatment approaches for HCC depend on the stage and the hepatic function, and includes surgical therapies (liver transplantation, resection, and ablation) and nonsurgical therapies, which may be liver-directed (percutaneous ethanol injection, radiofrequency ablation, trans-arterial embolization, external beam radiation therapy) or systemic therapies.

Until 2008, there was no effective systemic therapy for advanced HCC. Cytotoxic chemotherapy has not been used routinely as of low efficacy and poor functional status for patients with advanced HCC, who often have cirrhosis. Since the advent of sorafenib in 2008, there has been a surge of several targeted and immune therapies with various degree of effectiveness. In this chapter, systemic therapies for advanced HCC will be reviewed. Those include oral kinase inhibitors, antiangiogenic monoclonal antibodies, immune-therapeutic approaches and cytotoxic chemotherapies.

2. Kinase inhibitors

2.1. Sorafenib

Sorafenib is a multi-kinase inhibitor of vascular endothelial growth factor receptors (VEGFR), platelet-derived growth factor receptor (PDGFR) and Raf family kinases [2]. Sorafenib has shown to improve overall survival in comparison to placebo in advanced HCC, and it was the first drug to get Food and Drug Administration (FDA) approval as a first-line treatment for Child-Pugh score-A HCC. In the multicenter European SHARP trial, 602 inoperable HCC and Child-Turcotte-Pugh-A cirrhosis patients, were assigned to sorafenib (400 mg twice daily) or placebo [3]. The primary endpoint of the trial was overall survival, which was significantly longer in the sorafenib-treated group (10.7 vs. 7.9 months). Time to radiologic progression was also longer (5.5 vs. 2.8 months). Objective response rates were low at 2%.

Sorafenib was well tolerated in this trial. Diarrhea and hand-foot skin reaction were the only grade 3 or 4 adverse effects that occurred significantly more often in the treated group; (8 vs. 2%) and (8 vs. <1%) respectively. There were no differences in liver dysfunction or bleeding.

An exploratory analysis of SHARP trial showed that hepatitis C related HCC has the highest median overall survival advantage of 6.6 months (14 vs. 7.4 months). This is in comparison to 3.6 months (9.7 vs. 6.1 months) in those with HBV related cirrhosis and 2.3 months (10.3 vs. 8 months) in those with alcohol-related liver disease [4].

Hepatitis B virus is more prevalent in the Asian patients than in the Western population. Sorafenib was tested as a first-line treatment in Asian patients in a placebo-controlled phase III trial in which 226 patients with Child-Turcotte-Pugh A cirrhosis received sorafenib 400 mg twice daily or placebo [5]. Patients receiving sorafenib had significantly higher median overall survival (6.5 vs. 4.2 months). Grade 3 or 4 side effects were similar to SHARP trial.

Based on the results of SHARP trial, the FDA approved sorafenib monotherapy as first-line therapy for unresectable HCC.

It is worth mentioning that the patients enrolled in the above trials had mostly Child-Turcotte-Pugh A cirrhosis. This is not representative of the real practice where a significant number of patients have more advanced cirrhosis. FDA approval of sorafenib for HCC did not particularly specify the underlying cirrhosis state. Data regarding safety and efficacy of sorafenib in patients with Child-Turcotte-Pugh B or C cirrhosis are limited, and suggest that patients have poorer overall survival and overall worse side effect profile in comparison to patients with Child-Turcotte-Pugh A. Advanced progressive cirrhosis rather than sorafenib itself might be an explanation for such differences [6, 7].

Sorafenib is associated with several side effects such as hypertension, cardiotoxicity, arterial thromboembolism, bleeding, renal toxicity, hand-foot skin reaction and others. Sorafenib has been associated with potentially fatal liver toxicity. Liver function tests should regularly be monitored during treatment.

2.1.1. Combining sorafenib with doxorubicin

In a phase II trial, the combination of six cycles of doxorubicin with sorafenib 400 mg twice daily was compared to sorafenib and placebo [8]. Combination therapy was associated significantly longer median time to tumor progression (6.4 vs. 2.8 months) and median overall survival duration (13.7 vs. 6.5 months). The side effect profile was not significantly worse with combined therapy. However those results were not reproduced in the randomized phase III trial, Cancer and Leukemia Group B [CALGB] trial 80,802 [9]. The study was stopped early by the data monitoring safety board after a planned interim analysis suggested futility for the combination. In a preliminary report presented at the 2016 American Society of Clinical Oncology (ASCO) Gastrointestinal Cancers Symposium, median overall survival was not significantly better for the combination (9.3 vs. 10.5 months), nor was median progression-free survival (3.6 vs. 3.2 months), but toxicity was worse.

2.2. Lenvatinib

Lenvatinib is a multi-kinase inhibitor of VEGFRs, fibroblast growth factor receptors (FGFR), (PDGFR), c-Kit, and the RET proto-oncogene [10].

A randomized noninferiority trial, the REFLECT study, compared lenvatinib (12 mg once daily for body weight ≥60 kg, 8 mg daily for <60 kg) with sorafenib (400 mg daily for all patients) in 954 patients with unresectable HCC and no prior systemic therapy (99% Child-Turcotte-Pugh A) [11]. The predefined noninferiority margin (primary endpoint overall survival) was 1.08. Lenvatinib was noninferior to sorafenib (median overall survival 13.6 vs. 12.3 months, hazard ratio 0.92, 95% CI 0.79–1.06), the objective response rate was higher (24 vs. 9%), and median time to progression was longer (7.4 vs. 3.7 months, hazard ratio 0.66, 95% CI 0.57–0.77). Lenvatinib leads to higher grade 3 or 4 hypertension (23 vs. 14%), while sorafenib was associated with higher hand-foot skin reaction (11 vs. 3%).

Lenvatinib was approved in Japan in March 2018 for unresectable HCC. Lenvatinib is not approved by FDA yet.

Both sorafenib and lenvatinib can be used in the first-line treatment of advanced HCC. There are no data on second-line treatment after lenvatinib and whether lenvatinib is effective as a second line after sorafenib.

2.3. Regorafenib

Regorafenib is an antiangiogenic (including VEGFR-1, VEGFR-2, and VEGFR-3), anti-stromal, and an oncogenic tyrosine kinase inhibitor that is structurally similar to sorafenib [12].

In the randomized RESORCE trial, 573 patients who received sorafenib for at least 20 days at a dose of at least 400 mg daily and who had radiologic progression were randomly assigned to regorafenib (160 mg once daily for 3 weeks on and 1 week off) or placebo [13]. Regorafenib was associated with significantly higher median OS (10.6 vs. 7.8 months, hazard ratio for death 0.63) and disease control (objective response plus stable disease; 65 vs. 36%).

Treatment was relatively well tolerated; grade 3 or 4 hypertension, hand-foot skin disease and fatigue were more frequent with regorafenib. Sixty-eight percent of patients treated with regorafenib required dose modification for adverse events compared with 31% of the placebo group.

In April 2017, the FDA expanded the indications for regorafenib to include patients with HCC who had been previously treated with sorafenib.

Regorafenib is an alternative to nivolumab for second-line HCC treatment. There are no trials comparing regorafenib with nivolumab in this setting.

2.4. Cabozantinib

Cabozantinib is another inhibitor of several receptor tyrosine kinases, including the hepatocyte growth factor/c-MET and VEGFR [14]. Efficacy in patients with previously treated advanced HCC was shown in the placebo-controlled phase III CELESTIAL trial [15]. In a preliminary report, in the group of patients receiving second- or third-line treatment, median overall survival was significantly better with cabozantinib (10.2 vs. 8.0 months), and the difference was more pronounced when the analysis was limited to patients whose only prior therapy was sorafenib (median overall survival 11.3 vs. 7.2 months). The most common grade 3 or 4 adverse events with cabozantinib were palmar-plantar erythrodysesthesia (17 vs. 0 in the placebo group), hypertension (16 vs. 0%), increased aspartate aminotransferase (12 vs. 7%), fatigue (10 vs. 4%), and diarrhea (10 vs. 2%).

2.5. Axitinib

Axitinib is a selective kinase inhibitor that inhibits VEGFR. Axitinib was not superior to best supportive care alone in a randomized phase II trial comparing best supportive care plus axitinib (starting dose 5 mg twice daily) with placebo in 202 patients with advanced HCC who progressed on or were intolerant of one prior antiangiogenic therapy [16]. The difference in median overall survival (the primary endpoint), was not statistically significant (12.7 vs. 9.7).

2.6. Sunitinib

Sunitinib is another orally active multi-kinase inhibitor that targets a variety of tyrosine kinases in addition to VEGFR, including PDGFRs, KIT, RET, and FMS-like tyrosine kinase 3 (FLT3) [17].

Sunitinib was significantly inferior to sorafenib in a phase III trial that directly compared both drugs in 1073 previously untreated patients with advanced HCC [18]. The trial was closed prematurely when an interim analysis revealed that patients receiving sunitinib had significantly worse survival (median 7.9 vs. 10.2 months) and more frequent and severe treatment-related toxicity.

3. Antiangiogenic monoclonal antibodies

3.1. Bevacizumab

Bevacizumab is a monoclonal antibody directed against VEGFR that has some activity in advanced HCC. Efficacy was shown in a trial in which 46 patients with advanced nonmetastatic HCC received single-agent bevacizumab at a dose of either 5 or 10 mg/kg once every other week [19]. An objective response was documented in six (13%, one complete), and the median progression-free survival was 6.9 months. The most common grade 3 or 4 toxicities were hypertension (15%), thrombosis (6%), and major bleeding (11%).

Bevacizumab is also active in combination with capecitabine, with or without oxaliplatin [20, 21], and gemcitabine combined with oxaliplatin (GEMOX) [22]. Whether any of those combination regimens are better than bevacizumab alone is not clear and will require randomized trials.

3.2. Ramucirumab

Ramucirumab is a recombinant monoclonal antibody that binds to VEGFR-2. The REACH trial failed to show a significant survival advantage relative to placebo (median overall survival 9.2 vs. 7.6 months) in patients with advanced HCC who progressed on sorafenib [23]. An unplanned group analysis suggested a possible survival benefit in patients with a high initial level of alpha-fetoprotein (AFP) above 400 ng/mL) at diagnosis. A follow-up phase III trial in patients with AFP-elevated HCC is ongoing.

4. Immunotherapeutic approaches

4.1. Introduction

Immune-based approaches that focus on vaccination strategies, cytokines or non-specific T cell activation have been tested for many years in HCC without promising result. However, the recent advancement in immune-oncology with the FDA approval of many immune checkpoint inhibitors, sparked a great interest in the immune-based treatment approaches for patients with HCC. The strategy of adopting an immunocentric approach to HCC treatment may be potentially more efficacious and less toxic. Interestingly, what makes the immunotherapy appealing in liver cancer is that HCC is a high immunogenic cancer, due to high blood flow with unique vast tumor antigen repertoire because of mutations and aberrant expression profiles [24]. On the other hand, there is an inherently immunosuppressive microenvironment of the liver; "Tolerogenic Liver"; that helps evade the immune response. The liver's pathway to immune tolerance is multifactorial. T-cells are stimulated through a dual signaling pathway that requires the interaction of T cell receptors (TCR) with major histocompatibility complex (MHC)/peptide complexes on antigen presenting cells (APCs) and expression of co-stimulatory molecules on T cells and APCs. Down-regulation of MHC class I molecules on tumor cells induces impairment of tumor antigen processing and presentation [25]. In addition, a reduced expression of co-stimulatory molecules, such as B7-1 and B7-2, in HCC leads to T cell anergy [26]. Programmed cell death protein-1 (PD-1) overexpression in tumors promotes immune evasion and tumor growth by suppressing T-cell response [27]. PD-L1 is not the only immunosuppressive factor in the tumor microenvironment. HCC immune evasion can also be achieved through overexpression of MHC class II molecules in tumor cells, which leads to $CD4^+$ T cell anergy in the absence of co-stimulatory molecules (CMs) on T cells and APCs. A better understanding of the antigenic profile of HCC and tumor microenvironment has helped to develop a refined immunotherapeutic strategies in treatment of HCC [28].

4.2. Indirect immunological strategies

4.2.1. Checkpoint inhibitors

Checkpoint Inhibitors play critical roles in cancer immunology. Blockading the PD-1/PD-L1 pathway could modulate the tumor microenvironment, reactive T-cell and prime the endogenous antitumor immune responses. Treatment with checkpoints inhibitors have shown benefits in clinical trials of HCC. Common immune checkpoint proteins include cytotoxic T lymphocyte-associated antigen-4 (CTLA-4), PD-1, programmed cell death ligand one (PD-L1), lymphocyte activation gene three protein (LAG-3), B and T lymphocyte attenuator (BTLA), T-cell immunoglobulin and mucin-domain-containing (TIM-3), VISTA and OX40 [29, 30].

4.2.1.1. CTLA-4 inhibitors

CTLA-4 is constitutively expressed in activated T cells and NK cells [31]. CTLA-4 inhibitors prevent the binding of CTLA-4 to B7-1 and B7-2, thereby actively encourage the activation of T cells. CTLA-4 was the first checkpoint studied in HCC. Tremelimumab, an anti-CTLA-4 monoclonal antibody, was tested in a phase II study in a 21 patients with advanced HCC and hepatitis C. The disease control rate was (76.4%), median OS and PFS were 7.5 and 6.4 months respectively. Moreover, viral loads of HCC were significantly reduced. Although a short-lived remarkable rise in serum transaminases was observed after the first dose, no patients experienced immune-related adverse events or serious hepatotoxicity [32]. In another non-comparative clinical trial involving patients with advanced HCC, a combination therapy of tremelimumab and radiofrequency ablation increased the number of intratumoral $CD8^+$ T cells and reduced HCV viral loads [33].

4.2.1.2. PD-1 inhibitors

The PD-L1/PD-1 pathway is another mechanism of tumor-induced immune tolerance. PD-1 expression on effecter phase $CD8^+$ T cells is increased in patients with HCC compared to no HCC cirrhotic patients [34]. Moreover, there is frequent and early disease progression in patients with HCC with higher numbers of tumor-infiltrating and circulating PD-1 + $CD8^+$ T cells post hepatic resection [35]. Therefore, a supporting great rationale exists for using PD-1 and PD-L-1 blocking antibodies against HCC. Some PD-1 inhibitors, such as nivolumab, pembrolizumab, and pidilizumab, have been investigated for cancer treatment.

The CheckMate-040 phase I/II trial studied the safety and antitumor effect of nivolumab in 48 patients with advanced HCC [36]. The target population included patients with intermediate or advanced HCC and preserved liver function (Child-Turcotte-Pugh-A cirrhosis) who were candidates for systemic therapy and had progressed or were intolerant to sorafenib. In the escalation and expansion cohorts, objective tumor responses occurred in 15 and 20% of patients, respectively. There were durable responses that lasted for a median of 17 months. An additional 45% of patients had a stable disease associated with durability, lasting 6 months at minimum. Those responses were consistent across the different HCC risks, and both in sorafenib-naïve and sorafenib-exposed patients.

Overall, frequencies of grade 3/4 treatment-related AEs were 20%. Only 3% of patients discontinued nivolumab because of treatment-related adverse events, while no treatment-related deaths occurred. Elevated transaminases was the most frequent laboratory alteration (20%). However, only 5% of the patients had grade 3 or higher. Immune-related hepatitis requiring steroid therapy. CheckMate-040 showed that nivolumab might be effective with acceptable toxicity in HCC, regardless of hepatitis status. On September 22, 2017, and based on the outcome of CheckMate-040 study, the FDA granted accelerated approval to nivolumab for the treatment of hepatocellular carcinoma (HCC) as second-line therapy in patients who have been previously treated with sorafenib.

CheckMate-459 is an ongoing phase III study, (NCT02576509) that randomizes patients with advanced HCC to either nivolumab or sorafenib in the first-line setting [37].

The efficacy and safety of pembrolizumab in HCC has been investigated. The phase I/II study KEYNOTE-224 tested pembrolizumab in 104 patients with advanced HCC who progressed on sorafenib. The overall response rate was 16.3%. Durable response was seen with 94% of responders were estimated to have a response duration of 6 months or longer. The median PFS was 4.8 months, and the median OS was not been reached. The safety profile was generally comparable to that established for pembrolizumab monotherapy in other indications, and no viral flares were seen [38].

4.2.2. *Oncolytic immunotherapy*

Targeting tumor vasculature by oncolytic viruses (OVs) is an attractive strategy that offers several advantages. Oncolytic viruses are wild-type or engineered viruses that selectively target and replicate in cancer cells and cause lysis without harming normal tissues [39]. The underlying mechanism of the antitumor activity for oncolytic viruses involves direct killing of tumor cells by expanding in the cells and causing cell lysis. Different from normal cell, viruses can expand in cancer cells considerably due to the impairment of the tumor's defense mechanisms against viral infection. [40–43]. In addition,, OVs can initiate antitumor immune response by triggering key signals through oncolysis to dendritic cells (DCs) and other antigen-presenting cells (APCs) [44]. OVs have some advantages over other treatment modalities, those include: the low probability of generating resistance as OVs often target multiple oncogenic pathways; OVs replicate in a tumor-selective fashion with minimal systemic toxicities; and virus dose in the tumor increases over time due to in situ virus amplification, as opposed to classical drug pharmacokinetics that decreases with time [45]. The efficacy of an evolutionary cancer-favoring engineered vaccinia virus (CVV) was investigated in an animal model of metastatic HCC. In this animal study, the subjects were randomized into sorafenib, CVV, or sorafenib with CVV. Metastatic regions were interestingly rare in the CVV-treated groups (i.e., CVV or sorafenib with CVV) whereas metastatic regions existed in the sorafenib-treated group [46].

JX-594 is a thymidine kinase gene-inactivated oncolytic vaccinia virus engineered for the expression of transgenes encoding human granulocyte-macrophage-colony-stimulating factor (GM-CSF) and β-galactosidase, which increases antitumor immune responses [39, 47–49] This virus is safe in humans and extremely toxic to cancer cells.

Oncolytic viruses have produced enough therapeutic efficacy with great optimism in the future trials. Although the initial concerns of clinical investigators were for safety like a risk of viral infection or introduce oncogenic mutation, these have proven not to be a significant issue in these trials.

4.2.3. HCC vaccines

Cancer vaccination is performed by utilizing antigenic substances to stimulate tumor-specific immune responses that can remove cancer cells and prevent recurrences. HCC vaccines include cancer cells, antigen peptides, DCs, and DNA-based.

4.2.3.1. Antigen peptide vaccines

Peptide-based tumor-associated antigens (TAAs), such as alpha-fetoprotein (AFP), GPC3, SSX-2, NY-ESO-1, human telomerase reverse transcriptase (hTERT), HCA587, and melanoma antigen gene-A (MAGE-A), are excellent vaccine targets for the treatment of HCC [50].

AFP which normally originates from embryonic liver cells, can be overexpressed on HCC cell surfaces. However, immune responses to AFP are limited due to acquired immune tolerance during the development of the immune system. To overcome this tolerance, a research group investigated the use of a recombinant rat AFP to induce cross-reactions between xenografts and endogenous molecules in animals and observed modest cellular and humoral immune responses [51]. In a phase II trial of GPC3-derived peptide vaccine for HCC, 25 patients received 10 vaccinations over 1 year after surgery. The recurrence rate in patients who underwent both surgery and vaccination was significantly lower than the rate in 21 patients who underwent surgery only (24% vs. 48 and 52.4% vs. 61.9% at 1 and 2 years, $p = 0\ 047$ and 0.387, respectively), demonstrating the efficacy of the GPC3-derived vaccine [52].

4.2.3.2. Dendritic cell (DC) vaccines

DCs, were found to be the most powerful APCs in the body's immune system, and capable of stimulating naïve T cells and driving primary immune responses. A phase I/IIa comparative study with 30 patients with advanced HCC stratified into mature autologous DCs pulsed, and other control group received supportive treatment. The result demonstrated an improvement in overall survival with two patients (13.3%) partial radiological response was observed, and nine patients (60%) has stable disease. The study concludes using tumor antigen-pulsed DCs vaccine can be effective adjuvant therapy with other treatment modalities of HCC or palliative treatment option in advanced HCC where other treatment options are not applicable [53]. In addition, the safety and tolerance of DC vaccines have been confirmed in patients with HCC [54].

4.3. Direct immunological strategy

4.3.1. Adoptive cell therapy

Adoptive cell therapy (ACT) is an immunotherapeutic approach that attacks cancer cells using genetically engineered patients' lymphocytes. It functions by stimulating or loading autologous lymphocytes with cytokines or tumor antigens, cultivating them ex vivo and then re-infusing them into the patient [55–57]. Adoptive immunotherapy for HCC includes cytokine-induced killer (CIK) cells, tumor-infiltrating lymphocytes (TILs), natural killer (NK) cells, and chimeric antigen receptor (CAR) T cells. The effectiveness and safety of ACT in patients with HCC have been studied in many experiments, which paved the road for its clinical implication.

4.3.1.1. Cytokine induced killer cells (CIK)

CIK cells are a heterogeneous MHC independent cell population which are able to both recognize tumor antigens and kill cancer cells directly [58, 59]. In a phase III study of adjuvant CIK therapy after radical resection for HCC, patients were randomized to receive four cycles of CIK therapy or no treatment. The median time to recurrence (TTR) was 13.6 months in the CIK group and 7.8 months in the control group ($p = 0.01$), All adverse events were grade 1 or 2. There were no significant differences in incidence between the two groups, indicating the safety and efficacy with respect to prolonging TTR of CIK therapy in patients with HCC. However, there were no statistically significant differences between the groups in disease-free survival (DFS) and overall survival (OS) [60]. In addition, a meta-analysis of 693 patients with HCC demonstrated that a combination of dendritic cell- (DC-) CIK cells and TACE improves 1-and 2-year OS, overall response rate (ORR), disease control rate (DCR), and the quality of life [61].

4.3.1.2. Tumor infiltrating lymphocytes (TILs)

TILs are autologous tumor-infiltrating lymphocytes (TIL), which are derived from tumor tissues and are cultured and induced using IL-2 and anti-CD3 antibodies ex vivo [62–64]. Reinfusion of autologous TILs, which possess tumor-specific immunity, may target multiple tumor antigens. Low toxicity of autologous TILs was verified in a phase I study involving patients with HCC, suggesting a novel treatment option [65]. To date, TILs have not been well characterized, mainly due to difficulties in purifying and expanding them.

4.3.1.3. Natural killer cells (NKCs)

NK cells are component of innate immune system and can directly kill tumor cells and infected cells without preliminary sensitization or MHC restriction [66]. However, they lack the ability to target tumor cells and can injure normal liver tissues. In a previous series of experiments, the cytotoxicity of NK cells against HCC cells was enhanced by first generating a new hepatoma cell line, K562-mb15-41BBL, which achieved a more efficient stimulation of NK cells in vitro [67]. Furthermore, HCC cells exposed to 5 μmol/L sorafenib for 48 h showed high sensitivity to NK cells. Finally, NKG2D, an engineered NK-cell-activating receptor, was tested in vitro and in mice. All of the outcomes were positive in increasing the cytotoxicity of NK cells, providing the possibility of further clinical trials in HCC.

4.3.1.4. CAR-T cell

Chimeric antigen receptor redirected-T cells (CAR-T cells) are genetically modified T lymphocytes that specifically target tumor-associated antigens (TAAs) and kill cancer cells in an MHC-independent manner [68, 69]. CAR-T cells have achieved inspiring outcomes in patients with B cell malignancies with great therapeutic efficacy in leukemia and lymphoma therapy. CAR T therapy is being studied for solid tumors, such as HCC [70]. In some solid tumors with a tremendous phenotypic heterogeneity, CAR T cells could target the tumor antigen and cause antigen-positive cell death, while antigen-negative cancer cells may induce tumor relapse. However, Cart T cell structure engineering has been evolved significantly. Recently, CAR T cells with a transgenic "payload or TRUCK," also called the "fourth generation" CAR T cells, were designed [71]. This CAR T cells work by releasing inducible cytokines such as IL-12 which will augment T cell activation and further activate innate immune system to kill antigen negative cancer cells. Specific Tumor-associated antigens in HCC that recognized by cytotoxic T lymphocytes (CTLs) have been investigated. GPC3, which usually correlates with poor prognosis in HCC, has been demonstrated as a promising liver cancer-specific target in multiple studies, due to its overexpression in HCC and limited expression in normal tissues [72] GPC3-targeted CAR T cells could providing promising therapeutic intervention for GPC3-positive HCC. The ability of GPC3-targeted CAR T cells to eliminate GPC3-positive HCC cells was confirmed both in vivo and in vitro, and the survival of mice with HCC xenografts was prolonged with CAR T cell therapy in vivo [73]. In another study, T cells with two complementary CARs against GPC3 and asialoglycoprotein receptor 1 (ASGR1) decreased the risk of on-target, off tumor toxicities and demonstrated potent antitumor immune responses targeting $GPC3^{+}$ $ASGR1^{+}$ HCCs both in vivo and in vitro [74]. However, to date, the related studies conducted have been predominantly basic, and more clinical trials are required to prove the efficacy of CAR T in HCC.

4.4. Combination strategies

Combination therapies include combinations of different checkpoint inhibitors with TKIs, oncolytic viruses, small molecules and ablative therapies.

Combining anti-PD-1 with sorafenib has been studied in an animal model in HCC. The results showed efficacy only with the concomitant targeting of the hypoxic and immunosuppressive microenvironment with agents such as CXCR4 inhibitors, and not when combined with sorafenib alone [75]. According to these results, a potential future approach could be by careful titration of VEGF inhibition with the aim to block the VEGF pathway and contemporarily alleviate hypoxia by vascular normalization, enhancing immunotherapy efficacy [76].

Checkpoint inhibitors combinations have also been studied, as a way to improve synergy and overcome resistance. PD-L1 is not the only immunosuppressive factor in the tumor microenvironment. The regulatory T cells (Treg) stands out among the immunosuppressive cells of the tumor microenvironment. Anti-CTLA-4 agents deplete tumor-associated Treg via an FcεR dependant mechanism in preclinical models and have promising result in malignant melanoma [77].

5. Cytotoxic chemotherapies

Historically, traditional chemotherapeutic agents have not shown great efficacy in the treatment of HCC when used in the advanced disease stage, in particular in case of progression after locoregional therapy. Moreover, conventional cytotoxic chemotherapies have not provided a clinical benefit or prolonged survival for patients with advanced HCC. There are limited data supporting the use of cytotoxic chemotherapies in unresectable disease, and it should be used preferably in the context of a clinical trial [78].

6. Conclusions

Advanced HCC remains a deadly disease with limited systemic treatment options. The advent of sorafenib as first-line treatment ignited a plethora of trials testing various targeted and immunotherapeutic approaches. Currently, both regorafenib and nivolumab are FDA approved for second-line treatment among patients with advanced HCC who progressed

Agent	Type	MOA	FDA Approved	Line of treatment	Trial	Positive outcome	Ref.
Sorafenib	MKI	VEGFRs, PDGFR, TKI	Yes	First line	SHARP	OS, PFS	[3]
Lenvatinib	MKI	VEGFR, FGFR, PDGFRs, c-kit	No	First line	REFLECT	Non-inferior to sorafenib	[11]
Regorafenib	MKI	VEGFR, anti-stromal TKI	Yes	Second line	RESORCE	OS, DCR	[13]
Cabozantinib	MKI	VEGFR, MET, AXL c-KIT	No	Second or third line	CELESTIAL	OS	[15]
Nivolumab	IgG4 McA	Anti-PD-1	Yes	Second line	CheckMate-040	DCR, OS,PFS	[36]

List of abbreviations: MOA: mechanism of action, Ref: references, DCR: disease control rate, FGFR: fibroblast growth factor receptor, McA: monoclonal antibody, MKI: multi-tyrosine kinase inhibitor, OS: overall survival, PFS: progression free survival, PDGFR: platelet-derived growth factor receptor, PD-1: programmed death-1, TKI: trosine kinase inhibitor, VEGFRs: vascular endothelial growth factor receptors.

Table 1. Most common systemic agents for advanced HCC.

on sorafenib. The list of available treatment options (**Table 1**) is expected to increase with the encouraging results of several ongoing early phase trials, which eventually will lead to improvement in patients‚ survivals.

Author details

Mohammad Telfah, Mohammed Al-Jumayli and Anwaar Saeed*

*Address all correspondence to: asaeed@kumc.edu

Department of Medicine, Division of Medical Oncology, University of Kansas Medical Center Kansas City, Westwood, Kansas, USA

References

[1] SEER. Cancer Stat Facts: Liver and Intrahepatic Bile Duct Cancer. 2008-2014

[2] Chang YS et al. Sorafenib (BAY 43-9006) inhibits tumor growth and vascularization and induces tumor apoptosis and hypoxia in RCC xenograft models. Cancer Chemotherapy and Pharmacology. 2007;**59**(5):561-574

[3] Llovet JM et al. Sorafenib in advanced hepatocellular carcinoma. The New England Journal of Medicine. 2008;**359**(4):378-390

[4] Bruix J et al. Efficacy and safety of sorafenib in patients with advanced hepatocellular carcinoma: Subanalyses of a phase III trial. Journal of Hepatology. 2012;**57**(4):821-829

[5] Cheng AL et al. Efficacy and safety of sorafenib in patients in the Asia-Pacific region with advanced hepatocellular carcinoma: A phase III randomised, double-blind, placebo-controlled trial. The Lancet Oncology. 2009;**10**(1):25-34

[6] Pinter M et al. Sorafenib in unresectable hepatocellular carcinoma from mild to advanced stage liver cirrhosis. The Oncologist. 2009;**14**(1):70-76

[7] Abou-Alfa GK et al. Safety and efficacy of sorafenib in patients with hepatocellular carcinoma (HCC) and Child-Pugh A versus B cirrhosis. Gastrointestinal Cancer Research. 2011;**4**(2):40-44

[8] Abou-Alfa GK et al. Doxorubicin plus sorafenib vs doxorubicin alone in patients with advanced hepatocellular carcinoma: A randomized trial. Journal of the American Medical Association. 2010;**304**(19):2154-2160

[9] Abou-Alfa GK, Niedzwieski D, Knox JJ. Phase III randomized study of sorafenib plus doxorubicin versus sorafenib in patients with advanced hepatocellular carcinoma (HCC): CALGB 80802 (Alliance). Journal of Clinical Oncology. 2016;**34**(Suppl 4S; abstr 192)

[10] Ikeda K et al. Phase 2 study of lenvatinib in patients with advanced hepatocellular carcinoma. Journal of Gastroenterology. 2017;**52**(4):512-519

[11] Kudo M et al. Lenvatinib versus sorafenib in first-line treatment of patients with unresectable hepatocellular carcinoma: A randomised phase 3 non-inferiority trial. Lancet. 2018;**391**(10126):1163-1173

[12] Wilhelm SM et al. Regorafenib (BAY 73-4506): a new oral multikinase inhibitor of angiogenic, stromal and oncogenic receptor tyrosine kinases with potent preclinical antitumor activity. International Journal of Cancer. 2011;**129**(1):245-255

[13] Bruix J et al. Regorafenib for patients with hepatocellular carcinoma who progressed on sorafenib treatment (RESORCE): A randomised, double-blind, placebo-controlled, phase 3 trial. Lancet. 2017;**389**(10064):56-66

[14] Xiang Q et al. Cabozantinib suppresses tumor growth and metastasis in hepatocellular carcinoma by a dual blockade of VEGFR2 and MET. Clinical Cancer Research. 2014;**20**(11):2959-2970

[15] Abou-Alfa GK, Meyer T, Cheng A-L, et al. Cabozantinib (C) versus placebo (P) in patients (pts) with advanced hepatocellular carcinoma (HCC) who have received prior sorafenib: Results from the randomized phase III CELESTIAL trial (abstr). Journal of Clinical Oncology. 2018;**36**

[16] Kang YK et al. Randomized phase II study of axitinib versus placebo plus best supportive care in second-line treatment of advanced hepatocellular carcinoma. Annals of Oncology. 2015;**26**(12):2457-2463

[17] Faivre S et al. Safety and efficacy of sunitinib in patients with advanced hepatocellular carcinoma: An open-label, multicentre, phase II study. The Lancet Oncology. 2009; **10**(8):794-800

[18] Cheng A, Kang Y, Lin D, et al. Phase III trial of sunitinib versus sorafenib in advanced hepatocellular carcinoma (HCC) (Abstract 4000). Journal of Clinical Oncology. 2011; **29**(256s)

[19] Siegel AB et al. Phase II trial evaluating the clinical and biologic effects of bevacizumab in unresectable hepatocellular carcinoma. Journal of Clinical Oncology. 2008; **26**(18):2992-2998

[20] Sun W et al. Phase 2 trial of bevacizumab, capecitabine, and oxaliplatin in treatment of advanced hepatocellular carcinoma. Cancer. 2011;**117**(14):3187-3192

[21] Hsu CH et al. Efficacy and tolerability of bevacizumab plus capecitabine as first-line therapy in patients with advanced hepatocellular carcinoma. British Journal of Cancer. 2010;**102**(6):981-986

[22] Zhu AX et al. Phase II study of gemcitabine and oxaliplatin in combination with bevacizumab in patients with advanced hepatocellular carcinoma. Journal of Clinical Oncology. 2006;**24**(12):1898-1903

[23] Zhu AX et al. Ramucirumab versus placebo as second-line treatment in patients with advanced hepatocellular carcinoma following first-line therapy with sorafenib (REACH): A randomised, double-blind, multicentre, phase 3 trial. The Lancet Oncology. 2015;**16**(7):859-870

[24] Miamen AG, Dong H, Roberts LR. Immunotherapeutic approaches to hepatocellular carcinoma treatment. Liver Cancer. 2012;**1**(3-4):226-237

[25] Tsuchiya N et al. Potentiality of immunotherapy against hepatocellular carcinoma. World Journal of Gastroenterology. 2015;**21**(36):10314

[26] Fujiwara K et al. Decreased expression of B7 costimulatory molecules and major histocompatibility complex class-I in human hepatocellular carcinoma. Journal of Gastroenterology and Hepatology. 2004;**19**(10):1121-1127

[27] Henick BS, Herbst RS, Goldberg SB. The PD-1 pathway as a therapeutic target to overcome immune escape mechanisms in cancer. Expert Opinion on Therapeutic Targets. 2014;**18**(12):1407-1420

[28] Xie Y et al. Immunotherapy for hepatocellular carcinoma: Current advances and future expectations. Journalof Immunology Research. 2018;**2018**

[29] Hato T et al. Immune checkpoint blockade in hepatocellular carcinoma: Current progress and future directions. Hepatology. 2014;**60**(5):1776-1782

[30] Meng X et al. Predictive biomarkers in PD-1/PD-L1 checkpoint blockade immunotherapy. Cancer Treatment Reviews. 2015;**41**(10):868-876

[31] Vesely MD et al. Natural innate and adaptive immunity to cancer. Annual Review of Immunology. 2011;**29**:235-271

[32] Melero II et al. A clinical trial of Ctla-4 blockade with tremelimumab in patients with hepatocellular carcinoma and chronic hepatitis C. Immunology. 2012;**137**:54

[33] Duffy AG et al. Tremelimumab in combination with ablation in patients with advanced hepatocellular carcinoma. Journal of Hepatology. 2017;**66**(3):545-551

[34] Shi F et al. PD-1 and PD-L1 upregulation promotes $CD8^+$ T-cell apoptosis and postoperative recurrence in hepatocellular carcinoma patients. International Journal of Cancer. 2011;**128**(4):887-896

[35] Gao Q et al. Overexpression of PD-L1 significantly associates with tumor aggressiveness and postoperative recurrence in human hepatocellular carcinoma. Clinical Cancer Research. 2009;**15**(3):971-979

[36] El-Khoueiry AB et al. Nivolumab in patients with advanced hepatocellular carcinoma (CheckMate 040): An open-label, non-comparative, phase 1/2 dose escalation and expansion trial. The Lancet. 2017;**389**(10088):2492-2502

[37] Sangro B et al. A randomized, multicenter, phase 3 study of nivolumab vs sorafenib as first-line treatment in patients (pts) with advanced hepatocellular carcinoma (HCC): CheckMate-459. American Society of Clinical Oncology. 2016

[38] Zhu AX et al. KEYNOTE-224: Pembrolizumab in patients with advanced hepatocellular carcinoma previously treated with sorafenib. American Society of Clinical Oncology. 2018

[39] Parato KA et al. The oncolytic poxvirus JX-594 selectively replicates in and destroys cancer cells driven by genetic pathways commonly activated in cancers. Molecular Therapy. 2012;**20**(4):749-758

[40] Hammill AM, Conner J, Cripe TP. Oncolytic virotherapy reaches adolescence. Pediatric Blood & Cancer. 2010;**55**(7):1253-1263

[41] Bourke M et al. The emerging role of viruses in the treatment of solid tumours. Cancer Treatment Reviews. 2011;**37**(8):618-632

[42] Platanias LC. Mechanisms of type-I-and type-II-interferon-mediated signalling. Nature Reviews Immunology. 2005;**5**(5):375

[43] Guo ZS, Thorne SH, Bartlett DL. Oncolytic virotherapy: Molecular targets in tumor-selective replication and carrier cell-mediated delivery of oncolytic viruses. Biochimica et Biophysica Acta (BBA)-Reviews on Cancer. 2008;**1785**(2):217-231

[44] Kaufman HL, Kohlhapp FJ, Zloza A. Oncolytic viruses: a new class of immunotherapy drugs. Nature Reviews Drug Discovery. 2015;**14**(9):642

[45] Chiocca EA, Rabkin SD. Oncolytic viruses and their application to cancer immunotherapy. Cancer Immunology Research. 2014;**2**(4):295-300

[46] Yoo SY et al. Evolutionary cancer-favoring engineered vaccinia virus for metastatic hepatocellular carcinoma. Oncotarget. 2017;**8**(42):71489

[47] Breitbach CJ et al. A phase 2, open-label, randomized study of Pexa-Vec (JX-594) administered by intratumoral injection in patients with unresectable primary hepatocellular carcinoma. In: Gene Therapy of Solid Cancers. Springer; 2015. pp. 343-357

[48] Ady JW et al. Oncolytic immunotherapy using recombinant vaccinia virus GLV-1h68 kills sorafenib-resistant hepatocellular carcinoma efficiently. Surgery. 2014;**156**(2):263-269

[49] Wang J et al. Treatment of human hepatocellular carcinoma by the oncolytic herpes simplex virus G47delta. Cancer Cell International. 2014;**14**(1):83

[50] Sun T et al. Clinical research on dendritic cell vaccines to prevent postoperative recurrence and metastasis of liver cancer. Genetics and Molecular Research. 2015;**14**(4):16222-16232

[51] Zhang W et al. Immunotherapy of hepatocellular carcinoma with a vaccine based on xenogeneic homologous α fetoprotein in mice. Biochemical and Biophysical Research Communications. 2008;**376**(1):10-14

[52] Sawada Y et al. Phase II study of the GPC3-derived peptide vaccine as an adjuvant therapy for hepatocellular carcinoma patients. Oncoimmunology. 2016;**5**(5):e1129483

[53] El Ansary M et al. Immunotherapy by autologous dendritic cell vaccine in patients with advanced HCC. Journal of Cancer Research and Clinical Oncology. 2013;**139**(1):39-48

[54] Lee J-H et al. A phase I/IIa study of adjuvant immunotherapy with tumour antigen-pulsed dendritic cells in patients with hepatocellular carcinoma. British Journal of Cancer. 2015;**113**(12):1666

[55] Jixia Z, Chengyan Z, Pingli W. Advances in application of adoptive T-cell therapy for cancer patients. Journal of Zhejiang University (Medical Science). 2017;**46**(2):211-217

[56] Yeku O, Li X, Brentjens RJ. Adoptive T-cell therapy for solid tumors. In: American Society of Clinical Oncology Educational Book. American Society of Clinical Oncology. Meeting. NIH Public Access. 2017

[57] Baruch EN et al. Adoptive T cell therapy: an overview of obstacles and opportunities. Cancer. 2017;**123**(S11):2154-2162

[58] Longo V et al. Immunotherapeutic approaches for hepatocellular carcinoma. Oncotarget. 2017;**8**(20):33897

[59] Gao X et al. Cytokine-induced killer cells as pharmacological tools for cancer immunotherapy. Frontiers in Immunology. 2017;**8**:774

[60] Xu L et al. A randomized controlled trial on patients with or without adjuvant autologous cytokine-induced killer cells after curative resection for hepatocellular carcinoma. Oncoimmunology. 2016;**5**(3):e1083671

[61] Su Y et al. The efficacy and safety of dendritic cells co-cultured with cytokine-induced killer cell therapy in combination with TACE-predominant minimally-invasive treatment for hepatocellular carcinoma: a meta-analysis. Clinical Laboratory. 2016;**62**(4):599-608

[62] Toh U et al. Characterization of IL-2-activated TILs and their use in intrapericardial immunotherapy in malignant pericardial effusion. Cancer Immunology, Immunotherapy. 2006;**55**(10):1219-1227

[63] Yuan L et al. The preparation and study on hepatic targeting tendency of galactosyl-anti-CD3-McAb in mice. Hua Xi Yi Ke Da Xue Xue Bao (Journal of West China University of Medical Sciences). 2001;**32**(3):424-426

[64] Kikuchi T, Watanabe M, Ohno T. Cytological characteristics of human glioma-infiltrating lymphocytes stimulated with recombinant interleukin 2 and an anti-CD3 antibody. Cancer Science. 1991;**82**(3):339-345

[65] Jiang S-S et al. A phase I clinical trial utilizing autologous tumor-infiltrating lymphocytes in patients with primary hepatocellular carcinoma. Oncotarget. 2015;**6**(38):41339

[66] Narni-Mancinelli E, Vivier E, Kerdiles YM. The 'T-cell-ness' of NK cells: Unexpected similarities between NK cells and T cells. International Immunology. 2011;**23**(7):427-431

[67] Kamiya T, Chang Y-H, Campana D. Expanded and activated natural killer cells for immunotherapy of hepatocellular carcinoma. Cancer Immunology Research. 2016;**4**(7):574-581

[68] Abken H, Chmielewski M, Hombach AA. Antigen-specific T-cell activation independently of the MHC: Chimeric antigen receptor-redirected T cells. Frontiers in Immunology. 2013;**4**:371

[69] Li T, Wang H-T, Liu Z-G. Car technology and its application in treatment of multiple myeloma—Review. Zhongguo Shi Yan Xue Ye Xue Za Zhi. 2016;**24**(1):279-284

[70] Schuster SJ et al. Chimeric antigen receptor T cells in refractory B-cell lymphomas. New England Journal of Medicine. 2017;**377**(26):2545-2554

[71] Chmielewski M, Abken H. TRUCKs: The fourth generation of CARs. Expert Opinion on Biological Therapy. 2015;**15**(8):1145-1154

[72] Shirakawa H et al. Glypican-3 expression is correlated with poor prognosis in hepatocellular carcinoma. Cancer Science. 2009;**100**(8):1403-1407

[73] Gao H et al. Development of T cells redirected to glypican-3 for the treatment of hepatocellular carcinoma. Clinical Cancer Research. 2014;**20**(24):6418-6428

[74] Chen C et al. Development of T cells carrying two complementary chimeric antigen receptors against glypican-3 and asialoglycoprotein receptor 1 for the treatment of hepatocellular carcinoma. Cancer Immunology, Immunotherapy. 2017;**66**(4):475-489

[75] Chen Y et al. CXCR4 inhibition in tumor microenvironment facilitates anti-programmed death receptor-1 immunotherapy in sorafenib-treated hepatocellular carcinoma in mice. Hepatology. 2015;**61**(5):1591-1602

[76] Huang Y et al. Vascular normalizing doses of antiangiogenic treatment reprogram the immunosuppressive tumor microenvironment and enhance immunotherapy. Proceedings of the National Academy of Sciences. 2012;**109**(43):17561-17566

[77] Larkin J et al. Combined nivolumab and ipilimumab or monotherapy in untreated melanoma. New England Journal of Medicine. 2015;**373**(1):23-34

[78] Thomas MB et al. Systemic therapy for hepatocellular carcinoma: Cytotoxic chemotherapy, targeted therapy and immunotherapy. Annals of Surgical Oncology. 2008;**15**(4):1008-1014

5

Novel Techniques in the Surgical Management of Hepatocellular Carcinoma

Vasileia Ntomi, Anna Paspala and Dimitrios Schizas

Abstract

Hepatocellular carcinoma (HCC) is the most common primary liver malignancy with cirrhosis preceding its development in most cases. Surgical resection remains the primary therapeutic option despite the recent emergence of locoregional therapies. Novel surgical techniques are being proposed to overcome the limitations of traditional anatomical open liver resection. Laparoscopic resection is a safe and effective alternative to open liver resection, especially for left lateral or peripheral segment tumors. It is associated with less postoperative morbidity, intraoperative blood loss, and medial hospital stay with no difference in oncological outcomes. Robotic-assisted liver resection overcomes the technically difficult resection of tumors located at the posterosuperior segments with similar outcomes to laparoscopic resection. Associated liver partition and portal vein ligation for staged hepatectomy (ALPPS) procedure allows resection in patients with HCC, and associated major vascular resection or small future liver remnant (FLR) with long-term results yet to be announced. For patients with small solitary tumors or poor liver function, non-anatomical liver resection is a feasible therapeutic option due to minimal postoperative morbidity and similar oncological results of anatomical resection.

Keywords: hepatocellular carcinoma, laparoscopic, robotic, ALPPS, novel

1. Introduction

Hepatocellular carcinoma (HCC) is the fifth most common malignancy and the third leading cause of cancer-related deaths worldwide [1]. Cirrhotic patients have the highest risk of developing HCC [2]. Numerous factors contribute to cirrhosis which precedes HCC development, including viral hepatitis, heavy drinking, and aflatoxin exposure. Hepatitis C epidemic in the Western world and Hepatitis B epidemic in China have attributed to the incidence of

HCC [3]. However, HCC has a dismal prognosis, mainly due to the early recurrence; about 40% of patients that have undergone hepatectomy develop recurrence within the first year after surgery [2].

Although liver transplantation is considered as the ideal treatment, hepatic resection remains the only curative method of therapy for HCC. Other methods of potentially curative therapy are radiofrequency ablation (RFA), microwave ablation (MWA), high power focused ultrasound ablation (HIFU), and transarterial chemoembolization (TACE) [4, 5].

Novel surgical techniques are being proposed to overcome the limitations of traditional anatomical open liver resection. Laparoscopic and robotic resection as well as nonanatomical resection and ALPPS procedure have emerged as new and effective ways of surgical therapy for HCC.

The aim of this chapter is to analyze the aforementioned novel surgical techniques in the management of HCC and present the results from the relevant studies.

2. Laparoscopic liver resection for HCC

Laparoscopic surgery has become widely accepted as a feasible alternative to traditional open surgery for many surgical indications. The first laparoscopic hepatectomy was performed in 1992, for a benign tumor by Gagner et al. [6], and the first laparoscopic resection for HCC was reported in 1995 [7].

The liver presents many and significant technical challenges for minimally invasive techniques. Its mobilization is difficult, the space is limited, its vascular and biliary anatomy is complex and the parenchyma is fragile, friable and often fibrotic or cirrhotic [8]. Nevertheless, numerous studies have already shown the feasibility and safety of wedge resections, single-segment resections, and left lateral sectionectomies [9, 10].

The first international consensus conference on laparoscopic liver resection (LLR) was held in Louisville in 2008. It was suggested that the best indications for laparoscopic excision were solitary lesions less than 5 cm, located in the anterior segments. Also, the resection should be far from the hepatic hilum and the vena cava [11]. The second international consensus was held in Morioka, Japan in 2014, stating that anatomical resection for HCC is standard of care procedure, but the laparoscopic version needs to be standardized to increase propagation [12].

There are many reasons why laparoscopic major hepatectomy has not been widely accepted and performed yet. There are technical difficulties related to liver mobilization, vascular control, inability for manual palpation, access to posterosuperior liver segments, and intraoperative hazards such as gas embolism, massive bleeding, and bile duct injury [13, 14].

The benefits of laparoscopic surgery, though, have long been proven. Early postoperative ambulation, decreased respiratory complications, minimization of blood loss, minimal abdominal trauma, and less postoperative pain are some of the accepted benefits of laparoscopic surgery. For cirrhotic patients with HCC, the minimization of the surgical incision and the subsequent preservation of the abdominal wall circulation and lymphatic flow explains the decrease in postoperative liver failure and ascites formation [15].

The last decade, several meta-analyses of laparoscopic vs. open resection for HCC have been published [16–23]. These meta-analyses have analyzed and compared the results of many nonrandomized control trials and case-matched studies. Three categories of outcomes were used to compare the two operative techniques:

a. Operative outcomes, such as operative time, operative blood loss, and number of patients that needed transfusion.

b. Postoperative outcomes, such as morbidity, mortality, and hospital stay.

c. Oncologic results, such as pathologic resection margins, incidence of port-site recurrence, disease-free survival (DFS), and overall survival (OS).

Jiang et al. [16] reported the superiority of laparoscopic liver resection (LLR) concerning the reduced intraoperative blood loss and blood transfusion, the expansion of the pathologic resection margins, the increase of R0 resection, and the shorter length of hospital stay. Laparoscopic resection has similar OS, DFS, and recurrence rate as open liver resection (OLR).

Sotiropoulos et al. [17], in a recent meta-analysis of 44 studies, showed that laparoscopic resection is superior to open resection in terms of resection margin and R0 resection. It is possible that this difference in resection margin and R0 excision is due to the smaller size of tumors resected in the laparoscopic group. It was confirmed that the laparoscopic technique is strongly associated with less blood loss, fewer blood transfusions, less postoperative pain, faster recovery, and shorter hospital stay. Operative time and tumor recurrence were not statistically different between LLR and OLR as well as the long-term oncological results such as OS and DFS. These results confirm those of previous authors [15, 18, 21, 22]. Hand-assisted laparoscopic or laparoscopy-assisted resections (hybrid group) gain statistical advantage over the OLR group concerning the negative resection margin width and influence the results in favor of LLR. They, however, showed no difference as to the OS and 30-day mortality compared to the OLR group.

The main concerns about LLR are the inadequate tumor resection margins and the potential risk of port-site recurrence. Tumor recurrence is the main cause of death in patients with HCC. The adequate tumor-free margin is a prognostic indicator of HCC [23]. Due to the lack of tactile sensation in laparoscopic surgery, the tumor location is sometimes difficult to determine. Intraoperative ultrasonography is a useful tool for precise identification of lesions and its borders [24, 25]. Another concerning factor is the risk of tumor peritoneal dissemination and port-site metastases [26, 27]. Interestingly, there has not been any evidence so far of tumor peritoneal dissemination or port-site metastases [20, 22]. The use of a plastic bag to remove the specimen can help to prevent this complication.

Concern has also been raised about the safety of laparoscopic techniques in cirrhotic patients. A plethora of patients with HCC also suffer from cirrhosis. Portal hypertension is a major risk factor for the development of postoperative decompensation [28, 29]. The benefits of LLR can be attributed to the preservation of the abdominal wall collateral circulation and the preservation of the round ligament which may contain significant collateral veins [18]. In a study by Tranchart et al., LLR had lower rates of liver decompensation, with the occurrence of postoperative liver failure and ascites ranging from 7 to 8% in LLR vs. 26–36% in OLR [30]. One study from Japan showed lower rates of morbidity, ascites formation, and shorter hospital stay following LLR with no difference in survival [31]. A recent meta-analysis presented intraoperative and postoperative outcomes of patients with known cirrhosis undergoing resection for HCC, comparing results for OLR and LLR [32]. This meta-analysis showed wider resection margins, reduced intraoperative blood loss and transfusion need, as well as reduced morbidity rates and shorter lengths of stay with the laparoscopic approach. Another study by Sotiropoulos et al. [33] mentioned the difference in results concerning cirrhotic patients that undergo LLR vs. OLR. The operative time was longer as anticipated, but the blood loss and morbidity had no statistical difference from the noncirrhotic group. The mortality rate was significantly lower in the cirrhotic subgroup when LLR was performed. Although patients with preserved liver function are the best candidates for LLR, cirrhotic patients benefit from LLR in terms of shorter hospital stay, complication rate, and long-term oncologic outcomes.

Tumor recurrence after primary HCC has been shown to be 30–70% at 5 years, limiting the overall survival of these patients [34, 35]. Numerous studies have been published reporting the results of repeat laparoscopic liver resection (RLLR) in patients with recurrent HCC [36–38]. A recent systematic review by Machairas et al. demonstrates RLLR as a safe and promising approach for the treatment of recurrent HCC, with significant benefits in terms of short-term outcomes with the oncologic adequacy not compromised [39].

The conversion rate has decreased from 5–15% [9, 40] to 4%, indicative of the surgeons' growing experience, with the most common causes being bleeding and failure to progress secondary to difficult exposure.

Overall, LLR can facilitate a safe and feasible approach to the surgical management of HCC. Major laparoscopic hepatectomy still remains a technically demanding procedure and should only be performed by highly experienced hepatobiliary surgeons with training in laparoscopic surgery. Longer follow-up periods are needed for more definite conclusions about the survival probability of the LLR vs. the OLR groups.

3. Robotic liver resection for HCC

Robotic liver resection (RLR) has been incorporated into clinical practice with increasing frequency since 2003 when the first report of a robotic liver resection was published by Giulianotti et al. [41].

Robotic technology was developed to overcome the technical difficulties of laparoscopic surgery; precision of movement, three-dimensional vision, magnification of the operative field, motion scaling, tremor filtering, and seven degrees of movement mimicking the human hand provide steady and careful dissection as well as prompt and precise endosuturing in case of intraoperative bleeding. A major advantage of the robotic technology in liver surgery is the dissection of the hilum and the hepatocaval dissection in right hepatectomy [42] as well as the possibility of biliary reconstruction due to the microsuturing capacity of the robotic system [43].

All published liver resections were performed using the da Vinci Surgical System (Intuitive Surgical Inc., Sunnyvale, CA USA). The major disadvantage of robotic surgery is the high cost due to the longer operating time and the instruments required, in spite of the similar hospitalization costs [44]. The purchase and maintenance costs are significant, and that is the reason for the limited incorporation of the robotic system in many facilities.

A large series by Tsung et al. [45] compared RLR to LLR and with the exception of operative time, and they found no significant differences comparing operative and postoperative results of RLR and LLR. The R0 status did not change, and the oncologic margin was not compromised. It must be highlighted that using a minimally invasive technique, a greater percentage of minor and major hepatectomies was completed; 93% of RLRs were accomplished in a purely minimally invasive manner compared with 49.1% performed laparoscopically.

Chen et al. [46] compared RLR with OLR for HCC providing superior short-term outcomes for RLR (shorter length of stay and decreased need for patient-controlled analgesia) and similar long-term outcomes (DFS and OS) despite longer operative times for RLR. A substantial proportion of patients suffered from cirrhosis and half of patients underwent major hepatectomy. They reported a DFS in 1 year of 91.5% with the RLR, whereas DFS was 79.2%. Overall survival in 1 and 3 years did not differ between the two groups. The authors reported that the patients treated with RLR had significantly wider surgical margins compared with OLR. This matched comparison offers support for further RLR in patients with HCC, performed by experienced surgeons.

Another study by Lai et al. [47] presented the results of RLR vs. LLR for HCC. Robotic group had longer mean operating time (207.4 vs. 134.2 min). Both groups had similar blood loss (334.6 vs. 336 ml) and no difference in morbidity. Mortality rate was 0% in both groups. They reported a comparable 5-year DFS and 5-year OS between RLR and LLR (42 vs. 38% and 65 vs. 48%, respectively) in patients with HCC.

Salloum et al. [48] included 14 studies in their systematic review, with HCC comprising the majority of the malignant cases. Mortality was 0%, and overall morbidity ranged from 0 to 43.3%, results comparable to laparoscopy. The mean duration of LOS was similar in both techniques. There was no statistically significant difference between RLR and LLR concerning the surgical margins or R1 resections. No clear advantages of RLR over LLR were noted; therefore, it is difficult to establish the true indications for RLR. Nevertheless, RLR has the same advantages as LLR in terms of shorter LOS and postoperative return to normal activities. Also, it seems that the learning curve for RLR is shorter than that of LLR.

The most recent systematic review from Tsilimigras et al. [49] included 31 studies with HCC being the leading indication among malignancies, comparing RLR to LLR or OLR. Median operative time was 295.5 min, EBL was 224.5 ml, conversion rate was 5.9%, and complication rate was 17.6% in the RLR group. The complications were graded according to the Clavien-Dindo classification [50], with the most common complication being bile leak (2.9%). In minor resections, the complication rate was 14.8% compared with the major resections, where the complication rate was 17%. Most of the studies show no benefit of RLR over LLR concerning safety and feasibility and multicenter, and randomized, prospective trials are needed to validate the exact indications and benefits of RLR.

Buchs et al. [51], in a systematic review of eight studies, compared RLR to LLR with the majority of the malignant cases being HCC (50.3%). There were minor and major hepatectomy procedures, and tumor size ranged from 8 to 120 mm. In the RLR group, there was no mortality, and the overall complication rate was 23.3% which fell to 19% when only postoperative complications were considered. A reduction of the conversion rate during major hepatectomy was reported as well. Overall, there was no clear outcome difference between RLR and LLR.

Ocuin et al. [52] included 14 major series in their review with the most common indication for resection being HCC. The estimated blood loss (EBL) ranged from 50 to 413 ml and transfusion rates from 0 to 44%. An overall conversion rate of 7% and an overall complication rate of 21% were reported. No perioperative mortality was associated with RLR. Length of stay (LOS) varied from 4 to 12 days. One study by Ji et al. showed a shorter LOS following RLR than OLR (10 vs. 7 days) [53]. Most series reported a high R0 resection rate with no port site recurrences. Recurrence rates following RLR were similar to those reported for LLR [9].

In conclusion, robotic liver resection is an acceptable alternative to open surgery with the robotic approach allowing an increased proportion of major hepatectomies to be performed in a minimally invasive manner [54]. These encouraging results should prompt the expansion of the robotic approach by highly specialized surgeons in experience centers worldwide.

4. Associating liver partition and portal vein ligation for liver surgery (ALPPS) for HCC

Surgical resection is the only potential curative treatment for hepatocellular carcinoma (HCC). In many cases, a major hepatectomy is required to achieve tumor-free surgical margins. However, the volume and functional reserve of the future liver remnant (FLR) are essential to avoid post-hepatectomy liver failure (PHLF), which is a crucial and important cause of morbidity and mortality after extensive liver resection [55]. In recent decades, some new strategies, such as portal vein embolization (PVE), portal vein ligation (PVL), and two-staged hepatectomy (TSH) have been developed to induce regeneration of FLR, minimizing the risk of PHLF and finally expanding the resectability criteria in HCC and generally in liver tumors [56]. Makuuchi et al. first introduced portal vein embolization into clinical practice in 1980s [57]. In 2015, a systematic review and meta-analysis from Pandanaboyana et al. compared PVL and PVE to assess the percentile increase of the

FLR, morbidity, mortality, and tumor progression [58]. This meta-analysis revealed that the difference in the mean percentile increase in the FLR between those two techniques was not statistically significant, with similar results in morbidity, mortality, and disease progression.

In 2000s, Adam et al. first described the two-staged hepatectomy for liver malignancies in which a single surgical procedure was not possible [59]. The primary reason for the failure of TSH is tumor progression between two stages or an insufficient hypertrophy in FLR after the first stage of the procedure (portal vein occlusion).

An innovative, accelerated two-staged technique utilizing PVL and in situ split (ISS) of hepatic parenchyma was first described in 2012 by Schnitzbauer et al. [60]. In the same year, De Santibanes et al. named this procedure as ALPPS procedure (associating liver partition and portal vein ligation for staged hepatectomy) [61]. In 2007, ALPPS was first performed by chance by German surgeon Dr. Schlitt [62, 63]. In an attempt to perform an extended right hepatectomy for a perihilar cholangiocarcinoma, he intraoperatively realized that FLR was inadequate. He resected the liver adjacent to the falciform ligament after performing a left hepaticojejunostomy. The right portal vein was also ligated for the purpose of left lobe hypertrophy. Out of curiosity, on postoperative day 8, he performed a computed tomography (CT) scan. To his surprise, the left lateral section had extensively grown in size. He successfully removed the diseased liver in a second operation.

ALPPS indications are an FLR < 30% in patients with a normal liver or an FLR < 40% in patients with a cholestatic, steatotic or fibrotic liver [64]. Therefore, ALPPS can be performed for marginally resectable or locally advanced tumors with an inadequate FLR. This technique constitutes a surgical strategy for colorectal liver metastases, hilar cholangiocarcinoma, and hepatocellular carcinoma [64]. On the other hand, contradictions for ALPPS procedure include unresectable liver metastases in the FLR, unresectable extrahepatic metastases, severe portal hypertension, high anesthetic risks, and a poor condition of the patient prior to this major operation [64]. Patients with cirrhotic liver are less capable for hypertrophy of FLR after portal vein obstruction (PVL or PVE) than patients with healthy liver parenchyma. Vennarecci et al. reported that ALPPS for HCC is safe even when performing a major hepatectomy in a cirrhotic liver. They also mentioned that ALPPS induces a significant increase in FLR between the first and the second stage of the procedure and after hepatectomy, either in healthy or cirrhotic patients [65].

It has been reported that postoperative morbidity and mortality after ALPPS are 16–64 and 12–23%, respectively, with the main cause of morbidity being bile leakage and sepsis and the main cause of mortality being PHLF [66, 67]. In the latest systematic review and meta-analysis by Zhou et al., 719 patients were included, and the aim was to compare the regeneration efficiency, safety, and complication rates of ALPPS and TSH. The degree of FLR regeneration in ALPPS was significantly higher than that in TSH, and the interval of the two stages in ALPPS was obviously shorter than that in TSH. Bile fistulas were much more common after ALPPS with the reason being the liver splitting that is mandatory during this procedure.

Although ALPPS had lower 1-year DFS rate, no significant difference in the 90-day mortality rate was discovered comparing the two techniques [66]. ALPPS was associated with a higher completion rate, a lower probability of tumor progression during the stage interval, and a lower insufficient regeneration rate; these findings are similar to those of previous studies [56, 67, 68].

Many variations of the ALPPS technique have been recently mentioned in the literature with the aim of improving safety and extending indications of hepatectomy. Modifications, such as avoiding liver mobilization and hepatoduodenal skeletonization, seem to prevent tumor spreading, adhesions, overall invasiveness, and parenchymal ischemia [69–73]. In addition, anterior approaches, portal vein embolization (PVE) as an alternative to ligation, partial liver splitting, tourniquet application or ablation procedures replacing parenchymal transection, and laparoscopic approaches represent fundamental modifications to the original ALPPS procedure that aim to improve safety [15]. The result of these modifications is the reduction of morbidity and mortality in this innovative surgical procedure. Furthermore, prospective controlled studies are needed to confirm which of these modifications should be considered as a reliable and safe alternative strategy to classical ALPPS.

5. Anatomical vs. nonanatomical resection for HCC

The incidence of HCC continues to increase due to the dissemination of hepatitis B and C virus infection. Hepatic resection is the gold standard treatment for HCC [74]. Nevertheless, postoperative recurrence of HCC, 3 and 5 years after hepatectomy is 50–60% and 70–90%, respectively [75, 76].

It is known that HCC invades mainly the intrahepatic vascular system and spreads along the portal and hepatic vein branches, producing intrahepatic metastases [77, 78].

Since Makuuchi et al. introduced the concept of anatomical resection (AR), the advantages of anatomic resection for HCC have been suggested in many studies [79]. On the other hand, limited nonanatomic resection (NR) with a minimal safety margin may be preferred for patients with impaired liver function [80]. Tanaka et al. showed that microscopic vascular invasion was more important than tumor size as a predictive factor for local recurrence [81].

Anatomical liver resection is a plausible option for patients with HCC, as HCC tends to cause intrahepatic metastasis through vascular invasion, and its advantages in improved OS or DFS for HCC patients have widely been reported [82].

In a systematic review of Cucchetti et al., AR seemed to yield improved 5-year OS and DFS compared to NR [83]. Zhou et al. [84] and Bigonzi et al. [85] presented significantly improved 5-year OS with AR.

Nonanatomic resection is recommended for patients with impaired liver function [86, 87]. The plausible reason is that NR can preserve as much functional liver as possible, with surgical curability and hepatic function equally important [87, 88]. The preservation of hepatic functional reserve allows effective treatment options in HCC recurrence, which may also improve the long-term prognosis [87, 89].

The superiority of anatomical resection (AR) over nonanatomic resection (NR) for hepatocellular carcinoma (HCC) remains controversial. Marubashi et al. reported no significant differences in OS, DFS or recurrence within 2 years after hepatectomy between the AR and NR groups [90]. Likewise, Tanaka et al. reported no outstanding difference in the recurrence rates and OS between AR and NR patient groups; it was also stated that survival rates after recurrence and median survival time after recurrence were higher in the NR group compared to the AR group for patients with a solitary HCC confined to 1 or 2 liver segments [91]. Chen et al. reported in their meta-analysis that AR contributed to better DFS, but did not improve OS [92]. Thus, the superiority of AR over NR is still controversial. Furthermore, Yamamoto et al. reported that AR is associated with more perioperative risks. The same study revealed significantly greater intraoperative blood loss and longer postoperative hospital stay for the AR group [82].

In 2010, Yamashita et al. [80] published a retrospective study of 321 patients with HCC. About 120 patients underwent limited nonanatomic resection (NR) for a single HCC < 5 cm. In noncirrhotic patients (n = 215), both 5-year OS and DFS rates in the AR group were considerably better than those in the NR group (87 vs. 76% and 63 vs. 35%, respectively). In cirrhotic patients (n = 106), both 5-year OS and DFS in the AR group were worse than those in the NR group (48 vs. 72% and 28 vs. 43%, respectively).

According to their results, the width of the resection margin did not influence postoperative recurrence, and major hepatic resections did not improve patients' survival. The main disadvantage of AR in comparison with NR is the limitation of a repeat resection, which would be the most effective treatment for recurrence, because of its disadvantageous effects on remnant liver function [93, 94].

In conclusion, there is a need for more, large, prospective, multicenter studies to confirm the data about any possible superiority of nonanatomic resection for HCC.

6. Conclusion

Hepatocellular carcinoma is a malignancy with an increasing incidence and a dismal prognosis. Patients are often referred to specialists in an advanced stage of the disease. Surgery is the primary treatment and novel surgical techniques are developed offering better perioperative and oncological results (**Table 1**). Nevertheless, prospective, randomized controlled studies have to be designed for the confirmation of such possible advantages of those new surgical techniques.

Technique	Advantages	Limitations	Reference
Laparoscopic resection	• Early ambulation • Decreased respiratory complications • Minimal abdominal trauma • Less postoperative pain • Decrease in PHLF • Reduced blood loss • Shorter length of hospital stay • Increase of R0 resection	• Technical difficulties • Vascular control • Difficult access to posterosuperior segments • Massive bleeding • No manual palpation • Longer operative time	[13–17, 23, 26, 27]
Robotic resection	• Precision of movement • 3-dimensional vision • 7 degrees of movement • Precise endosuturing • Dissection of the hilum • Biliary reconstruction • Shorter length of stay	• High cost • Longer operative time • Specialized surgeons	[42–44, 46, 54]
ALPPS	• Increase in FLR • Application to cirrhotic patients • Marginally resectable tumors • Locally advances tumors	• Severe portal hypertension • High risk patients • High rates of post-operative morbidity and mortality • Bile leakage • Sepsis	[64–67]
Nonanatomical resection	• Repeat resection • Impaired liver function • No difference in recurrence rates • Less intra-operative blood loss • Cirrhotic patients	• Worse 5-year OS and DFS • Width of resection margin • Microscopic vascular invasion	[80, 81, 83–85, 90, 91, 93, 94]

Table 1. Advantages and limitations of novel surgical techniques for hepatocellular carcinoma management.

Author details

Vasileia Ntomi[1], Anna Paspala[1] and Dimitrios Schizas[2*]

*Address all correspondence to: schizasad@gmail.com

1 Third Department of Surgery, National and Kapodistrian University of Athens, Attikon University Hospital, Athens, Greece

2 First Department of Surgery, National and Kapodistrian University of Athens, Laikon General Hospital, Athens, Greece

References

[1] Torre L, Bray F, Siegel RL, et al. Global cancer statistics, 2012. CA: A Cancer Journal for Clinicians. 2015 Mar;**65**(2):87-108. DOI: 10.3322/caac.21262

[2] Llovet JM, Burroughs A, Bruix J. Hepatocellular carcinoma. Lancet. 2003 Dec;**362**(9399): 1907-1917. DOI: 10.1016/S0140-6736(03)14964-1

[3] El-Serag HB. Hepatocellular carcinoma. The New England Journal of Medicine. 2011 Sep;**365**(12):1118-1127. DOI: 10.1056/NEJMra1001683

[4] Shen JY, Li C, Wen TF, et al. Liver transplantation versus surgical resection for HCC meeting the Milan criteria: A propensity score analysis. Medicine (Baltimore). 2016 Dec;**95**(52):e5756

[5] Crocetti L, Bargellini I, Cioni R. Loco-regional treatment of HCC: Current status. Clinical Radiology. 2017 Aug;**72**(8):626-635. DOI: 10.1016/j.crad.2017.01.013

[6] Gagner M, Rheault M, Dubuc J. Laparoscopic partial hepatectomy for liver tumor. Surgical Endoscopy. 1992;**6**:97-98

[7] Hashizume M, Takenaka K, Yanaga K, et al. Laparoscopic hepatic resection for hepato_ cellular carcinoma. Surgical Endoscopy. 1995;**9**(12):1289-1291

[8] Beard RE, Tsung A. Minimally invasive approaches for surgical management of primary liver cancers. Cancer Control. 2017 Jul–Sep;**24**(3):1073274817729234. DOI: 10.1177/ 1073274817729234

[9] Nguyen KT, Gamblin TC, Geller DA. World review of laparoscopic liver resection-2, 804 patients. Annals of Surgery. 2009 Nov;**250**(5):831-841. DOI: 10.1097/SLA.0b013e3181b0c4df

[10] Nguyen KT, Laurent A, Dagher I, et al. Minimally invasive liver resection for metastatic colorectal cancer: A multi-institutional, international report of safety, feasibility, and early outcomes. Annals of Surgery. 2009 Nov;**250**(5):842-848

[11] Buell JF, Cherqui D, Geller DA, et al. The international position on laparoscopic liver surgery: The Louisville statement, 2008. Annals of Surgery. 2009 Nov;**250**(5):825-830

[12] Wakabayashi G, Cherqui D, Geller DA, et al. Recommendations for laparoscopic liver resection: A report from the second international consensus conference held in Morioka. Annals of Surgery. 2015 Apr;**261**(4):619-629. DOI: 10.1097/SLA.0000000000001184

[13] Buell JF, Thomas MT, Rudich S, et al. Experience with more than 500 minimally invasive hepatic procedures. Annals of Surgery. 2008 Sep;**248**(3):475-486. DOI: 10.1097/ SLA.0b013e318185e647

[14] Vibert E, Perniceni T, Levard H, et al. Laparoscopic liver resection. The British Journal of Surgery. 2006 Jan;**93**(1):67-72. DOI: 10.1002/bjs.5150

[15] Chen K, Pan Y, Zhang B, et al. Laparoscopic versus open surgery for hepatocellular carcinoma: A meta-analysis of high-quality case-matched studies. Canadian Journal of Gastroenterology and Hepatology. 2018 Mar;**2018**:1746895. DOI: 10.1155/2018/1746895

[16] Jiang B, Yan XF, Zhang JH. Meta-analysis of laparoscopic versus open liver resection for hepatocellular carcinoma. Hepatology Research. 2018 Jul;**48**(8):635-663. DOI: 10.1111/hepr.13061

[17] Sotiropoulos GC, Prodromidou A, Kostakis ID, et al. Meta-analysis of laparoscopic *vs.* open liver resection for hepatocellular carcinoma. Updates in Surgery. 2017 Sep;**69**(3):291-311. DOI: 10.1007/s13304-017-0421-4

[18] Yin Z, Fan X, Ye H, et al. Short- and long-term outcomes after laparoscopic and open hepatectomy for hepatocellular carcinoma: A global systematic review and meta analysis. Annals of Surgical Oncology. 2013 Apr;**20**(4):1203-1215. DOI: 10.1245/s10434-012-2705-8

[19] Xiong JJ, Altaf K, Javed MA, et al. Meta-analysis of laparoscopic *vs* open liver resection for hepatocellular carcinoma. World Journal of Gastroenterology. 2012 Dec;**18**(45):6657-6668. DOI: 10.3748/wjg.v18.i45.6657

[20] Li N, Wu YR, Wu B, et al. Surgical and oncologic outcomes following laparoscopic versus open liver resection for hepatocellular carcinoma: A meta-analysis. Hepatology Research. 2012;**42**(1):51-59. DOI: 10.1111/j.1872-034X.2011.00890.x

[21] Fancellu A, Rosman AS, Sanna V, et al. Meta-analysis of trials comparing minimally invasive and open liver resections for hepatocellular carcinoma. The Journal of Surgical Research. 2011 Nov;**171**(1):e33-e45. DOI: 10.1016/j.jss.2011.07.008

[22] Zhou YM, Shao WY, Zhao YF, et al. Meta-analysis of laparoscopic versus open resection for hepatocellular carcinoma. Digestive Diseases and Sciences. 2011 Jul;**56**(7):1937-1943. DOI: 10.1007/s10620-011-1572-7

[23] Masutani S, Sasaki Y, Imaoka S, et al. The prognostic significance of surgical margin in liver resection of patients with hepatocellular carcinoma. Archives of Surgery. 1994 Oct;**129**(10):1025-1030

[24] Silberhumer GR, Steininger R, Laengle F, et al. Intraoperative ultrasonography in patients who undergo liver resection or transplantation for hepatocellular carcinoma. Surgical Technology International. 2004;**12**:145-151

[25] Arii S, Tanaka S, Mitsunori Y, et al. Surgical strategies for hepatocellular carcinoma with special reference to anatomical hepatic resection and intraoperative contrast-enhanced ultrasonography. Oncology. 2010 Jul;**78**(Suppl 1):125-130. DOI: 10.1159/000315240

[26] Ishida H, Murata N, Yamada H, et al. Influence of trocar placement and CO(2) pneumoperitoneum on port site metastasis following laparoscopic tumor surgery. Surgical Endoscopy. 2000 Feb;**14**(2):193-197

[27] Bouvy ND, Marquet RL, Jeekel H, et al. Impact of gas(less) laparoscopy and laparotomy on peritoneal tumor growth and abdominal wall metastases. Annals of Surgery. 1996 Dec;**224**(6):694-700

[28] Bruix J, Castells A, Bosch J, et al. Surgical resection of hepatocellular carcinoma in cirrhotic patients: Prognostic value of preoperative portal pressure. Gastroenterology. 1996 Oct;**111**(4):1018-1022

[29] Powell-Jackson P, Greenway B, Williams R. Adverse effects of exploratory laparotomy in patients with unsuspected liver disease. The British Journal of Surgery. 1982 Aug;**69**(8):449-451

[30] Tranchart H, Di Giuro G, Lainas P, et al. Laparoscopic resection for hepatocellular carcinoma: A matched-pair comparative study. Surgical Endoscopy. 2010 May;**24**(5):1170-1176. DOI: 10.1007/s00464-009-0745-3

[31] Yamashita Y, Ikeda T, Kurihara T, et al. Long-term favorable surgical results of laparoscopic hepatic resection for Hepatocellular carcinoma in patients with cirrhosis: A single-center experience over a 10-year period. Journal of the American College of Surgeons. 2014 Dec;**219**(6):1117-1123. DOI: 10.1016/j.jamcollsurg.2014.09.003

[32] Twaij A, Pucher PH, Sodergren MH, et al. Laparoscopic vs open approach to resection of Hepatocellular carcinoma in patients with known cirrhosis: Systematic review and meta-analysis. World Journal of Gastroenterology. 2014 Jul;**20**(25):8274-8281. DOI: 10.3748/wjg.v20.i25.8274

[33] Sotiropoulos GC, Prodromidou A, Machairas N. Meta-analysis of laparoscopic vs. open liver resection for hepatocellular carcinoma: The European experience. JBUON. 2017 Sep–Oct;**22**(5):1160-1171

[34] Llovet JM, Schwartz M, Mazzaferro V. Resection and liver transplantation for hepatocellular carcinoma. Seminars in Liver Disease. 2005;**25**(2):181-200

[35] Zhou Y, Sui C, Li B, et al. Repeat hepatectomy for recurrent hepatocellular carcinoma: A local experience and a systematic review. World Journal of Surgical Oncology. 2010 Jul;**8**:55. DOI: 10.1186/1477-7819-8-55

[36] Ahn KS, Han HS, Yoon YS, et al. Laparoscopic liver resection in patients with a history of upper abdominal surgery. World Journal of Surgery. 2011 Jun;**35**(6):1333-1339. DOI: 10.1007/s00268-011-1073-z

[37] Shelat VG, Serin K, Samim M, et al. Outcomes of repeat laparoscopic liver resection compared to the primary resection. World Journal of Surgery. 2014 Dec;**38**(2):3175-3180. DOI: 10.1007/s00268-014-2728-3

[38] Zhang J, Zhou ZG, Huang ZX, et al. Prospective, single-center cohort study analyzing the efficacy of complete laparoscopic resection on recurrent hepatocellular carcinoma. Chinese Journal of Cancer. 2016 Mar;**35**:25. DOI: 10.1186/s40880-016-0088-0

[39] Machairas N, Papaconstantinou D, Stamopoulos P, et al. The emerging role of laparoscopic liver resection in the treatment of recurrent hepatocellular carcinoma: A systematic review. Anticancer Research. 2018 May;**38**(5):3181-3186. DOI: 10.21873/anticanres.12582

[40] Vigano L, Tayar C, Laurent A, et al. Laparoscopic liver resection: A systematic review. Journal of Hepato-Biliary-Pancreatic Surgery. 2009;**16**(4):410-421. DOI: 10.1007/s00534-009-0120-8

[41] Giulianotti PC, Coratti A, Angelini M. Robotics in general surgery: Personal experience in a large community hospital. Archives of Surgery. 2003 Jul;**138**(7):777-784. DOI: 10.1001/archsurg.138.7.777

[42] Giulianotti PC, Coratti A, Sbrana F, et al. Robotic liver surgery: Results for 70 resections. Surgery. 2011 Jan;**149**(1):29-39. DOI: 10.1016/j.surg.2010.04.002

[43] Giulianotti PC, Sbrana F, Bianco FM, et al. Robot-assisted laparoscopic extended right hepatectomy with biliary reconstruction. Journal of Laparoendoscopic & Advanced Surgical Techniques. Part A. 2010 Mar;**20**(2):159-163. DOI: 10.1089/lap.2009.0383

[44] Turchetti G, Palla I, Pierotti F, et al. Economic evaluation of da Vinci-assisted robotic surgery: A systematic review. Surgical Endoscopy. 2012 Mar;**26**(3):598-606. DOI: 10.1007/s00464-011-1936-2

[45] Tsung A, Geller DA, Sukato DC, et al. Robotic versus laparoscopic hepatectomy: A matched comparison. Annals of Surgery. 2014 Mar;**259**(3):549-555. DOI: 10.1097/SLA.0000000000000250

[46] Chen PD, Wu CY, Hu RH, et al. Robotic versus open hepatectomy for hepatocellular carcinoma: A matched comparison. Annals of Surgical Oncology. 2017 Apr;**24**(4):1021-1028. DOI: 10.1245/s10434-016-5638-9

[47] Lai EC, Tang CN. Long-term survival analysis of robotic versus conventional laparoscopic hepatectomy for hepatocellular carcinoma: A comparative study. Surgical Laparoscopy, Endoscopy & Percutaneous Techniques. 2016 Apr;**26**(2):162-166. DOI: 10.1097/SLE.0000000000000254

[48] Salloum C, Lim C, Malek A, et al. Robot-assisted laparoscopic liver resection: A review. Journal of Visceral Surgery. 2016 Dec;**153**(6):447-456. DOI: 10.1016/j.jviscsurg.2016.08.005

[49] Tsilimigras DI, Moris D, Vagios S, et al. Safety and oncologic outcomes of robotic liver resections: A systematic review. Journal of Surgical Oncology. 2018 Jun;**117**(7):1517-1530. DOI: 10.1002/ jso.25018

[50] Dindo D, Demartines N, Clavien PA. Classification of surgical complications: A new proposal with evaluation in a cohort of 6336 patients and results of a survey. Annals of Surgery. 2004 Aug;**240**(2):205-213

[51] Buchs NC, Oldani G, Orci LA, et al. Current status of robotic liver resection: A systematic review. Expert Review of Anticancer Therapy. 2014 Feb;**14**(2):237-246. DOI: 10.1586/14737140.2014.863155

[52] Ocuin LM, Tsung A. Robotic liver resection for malignancy: Current status, oncologic outcomes, comparison to laparoscopy, and future applications. Journal of Surgical Oncology. 2015 Sep;**112**(3):295-301. DOI: 10.1002/jso.23901

[53] Ji WB, Wang HG, Zhao ZM, et al. Robotic-assisted laparoscopic anatomic hepatectomy in China: Initial experience. Annals of Surgery. 2011 Feb;**253**(2):342-348. DOI: 10.1097/SLA.0b013e3181ff4601

[54] Milone L, Daskalaki D, Fernandes E, et al. State of the art in robotic hepatobiliary surgery. World Journal of Surgery. 2013 Dec;**37**(12):2747-2755. DOI: 10.1007/s00268-013-2276-2

[55] Kishi Y, Abdalla EK, Chun YS, et al. Three hundred and one consecutive extended right hepatectomies: Evaluation of outcome based on systematic liver volumetry. Annals of Surgery. 2009 Oct;**250**(4):540-554. DOI: 10.1097/SLA.0b013e3181b674df

[56] Zhang GQ, Zhang ZW, Lau WY, et al. Associating liver partition and portal vein ligation for staged hepatectomy (ALPPS): A new strategy to increase resectability in liver surgery. International Journal of Surgery. 2014;**12**(5):437-441. DOI: 10.1016/j.ijsu.2014.03.009

[57] Makuuchi M, Thai BL, Takayasu K, et al. Preoperative portal embolization to increase safety of major hepatectomy for hilar bile duct carcinoma: A preliminary report. Surgery. 1990 May;**107**(5):521-527

[58] Pandanaboyana S, Bell R, Hidalgo E, et al. A systematic review and meta-analysis of portal vein ligation versus portal vein embolization for elective liver resection. Surgery. 2015 Apr;**157**(4):690-698. DOI: 10.1016/j.surg.2014.12.009

[59] Adam R, Laurent A, Azoulay D, et al. Two-stage hepatectomy: A planned strategy to treat unresectable liver tumors. Annals of Surgery. 2000 Dec;**232**(6):777-785

[60] Schnitzbauer AA, Lang SA, Goessmann H, et al. Right portal vein ligation combined with in situ splitting induces rapid left lateral liver lobe hypertrophy enabling 2-staged extended right hepatic resection in small-for-size settings. Annals of Surgery. 2012 Mar;**255**(3):405-414. DOI: 10.1097/SLA.0b013e31824856f5

[61] de Santibañes E, Clavien PA. Playing play-doh to prevent postoperative liver failure: The "ALPPS" approach. Annals of Surgery. 2012 Mar;**255**(3):415-417. DOI: 10.1097/SLA.0b013e318248577d

[62] Donati M, Basile F, Oldhafer KJ. Present status and future perspectives of ALPPS (associating liver partition and portal vein ligation for staged hepatectomy). Future Oncology. 2015;**11**(16):2255-2258. DOI: 10.2217/fon.15.145

[63] Cai X, Tong Y, Yu H, et al. The ALPPS in the treatment of hepatitis B-related hepatocellular carcinoma with cirrhosis: A single-center study and literature review. Surgical Innovation. 2017 Aug;**24**(4):358-364. DOI: 10.1177/1553350617697187

[64] Alvarez FA, Ardiles V, Sanchez Claria R, et al. Associating liver partition and portal vein ligation for staged hepatectomy (ALPPS): Tips and tricks. Journal of Gastrointestinal Surgery. 2013 Apr;**17**(4):814-821. DOI: 10.1007/s11605-012-2092-2

[65] Vennarecci G, Laurenzi A, Levi Sandri GB, et al. The ALPPS procedure for hepatocellular carcinoma. European Journal of Surgical Oncology. 2014 Aug;**40**(8):982-988. DOI: 10.1016/j.ejso.2014.04.002

[66] Zhou Z, Xu M, Lin N, et al. Associating liver partition and portal vein ligation for staged hepatectomy versus conventional two-stage hepatectomy: A systematic review and meta-analysis. World Journal of Surgical Oncology. 2017 Dec 19;**15**(1):227. DOI: 10.1186/s12957-017-1295-0

[67] Schadde E, Schnitzbauer AA, Tschuor C, et al. Systematic review and meta-analysis of feasibility, safety, and efficacy of a novel procedure: Associating liver partition and portal vein ligation for staged hepatectomy. Annals of Surgical Oncology. 2015 Sep;**22**(9):3109-3120. DOI: 10.1245/s10434-014-4213-5

[68] Bertens KA, Hawel J, Lung K, et al. ALPPS: Challenging the concept of unresectability—A systematic review. International Journal of Surgery. 2015 Jan;**13**:280-287. DOI: 10.1016/j.ijsu.2014.12.008

[69] Tanaka K. Modified ALPPS procedures: More safety through less invasive surgery. Langenbeck's Archives of Surgery. 2017 Jun;**402**(4):563-574. DOI: 10.1007/s00423-017-1588-3

[70] Dokmak S, Belghiti J. Which limits to the ALPPS approach? Annals of Surgery. 2012 Sep;**256**:e6; author reply e16-7. DOI: 10.1097/SLA.0b013e318265fd64

[71] Ardiles V, Schadde E, Santibanes E, et al. Commentary on happy marriage or dangerous liaison: ALPPS and the anterior approach. Annals of Surgery. 2014 Aug;**260**(2):e4. DOI: 10.1097/SLA.0000000000000735

[72] Alvarez FA, Ardiles V, de Santibañes M, et al. Associating liver partition and portal vein ligation for staged hepatectomy offers high oncological feasibility with adequate patient safety: A prospective study at a single center. Annals of Surgery. 2015 Apr;**261**(4): 723-732. DOI: 10.1097/SLA.0000000000001046

[73] Hernandez-Alejandro R, Bertens KA, Pineda-Solis K, et al. Can we improve the morbidity and mortality associated with the associating liver partition with portal vein ligation for staged hepatectomy (ALPPS) procedure in the management of colorectal liver metastases? Surgery. 2015 Feb;**157**(2):194-201. DOI: 10.1016/j.surg.2014.08.041

[74] Kudo M, Matsui O, Izumi N, et al. JSH consensus-based clinical practice guidelines for the management of hepatocellular carcinoma: 2014 update by the liver cancer study group of Japan. Liver Cancer. 2014 Oct;**3**(3-4):458-468. DOI: 10.1159/000343875

[75] Colecchia A, Schiumerini R, Cucchetti A, et al. Prognostic factors for hepatocellular carcinoma recurrence. World Journal of Gastroenterology. 2014 May;**20**(20):5935-5950. DOI: 10.3748/wjg.v20.i20.5935

[76] Shim JH, Jun MJ, Han S, et al. Prognostic nomograms for prediction of recurrence and survival after curative liver resection for hepatocellular carcinoma. Annals of Surgery. 2015 May;**261**(5):939-946. DOI: 10.1097/SLA.0000000000000747

[77] Cucchetti A, Zanello M, Cescon M, et al. Improved diagnostic imaging and interventional therapies prolong survival after resection for hepatocellular carcinoma in cirrhosis: The university of bologna experience over 10 years. Annals of Surgical Oncology. 2011 Jun;**18**(6):1630-1637. DOI: 10.1245/s10434-010-1463-8

[78] Tanaka S, Mogushi K, Yasen M, et al. Surgical contribution to recurrence-free survival in patients with macrovascular-invasion-negative hepatocellular carcinoma. Journal of the American College of Surgeons. 2009 Mar;**208**(3):368-374. DOI: 10.1016/j.jamcollsurg.2008.10.031

[79] Makuuchi M, Hasegawa H, Yamazaki S. Ultrasonically guided subsegmentectomy. Surgery, Gynecology & Obstetrics. 1985 Oct;**161**(4):346-350

[80] Yamashita Y, Taketomi A, Itoh S, et al. Longterm favorable results of limited hepatic resections for patients with hepatocellular carcinoma: 20 years of experience. Journal of the American College of Surgeons. 2007 Jul;**205**(1):19-26. DOI: 10.1016/j.jamcollsurg.2007.01.069

[81] Vauthey JN, Lauwers GY, Esnaola NF, et al. Simplified staging for hepatocellular carcinoma. Journal of Clinical Oncology. 2002 Mar;**20**(6):1527-1536. DOI: 10.1200/JCO.2002.20.6.1527

[82] Yamamoto T, Yagi S, Uryuhara K, et al. Clinical factors that affect the outcomes after anatomical versus non-anatomical resection for hepatocellular carcinoma. Surgery Today. 2017 Feb;**47**(2):193-201. DOI: 10.1007/s00595-016-1397-2

[83] Cucchetti A, Cescon M, Ercolani G, et al. A comprehensive meta-regression analysis on outcome of anatomic resection versus nonanatomic resection for hepatocellular carcinoma. Annals of Surgical Oncology. 2012 Nov;**19**(12):3697-3705. DOI: 10.1245/s10434-012-2450-z

[84] Zhou Y, Xu D, Wu L, et al. Meta-analysis of anatomic resection versus non anatomic resection for hepatocellular carcinoma. Langenbeck's Archives of Surgery. 2011 Oct;**396**(7):1109-1117. DOI: 10.1007/s00423-011-0784-9

[85] Bigonzi E, Cucchetti A, Pinna AD. Meta-analysis of anatomic resection versus non-anatomic resection for hepatocellular carcinoma: Are they comparing apples with oranges? Langenbeck's Archives of Surgery. 2012 Jan;**397**(1):141-142. DOI: 10.1007/s00423-011-0816-5

[86] Yune Y, Kim S, Song I, et al. Comparative analysis of intraoperative radiofrequency ablation versus non-anatomical hepatic resection for small hepatocellular carcinoma: Short-term result. Korean Journal of Hepato-Biliary-Pancreatic Surgery. 2015 Nov;**19**(4):173-180. DOI: 10.14701/kjhbps.2015.19.4.173

[87] Huang X, Lu S. A meta-analysis comparing the effect of anatomical resection vs. non-anatomical resection on the long-term outcomes for patients undergoing hepatic resection for hepatocellular carcinoma. HPB: The Official Journal of the International Hepato Pancreato Biliary Association. 2017 Oct;**19**(10):843-849. DOI: 10.1016/j.hpb.2017.06.003

[88] Zhang YM, Wang J. Progress of clinical application of anatomic resection and nonanatomic resection. Zhonghua Wai Ke Za Zhi. 2016 Dec;**54**(12):947-950. DOI: 10.3760/cma.j.issn.0529-5815.2016.12.016

[89] Cucchetti A, Cescon M, Trevisani F, et al. Current concepts in hepatic resection for hepatocellular carcinoma in cirrhotic patients. World Journal of Gastroenterology. 2012 Nov;**18**(44):6398-6408. DOI: 10.3748/wjg.v18.i44.6398

[90] Marubashi S, Gotoh K, Akita H, et al. Anatomical versus non-anatomical resection for hepatocellular carcinoma. The British Journal of Surgery. 2015 Jun;**102**(7):776-784. DOI: 10.1002/bjs.9815

[91] Tanaka K, Shimada H, Matsumoto C, et al. Anatomic versus limited nonanatomic resection for solitary hepatocellular carcinoma. Surgery. 2008 May;**143**(5):607-615. DOI: 10.1016/j.surg.2008.01.006

[92] Chen J, Huang K, Wu J, et al. Survival after anatomic resection versus nonanatomic resection for hepatocellular carcinoma: A meta-analysis. Digestive Diseases and Sciences. 2011 Jun;**56**(6):1626-1633. DOI: 10.1007/s10620-010-1482-0

[93] Nagasue N, Yamanoi A, el-Assal ON, et al. Major compared with limited hepatic resection for hepatocellular carcinoma without underlying cirrhosis: A retrospective analysis. The European Journal of Surgery. 1999 Jul;**165**(7):638-646. DOI: 10.1080/11024159950189681

[94] Minagawa M, Makuuchi M, Takayama T, et al. Selection criteria for repeat hepatectomy in patients with recurrent hepatocellular carcinoma. Annals of Surgery. 2003 Nov;**238**(5):703-710. DOI: 10.1097/01.sla.0000094549.11754.e6

6

Living Donor Liver Transplantation for Hepatocellular Carcinoma

Chih-Che Lin,
Ahmed Mohammed Abdel Aziz Elsarawy and
Chao-Long Chen

Abstract

Hepatocellular carcinoma (HCC) is a major worldwide health problem, which is expected to increase steadily due to different underlying liver diseases. Surgical treatment modalities including liver transplantation (LT) or liver resection (LR) are the mainstay options for early cases of HCC. Liver transplantation for well-selected cases provides excellent survival outcomes comparable to nonmalignant indications of LT. Living donor liver transplantation (LDLT) is an alternative option or even the sole one in the current era of organ shortage problem and in some Asian countries where deceased organ donation is markedly reduced due to various reasons. The adoption of LDLT for HCC treatment elicited many dynamic changes and debates to the dilemma of LT as a whole. In this chapter, we focus on different perspectives of LDLT for HCC, including selection criteria evolution, controversial topics, ethical considerations, operative highlights, and other points.

Keywords: hepatocellular carcinoma, living donor, liver, transplantation, criteria, loco-regional therapy

1. Introduction

Hepatocellular carcinoma (HCC) is the sixth most common cancer and the third leading cause of deaths globally. The selection of treatment modalities for HCC is challenging because it depends not only on the stage of tumor and the patient's performance but also on the underlying liver function. Though the staging systems of HCC are clinically useful for treatment allocation, the decision making should be tailored to each patient, taking into account morphological, pathological, and biological tumor criteria. Liver resection (LR) or liver transplantation (LT) can be adopted as a surgical curative therapy for early disease. Ablative therapies such as radiofrequency ablation (RFA) and percutaneous ethanol injection (PEI) can also cure small tumors. Transarterial chemoembolization (TACE), transarterial radio embolization (TARE), and external beam radiation therapy (EBRT) can control locally advanced disease that is no longer amenable to cure [1].

Liver transplantation has been considered theoretically the best treatment for HCC since it cures the cancer and its underlying pathology. Milan criteria (MC) were the cornerstone for LT because patient selection according to them resulted in survival outcome comparable to LT for nonmalignant cases. More cases of HCC were subjected to LT with the changes made in 2002 in western countries when additional points were added to the model for end-stage liver disease (MELD) scoring system for HCC patients that are within MC. However, the protracted waiting list for deceased donor liver transplantation (DDLT) took many patients beyond MC and hence lost their chance of LT [2].

The incorporation of living donor liver transplantation (LDLT) into the treatment roadmaps of HCC not only gave a new horizon to more patients, but also elicited many dynamic scientific debates and opened different perspectives for the field of LT in general and the treatment of HCC in particular. Thanks to the extensive research and experience of many groups working on LDLT, especially the Asian transplantation groups, most LT centers now are achieving excellent results.

Specifically to the treatment of HCC, LDLT has several major advantages including: avoidance of prolonged waiting times, allowing elective timing of transplantation under best circumstances both for the patient and the tumor burden, not consuming the public donor pool that may reduce the chance of LT for nonmalignant cases awaiting transplant, and providing organ replacement therapy in parts of the world where brain death and deceased donation are less commonly accepted [3].

In addition to the conventional hepatitis virus-related HCC, a steadily increasing burden of HCC will be witnessed with the emergence of alcohol-related cirrhosis and nonalcoholic steatohepatitis (NASH) as potential major causes of HCC, adding more burden to the transplantation demands and worsening the worldwide problem of organ shortage. It has been recognized that fine-tuning and timing of liver transplantation for HCC are only possible with live organ donation. For these reasons, the need for implementation and optimization of LDLT program will continue in the near future [4–6].

In the following sections, we will discuss basic concepts, criteria evolution, ethical considerations, and controversial topics regarding LDLT for HCC treatment, some of them are commonplace among LDLT and DDLT. The technical details of the procedure of LDLT in general are beyond the scope of this chapter. However, surgical details that are related to the oncologic outcome of the patients with HCC are highlighted.

2. Current practice of LDLT for HCC

HCC represents more than 90% of primary liver cancers and It has a well-remarked geographic distribution. Around 85% of cases occur in East Asia, sub-Saharan Africa, and Melanesia. The great burden of HCC is most prevalent among the less developed world. In developed regions, the incidence is low, except for Southern Europe where the incidence is significantly higher [7, 8].

By and large, LDLT has emerged as an alternative to DDLT and it is the only option for patients with HCC in many Asian countries, where the problem of organ shortage is commonly faced. It also provides a suitable option for patients exceeding the MC in western countries such as the United States and Europe, and in the absence of legislative regulations and setup for DDLT in some developing countries especially in the Middle East and North Africa [9–11].

At the beginning of this century, it was estimated that LDLT would represent a significant proportion of the patients transplanted with HCC. Unfortunately, the risks of death and major complications for the healthy donors at the early experience (0.3 and 2%, respectively) reduced its practice on a wide scale. With the cumulative experiences over the past two decades, LDLT is now practiced smoothly in centers of excellence with experience of hepatobiliary surgery and transplantation medicine [7, 12].

2.1. Western experience

Since 2002, HCC patients who are within Milan criteria gain additional points under the MELD organ allocation policy. This resulted in shorter waiting time for HCC patients in many regions of the United States, obviating the need for LDLT. In some regions, however, longer waiting times with higher dropout rates support the use of LDLT for cases of HCC within the Milan criteria and in candidates who do not meet criteria for waiting list priority [13].

The situation of LDLT within the western experience can be configured from the 2012 release of European Association of Study of the Liver (EASL) guidelines, that mentioned "Living donor liver transplantation is an alternative option in patients with a waiting list exceeding 6–7 months, and offers a suitable setting to explore extended indications within research programs" [7].

In the United States, approximately 7000 new patients with HCC are put on the waiting list for LT every year, 10–15% of whom die during the waiting period. In Europe and the United States, the dropout rate at various centers ranges between 15 and 35%. From this perspective, LDLT offer a survival advantage to a significant proportion of HCC patients in the western world [14].

2.2. Eastern experience

The liver transplantation setup in Asia differs from that in the West, in the fact that no priority is given to HCC patients. This setup is formulated to avoid the inevitable shift of most of the deceased grafts to the persistently increasing HCC cases on the expense of nonmalignant cases waiting LT. The resultant wait-list lead Asian centers to practice various approaches to cover the needs, including bridging treatment for HCC, salvage transplantation after prior hepatectomy and LDLT for HCC. Shortage of donors in Asian countries is attributed to many factors including cultural and religious beliefs [10, 15].

3. Basic concepts

3.1. Philosophy

The most prominent advantage of LDLT for HCC treatment is the reduction of waiting time on the list for all cases including other etiologies of liver failure with nearly no effect on public donor pool. Living donor liver grafts are dedicated gifts to the recipients and are generally of good quality taking into account that most of living donors are healthy young individuals [15, 16].

The concept of "gifting" allowed LDLT for HCC patients who are beyond MC or any other proposed criteria and opened the door for liberal expansion. This concept is not accepted in the wait list of DDLT in which the procedure is conditioned to the "within criteria" cases only. The concept of "gifting" must not be taken for granted in the case of LDLT. Since the risk of a living donor is taken, selection criteria must be adopted for HCC patients with optimization of the pretransplantation conditions to ensure a high survival outcome. In other words, the readily available willing donor does not justify the ultramajor procedure of transplantation in the absence of a survival benefit for the recipient. In addition, donor safety remains the other pillar of a sound decision of LDLT [17].

3.2. Indications

LDLT is indicated in HCC patients, who are within accepted universal or regional criteria for transplantation. In view of organ scarcity, the indications can be described currently to be result-oriented in terms of overall and recurrence-free survival. Consequently, there is marked variation between different regions and institutions for applied indications. In essence, cases fitting Milan criteria are indicated for LDLT if waiting list would be >7 months or if there is a willing available donor. Milan criteria form the solid base of morphological indications for HCC. As discussed later, LDLT has allowed transplantation for patients who are outside Milan criteria according to the dynamically changing criteria in different institutions [18, 19].

3.3. Contraindications

Likewise, there is heterogeneity in the contraindications between different regions according to criteria limits for patient selection. However, there is a body of evidence that LDLT is absolutely contraindicated in the following conditions: cases of HCC that show major vascular invasion as evidenced by pretransplant imaging, the presence of extrahepatic metastases including suspicious porta hepatis nodal disease and cases with ruptured HCC. Absolute contraindications of LDLT in nonmalignant cases hold true for HCC and include cases with uncontrolled systemic infection or lethal uncontrolled medical comorbidities [20].

4. Terminology

With the implementation of LDLT programs and better understanding of the clinical course and biological nature of HCC, various clinical settings have emerged. In addition, the current progress of the interventional anticancer therapies enforced the armamentarium of the HCC management for all clinical scenarios. The following are different settings rather than different types of LDLT.

4.1. Primary LDLT

It is the procedure of LDLT performed upfront for the treatment of the cancer and underlying primary liver disease. In this setting, no previous liver resection is performed but initial ablative loco-regional therapies like RFA or PEI may have been performed. It is carried out for nonresectable HCC cases fitting the standard Milan criteria, UCSF criteria or other established and justified criteria for individual institutions. According to Barcelona Clinic Liver Cancer (BCLC) guidelines, primary LDLT is conducted for early cases of HCC with poor liver functions that cannot tolerate initial resection or ablation [7].

4.2. Salvage LDLT

In this setting, LT is performed when there is tumor recurrence or deterioration of liver functions after initial hepatectomy. The integral point in salvage LDLT is that it is performed aiming at a similar outcome to nonrecurrent cases. The pretransplant setting in the case of salvage LT after previous hepatectomy differs from that of primary LT in the availability of tissue pathology, so that almost all factors that determine tumor's behavior (grade, the presence or absence of microvascular invasion, the grade of necrosis in response to loco-regional therapy) are determined beforehand. That is why the predictive power of outcome of salvage LT should be more precise. Very importantly, we should consider that patients who have "within criteria" recurrence after hepatectomy, and hence amenable to salvage LT, are not more than 25% in some series. This means that nearly 70% of cases may miss the chance of a curative LT at all. The transplantability at the time of recurrence has been found to be an important variable determining the final outcome [21]. Noteworthy that when salvage LT is considered due to transplantable recurrence, the recurrence pattern should be evaluated before embarking into LT even if the liver functions and tumor burden are amenable to LT. Intrahepatic recurrent tumors after hepatectomy originates from either primary tumor metastases or de novo tumor foci. The interval and histopathological analysis of hepatectomy specimens give a clue to the pattern of recurrence. Tumors recurring in the first 12 months are most likely tumor metastases within the liver, while those arising after 12 months represent newly developed tumor foci. At histopathological analysis of hepatectomy, the presence of satellite nodules and portal vein invasion herald tumor metastases and early recurrence. The transplantation team should not rush to salvage LDLT except after considering the biological aggressiveness of the recurrent tumor and the likelihood of re-recurrence into the implanted neo-liver [22].

4.3. Sequential LDLT and preemptive LDLT

They are new categories with no consensus, performed in some centers within institutional protocols. In preemptive LDLT, cases that underwent initial hepatectomy and showed adverse histopathological criteria like microvascular invasion or satellite tumor nodules are prepared for LDLT without unnecessary waiting for the inevitable expected recurrence [21, 23, 24].

In sequential LDLT, pretransplant loco-regional therapy (LRT) is administered aiming at complete pathological necrosis of the index tumor before LDLT for cases within accepted criteria. Moreover, LDLT is performed after a scheduled short interval due to donor availability. The exact duration of the interval is not yet determined. Some centers perform LDLT after 3 months from the time of pretransplant therapy. This concept developed from the cumulative experience of histopathological assessment of explanted livers and the impact of pathological necrosis on post LT outcomes. HCC patients who achieve pathological necrosis ≥60% have significantly better overall survival and recurrence-free survival [25].

> *The employment of salvage LDLT is sometimes controversial. Some transplant surgeons, in view of certain radiological, pathological and biological hallmarks, don't prefer to wait for the inevitable recurrence or deterioration of patient or liver conditions to occur (preemptive LDLT). Some argue that the readily available donor associated with vigilant surveillance can always tailor the transplantation in the right time for the best outcome (salvage LDLT).*

5. Evolution of selection criteria

Over the previous two decades, criteria of LT had been expanded and modified from morphological and nonmorphological perspectives. Nevertheless, Milan criteria (MC) keep their place as the gold standard for LT. The long-term outcome and prognostic impact of LT within MC had been reproducibly studied with consistent excellent results [19, 26].

5.1. Why the criteria for LDLT had been expanded?

The MC advocated by Mazzaferro et al. [27] in 1996 are considered the base upon which several centers around the world validated their experiences in liver transplantation. These first clear-cut criteria were published in the *New England journal of medicine* as a practice changing and ground breaking progress in HCC treatment. That is because MC provided posttransplant survival rates of 75–95% at 2 years and 70–80% at 5 years in several studies. Indeed, a meta-analysis of published data has confirmed the survival advantage of MC and its association with a low risk of selecting patients with aggressive tumors [19, 27–29].

However, Milan criteria have been expanded and modified steadily for the following reasons:

1. They were considered too restrictive and many reports showed similar outcomes for cases beyond Milan [13, 30].

2. The growing evidence of the clear contribution of nonmorphological tumor characteristics to the outcome of patients after transplantation. So, the static "morphological" Milan criteria were expanded and modified. The other pathological and biological tumor criteria include: micro-vascular invasion, alpha-feto protein (AFP) level, deoxy-gamma carboxy prothrombin (dGCP) level and tumor avidity on PET scan [31–35].

3. The observation of two incorrectly estimated groups: an underestimated group that had been transplanted within MC but showed worse outcome and an overestimated group that was beyond MC and had comparable outcome after LDLT [35, 36].

5.2. Selection criteria according to different centers of excellence (Table 1) [27, 37–45]

Selection criteria of liver transplantation in different series and centers of excellence			
Criteria	**Parameters**	**Type of parameters**	**Over-all survival**
Milan	Solitary tumor ≤ 5 cm[T1], up to 3 tumors non >3 cm, no macrovascular invasion	Morphological only	85% (4-year)
UCSF	Solitary HCC ≤ 6.5 cm, or ≤ 3 nodules with the largest lesion ≤ 4.5 cm and a total tumor diameter ≤ 8 cm	Morphological only	75% (5-year)
Modified Milan (Up to 7)	Tumor number + size of the largest tumor (cm) ≤ 7	Morphological only	71% (5-year)
Toronto	Any tumor size or number, if pretransplant tumor biopsy showed no poor differentiation, no major vascular invasion, no extrahepatic disease	Morphological-pathological	72% (5-year)
Kyoto University	≤ 10 tumors, all ≤ 5 cm and the serum level of des. Gama carboxy prothrombin (d.GCP) ≤ 400 mIU/ml	Morphological-biological	87% (5-year)
Kyushu University	HCC ≤ 5 cm and a serum d.GCP ≤ 300 mIU/ml. It had been refined by adding neutrophil to lymphocyte ratio (NLR) >4	Morphological-biological	83% (5-year)
Tokyo University	5-5 rule: HCC not larger than 5 cm and no more than 5 nodules	Morphological only	75% (5-year)
Asan Medical Center	HCC not larger than 5 cm, 6 or fewer nodules without gross vascular invasion	Morphological only	82% (5-year)
Hangzhou	HCC ≥ 8 cm if serum alpha-fetoprotein level ≤ 400 ng/ml and only grade I or II	Morphological, biological, and pathological	72.% (5-year)

Table 1. Different selection criteria for liver transplantation adopted in most of transplantation in the world. Note that the main western criteria (Milan, UCSF, UP to 7) depend largely on morphology. Eastern-based criteria (Kyoto-Kyushu-Hangzhou) had modified by incorporating biological behavior of the tumors. The Toronto criteria are unique in its sole dependence on pretransplant biopsy.

Milan criteria were based on preoperative imaging and validated in many institutions all over the world [27]. In 2001, Yao et al. in the University of California San Francisco (UCSF) expanded the morphological criteria based on pathological assessment of explanted livers and then they prospectively validate their criteria based on pretransplant imaging in 2007 [37, 46]. Though this set of criteria is applied successfully in many regions, it has not been applied on a wide scale because they allow transplantation for large HCCs (6.5 cm, representing a tumor volume of 144 cm^3), which had been associated with worse outcomes in some studies. UCSF criteria (like Milan criteria) also exclude all patients with more than three lesions, some of whom may have the same outcome as those within criteria [47]. The 3- and 5-year survival rates after LDLT based on the UCSF criteria range between 78–96% and 66–90%, respectively, in different centers [28]. This wide variation of survival outcomes may also be attributed to variations of the surgical outcome and early mortality.

It should be emphasized that there are no consensus criteria for LDLT allocation. Each individual institution adopts one of the current criteria, tailoring treatment to their unique patient and general circumstances. Most of centers with high experience in LDLT for HCC currently focus on modification rather than numerical expansion of the number and size of tumors. The incorporation of biological factors (tumor markers, inflammatory markers) or available pathological factors from previous hepatectomy help select best candidates and hence predict the outcome and protect against recurrence [29, 35, 48].

6. Preoperative evaluation

Liver transplantation under optimal circumstances is a clear benefit of LDLT. The procedure can be carried out in a timely fashion after exhaustive assessment of tumor burden by different imaging modalities and biological markers. The tumor burden can then be manipulated by pretransplant therapies using the different loco-regional treatment options. Preoperative evaluation of the donor is not much different from the nonmalignant cases of LDLT except for some additional ethical perspectives as discussed previously. For the recipient, the details of preoperative assessment are beyond the scope of this chapter. However, we consider some important points in the pretransplant setting.

6.1. Imaging

Preoperative imaging of the recipient aims at assessment of tumor burden and suitable metastatic workup, for occult HCC or other cancer types. Dynamic CT or MRI with arterial enhancement is the standard of care according to high level of evidence. Extrahepatic staging should include CT chest and CT or MRI of abdomen and pelvis [12, 23].

The discrepancy between preoperative imaging and real tumor burden in explanted livers had been investigated in many centers. The state-of-the-art imaging modalities are not 100% accurate. CTA and MRI were both accurate to determine whether patients fit within the Milan or UCSF criteria, but CTA was slightly better than MRI to evaluate tumor number and size [49]. In the current era of pretransplant invasive therapies, the liver background became more confusing due to the presence of regenerative nodules, necrotized tumors, and other small tumors [35].

The incidental finding of pulmonary nodule(s) on pretransplant CT warrants appropriate evaluation. Many studies had determined a cutoff point to the size of pulmonary lesion at 5 mm. A lesion < 5 mm is less likely to be malignant and if remained stable or showed regression over a period of 3–6 months, liver transplantation is performed. For a lesion > 5 mm, a biopsy is needed to rule out malignant nature that contraindicates transplantation. If this lesion was the same in repeated images over previous 2 years, the possibility of infection is most likely and management is done accordingly. Video-assisted thoracic surgery (VATS) is perfectly employed for an excision biopsy of these small pulmonary nodules [50].

6.2. Alpha-feto protein (AFP)

This biological tumor marker plays important role in the assessment of tumor burden and aggressiveness although many other markers have been used in clinical practice over the past two decades. The AFP value has its clinical significance either in the preoperative or the posttransplant settings. In addition, the dynamic changes to its value in relation to downstaging therapy had been explored. An important question in the preoperative setting is its role as an exclusion tool, either alone or in combination of other radiological, biological, or pathological markers.

Some studies check the cutoff level above which patients should not undergo LT. At an AFP level >1000 ng/ml, approximately 5% of patients would be excluded from LT with 20% reduction in the rate of HCC recurrence. If a lower cut-off level is applied, this would result in a greater reduction in the recurrence rate but at the expense of excluding many more patients from LT who might not have tumor recurrence and would have benefited from LT. Also, patients who had decline of an initial AFP level >1000 ng/ml after loco-regional therapy had a more favorable prognosis after LT. Alpha feto-protein level <1000 has thus been combined to the UCSF criteria for patient selection in some centers [51].

More recently, a prospective multicenter study has explored the use of a combination of total tumor volume (TTV) ≤ 115 cm^3 and AFP ≤ 400 ng/ml as an exclusion tool from LT in centers with a median waiting time of 8 months. This study took an advantage from a previous observation of the inferior survival outcome of patients who are within MC but have the AFP level ≥400 ng/ml. In this study, patients who were beyond MC but within TTV/AFP had survival outcome similar to cases within MC [29].

Many other biomarkers can be evaluated in the pretransplant setting to predict the posttransplant outcome. A recent study in our center showed that repeated measurement of serum levels of novel biomarkers including fibroblast growth factor-2 (FGF-2), survivin, Ki67, endostatin, and vascular endothelial growth factor (VEGF), before and after LDLT for HCC, could predict HCC recurrence [52].

6.3. Fludro-deoxy glucose-positron emission tomography (FDG-PET) scan

Pretransplant 18F-FDG uptake on PET scan in liver transplant candidates with HCC is a useful additional parameter for the evaluation of tumor biology. Positive preoperative PET scans are significantly associated with an increased risk of posttransplant HCC recurrence and inferior outcome, an observation that relates a positive PET status with the presence of microvascular invasion in explant tumor pathology [31]. In a recent Korean study, the combination of the positive FDG-PET study and AFP level >200 ng/ml could predict tumor recurrence more precisely after LDLT than Milan criteria [35]. More recently, a retrospective study at our center has showed that the combination of UCSF criteria with the FDG-PET status can predict tumor recurrence after LDLT and that tumor recurrence is earlier in cases with positive FDG-PET results. On the basis of the maximal standardized uptake value (SUVmax), high-risk group cases (positive study with $SUV_{max} \geq 5$) had worse recurrence-free survival compared with low-risk cases (positive study with $SUV_{max} < 5$) [53].

6.4. Donor characteristics

In addition to the previously discussed controversy of impact of donor type (living or deceased) on HCC recurrence, other donor factors have been studied. A recent review of the American Scientific Registry of Transplant Recipients (SRTR) that involved 9724 patients revealed that the following donor factors were independently associated with high risk of HCC recurrence after transplantation: high BMI, history of DM, and severe graft steatosis. All the previous factors are evident at the time of organ allocation and must be considered before transplantation [54].

7. Loco-regional therapy (LRT)

The pretransplant therapies are implemented heavily for HCC, being an essential component of HCC treatment algorithms in most of treatment guidelines. Earlier in the treatment of HCC roadmaps, they were considered "bridging" tools to keep the patient chances of LT during the waiting time. Currently, a realized value of LRT is their ability to probe the tumor's internal milieu, acting as a selecting tool based on the degree of tumor's response as an indicator of its aggressiveness. So, adopting such therapies gives the time to observe the tumor's behavior before the ultramajor costly step of liver transplantation [55]. Bypassing such an observation period in the setting of multifocal or locally advanced tumor risks transplanting patients with systemic disease.

7.1. HCC downstaging before liver transplantation

The difference between downstaging and neoadjuvant therapies is that in the former the tumor status is beyond the proposed criteria for transplantation and LRT is administered to reduce the tumor burden and to render the case fit for transplantation. In neoadjuvant therapy, the patient is already within criteria but treatment is given to prevent tumor progression to the "beyond criteria" state while waiting for the donor and to induce tumor necrosis aiming at better long-term outcome [56].

In different series from Asian centers, more than 30% of patients who were beyond Milan/ UCSF criteria were effectively downstaged to the "within criteria" state with a 5-year survival rate similar to the initially fit cases [57, 58]. A meta-analysis explored the effect of downstaging to Milan criteria, and the success rate exceeded 40%. However, the recurrence rate was as high as 16% [59].

TACE and RFA are the main tools of downstaging. TACE mediates its effect by inducing complete pathological necrosis with response rates ranging between 27 and 57%. RFA is used For accessible lesions to induce coagulative necrosis, either alone or in combination with liver resection [60]. In LDLT, timing of transplantation after a period of waiting from the time of LDLT is possible. Most centers wait for a period of 3–6 months to evaluate tumor progression as an indicator of aggressiveness before embarking into LDLT.

Though widely applicable in most HCC guidelines, there are no unified criteria either for selecting cases for downstaging or for determining them as good responders and hence listing them for LT. This fact highlights the wide variation of transplantation criteria among different regions and centers. As a rule of thumb, the criteria to enter a downstaging program should include patients who have well-defined and acceptable chances of good outcomes after transplantation if the downstaging goal is achieved [56]. In our center, not only we apply downstaging for cases beyond UCSF criteria, but also we consider cases with high AFP or high FDG uptake on PET scan for downstaging. In our early experience, patients were downstaged to fit Milan criteria. Our initial results of 35 patients were encouraging with a 5-year survival rate of 90% and those patients are still disease-free up to date, after follow-up of 10 years. Since July 2006, our criteria were extended to UCSF criteria. In our experience of 161 HCC patients, 51 (31.6%) were successfully downstaged to fit the UCSF criteria. The overall 1- and 5-year survival rates for downstaged cases were 94.1 and 92.7%, respectively. The recurrence rate was 9.2%. The survival rates were similar for different pretransplantation downstaging procedures [57].

8. Operative/surgical highlights

The first successful case of liver transplantation in Asia was performed by Chen in 1984 in Chang Gung Memorial Hospital, Taiwan. From the cumulative experience at our center, we would like to emphasize that a sound surgical procedure is mandatory for the best outcome. It has been postulated that the experience of the transplant team is an important factor that independently affects the outcome though the learning curve of liver transplant can be steep and painful in some centers launching an LDLT program. In essence, we prefer not to correct recipient coagulopathy before surgery, because many studies showed no value of preoperative correction. Donor hepatectomy should be accomplished with minimal blood loss, obviating the need for blood transfusion. The routine use of microsurgical procedure is performed in our center for arterial anastomosis as well as biliary reconstruction. Surgical outcome largely affects survival and hence final outcome. Early postoperative vascular complications are the main reasons of graft loss and in-hospital mortality and must be managed vigorously [49, 61–64].

8.1. Timing of donor and recipient surgeries

In nonmalignant cases of LDLT, the recipient surgery is usually begun after the donor surgery commenced till confirmation of feasible biliary anatomy by cholangiography. In the early experience of LDLT for HCC, some surgeons preferred to confirm resectability of the liver containing cancer and the absence of lymph node metastases through a smaller incision before proceeding with graft harvesting from the donor [65, 66]. However, the current imaging modalities surpass this step and allow precise decision in advance. Most experienced centers largely depend on high quality CT or MRI images and the timing is adopted like nonmalignant cases of end-stage liver failure.

8.2. Safety margin

A proper safety margin is an integral part of the sound oncological surgical procedure. Some peripheral lesions may be found in very close proximity to or even adherent to parietal peritoneum, diaphragm, omentum, or less commonly small or large bowl loops. A previous hepatectomy increases the adhesions with the aforementioned structures. It is thus convenient to take a proper safety margin through excision of parts of peritoneum and diaphragmatic muscle. Very infrequently, small or large bowl resection and anastomosis may be required. Re-exploration for additional safety margin after final pathological assessment is a very hazardous procedure for such a frail patient, but may be warranted in some conditions according to institutional experience.

8.3. Management of nodal disease

In a recent review from the International Registry of Hepatic Tumors in Liver Transplantation, the incidence of lymph node metastases in cirrhotic patients with HCC undergoing LT was 6.5%. Hilar lymph node (LN) involvement in cases of HCC constitutes a contraindication for liver transplantation because of dismal prognosis. Recent imaging techniques are able to identify enlarged suspicious lymph nodes in the pretransplant setting. However, the frequent presence of LN enlargement due to chronic inflammation in cases of hepatitis C-induced cirrhosis may make the diagnosis less clear. It is convenient to perform frozen section evaluation for suspicious nodes unexpectedly encountered during recipient operation. The decision to proceed or abort the procedure in the case of inconclusive frozen section analysis or the unavailability of frozen section depends largely on the experience of the transplant team. According to a meta-analysis study, systematic hilar lymphadenectomy during LT for HCC should routinely be undertaken, especially in the context of coexisting hepatitis C or secondary biliary cirrhosis. Some centers recommend harvesting of at least four lymph nodes at the time of liver transplantation but the debate remains open with no available consensus on the extent of such lymphadenectomy [67, 68].

8.4. The middle hepatic vein (MHV)

The MHV is a controversial topic within the LDLT procedure in general. In the case of LDLT for HCC, this issue should be taken more seriously. It has been postulated that the resultant venous congestion from improper management of tributaries of MHV is a possible factor favoring tumor recurrence. Congestion of the graft leads to impediment of portal inflow with subsequent ischemia in the congested region and compensatory accelerated regeneration of the well-drained areas of the graft. Consequently, the cellular changes in response to both processes may enhance tumor recurrence [69].

8.5. IVC management (see Figure 1)

The observation of HCC recurrence after LDLT in the hepatic vena-caval wall has shed light on the possibility of microvascular infiltration with consequent local and distant recurrence. This finding triggered the concept of aggressive en-bloc caval resection and reconstruction during LDLT. This step is also justified by another two facts: first, it prevents a positive margin of latent cancer in caval branches; second, the least amount of manipulation of the native liver with HCC should be employed to avoid and control distant metastasis after LDLT [70].

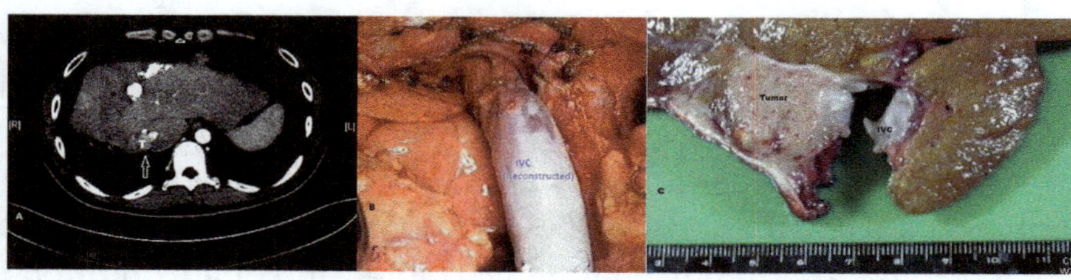

Figure 1. A case of HCC subjected to LDLT. The tumor (T) was intimately adherent to the IVC wall without apparent invasion in pretransplant CT angiography (A; arrow). During the recipient operation, the liver was explanted en-bloc with the IVC segment adjacent to the tumor. Reconstruction of the IVC was carried out using cryo-preserved iliac v. graft (B). Final gross pathology shows no intraluminal transgression by the tumor (C).

8.6. Complications of LDLT of the manipulated liver, i.e., after loco-regional therapy

Extensive adhesions are commonly encountered following previous liver resection in case of salvage liver transplantation. Tough vascular adhesions usually form between a large hepatectomy site and small intestine and omentum. Sharp dissection and meticulous hemostatic control would reduce the difficulty of subsequent transplantation and decrease the incidence of postoperative complications [71]. Laparoscopic liver resection is now performed on a wide scale in many centers. One of the most prominent advantages of laparoscopic initial hepatectomy is the marked reduction of adhesions as evidenced in subsequent liver transplantation in many series thus facilitating the procedure [72].

Intimal dissection (ID) of the recipient hepatic artery has emerged as a grave complication that may occur after TAE or TACE. Intimal dissection if not discovered and managed properly may end up in graft loss. Gentle handling of HA is mandatory during LT to prevent aggravation or precipitation of dissection in the fragile HA. Once this complication is suspected intraoperatively, microscopic assessment is needed for proper decision. Either trimming and discarding the dissected segment or discarding the whole native HA and reconstruction may be considered, hence the importance of microvascular expertise in the LDLT team [73].

9. Ethical considerations

Two main ethical pillars of the decision of LDLT for management of HCC must be considered. First, donor safety and optimizing his or her care is no different in LDLT for HCC compared to that for nonmalignant cases of liver failure. Second, the procedure must provide an acceptable outcome to the recipient compared to DDLT. From the ethical point of view, LDLT is justified, as long as the proposed regional criteria are strictly followed, being MC or any scientifically justified institutional expanded or modified criteria. Noteworthy that there is no consensus about what risk to the living donor might be considered acceptable for a given risk of recurrence [13, 74].

With increased awareness and patient education facilities, the ethical responsibilities regarding patient counseling became more complex. It is not all about the perioperative complications. Recently, ethical considerations took a very different perspective, that is offering LDLT to high-risk patients and excluding others who are low-risk patients based on imaging criteria only. As mentioned earlier, two wrongly estimated groups are revealed: cases within criteria that have aggressive biological behavior and cases beyond criteria with indolent tumors. Two ethical situations subsequently ensued; the first is the risk of recurrence of biologically aggressive tumors even when strict criteria are adhered to, i.e., the underestimated group. The second is about the loss of chance of LT in the other group. The transplantation team should never rush to transplantation in response to family pressure and readily available donor without proper discussion of all that issues [35].

When the partial graft fails for any reason, a special—but very uncommon—ethical situation is encountered because normally it requires an urgent deceased donor retransplantation. It has been established that if LDLT was used in a situation where a deceased donor is contraindicated, such as exceeding the accepted criteria for deceased donation, the patient should not be retransplanted because he/she would not be transplanted initially if on wait-list for DDLT [12, 66]. Finding another living donor must be balanced against the expected outcome of the procedure. There are no clear-cut decisions to such situations and the institutional experience would tailor the right decision.

When talking about salvage LDLT, the patient may be reluctant to undergo the procedure even with the availability of a donor. Some patients may argue that they want to be alive more but do not want to harm anyone. In these circumstances, the transplant team should alert the patient about how long can he/she delay the procedure without a considerable risk of tumor progression or being transferred into the nontransplantable state. A study from Japan revealed that patients who receive downstaging therapy can wait no more than 12 months. However, the exact duration is not determined and the management plan should be tailored to each case [75].

10. Controversial topics

The increasing number of HCC cases, the parallel progress in expertise of LDLT, and the dynamic changes in the selection criteria all enriched the liver transplantation community with many important topics and debates. A lot of studies were carried out to find answers or to reach a consensus in many of these topics. However, the retrospective nature of most studies, the different reporting methodologies and small sample sizes are all flaws that hampered the appearance of high level of evidence to address all topics.

10.1. What is the best treatment option of early HCC? Resection or liver transplantation? Primary or salvage approach?

- The surgical decision can be either LR or LT in 20–25% of cases of HCC amenable for surgery. Liver transplantation is hypothetically superior to resection because it removes the cancer and its underlying pathology. For many patients it is not possible to perform resection because of the tumor size, anatomical location of the tumor, or poor liver function, and liver transplantation is the only surgical option [76]. However, even in many Asian centers which perform LDLT on regular basis, up to 50% of early HCC cases may not have suitable donors or be concerned about the risk to donor. So, many Asian centers adopt the policy of offering LR to patients with resectable tumors with compensated cirrhosis and deferring LT to the salvage setting [13, 23, 77, 78].
- The controversy regarding LR or LT in HCC patients is largely confined to early cases with a well-preserved liver function. There are no randomized controlled trials that addressed this issue through a head-to-head comparison. Given that organ shortage for LT is a persistent challenge worldwide and also the presence of underserved areas with deficient LT programs, the identification of cases that would obtain similar survival outcomes when either submitted to LR or to LT is of paramount importance [79, 80].
- The strategy of offering LR for simultaneously resectable and transplantable cases was based on the observation from many studies that 20–30% of HCC cases that had LR may not witness recurrence for >5 years. In addition, with vigilant surveillance programs, most of recurrent cases would fit into the MC and can be transplanted under optimal conditions due to the availability of the living donor, with no negative impact on the outcome. This obviates many patients the downside of early immunosuppression [5]. In addition, the mortality rate of LR at an experienced center is less than 2–5%, and overall survival rates were comparable to primary LT [4, 24].
- **The Barcelona Clinic Liver Cancer approach**: Resection is the treatment of choice in patients with very early stage HCC and normal bilirubin levels as well as the absence of portal hypertension. If the liver functions are impaired, LT is recommended as a primary treatment approach. In the early stage of HCC, it has been found that the 10-year outcome after LT is superior to LR in view of the latter's well-known higher recurrence risk. So, the choice of primary LT is recommended. The same approach is adopted by the American Association of Study of Liver Disease (AASLD) guidelines that prefer liver resection for very early cases with the optimal liver profile [7, 78, 81, 82].

- A meta-analysis of studies that involved patients within MC revealed a survival advantage for LT over LR [83]. In a more recent meta-analysis that involved 1572 patients in whom both LR and LT are feasible, the authors did not find any survival advantage of LT compared with LR. They concluded—based on low quality evidence—that LR is preferable to LT in patients who are feasible for both options [84].

- Conclusion: the overall survival advantage of LT is unclear, though recurrence-free survival is definitely better with LT. The main drawback for LT—especially LDLT—is the relatively increased mortality in the early postoperative period. In high volume centers where LDLT is performed at high rates, perioperative mortality is reduced significantly. So, a clear overall survival advantage for LT may be evident [85]. For a definite evidence-based conclusion, a randomized controlled trial comparing LT and LR is needed, a condition that is very difficult due to practical and ethical restrictions. Proper patient selection and optimization of criteria according to the pretransplant setting (primary or secondary) would help make a treatment roadmap.

10.2. Living donor or deceased donor for HCC?

One of the most critical controversies in the transplantation field is the possibility of an increased rate of recurrence of HCC after LDLT compared to DDLT.

Several hypotheses have been postulated to figure out this possibility:

- The fast tract effect: due to the shortened waiting time for LDLT, progression of HCC with aggressive tumor biology might not be recognized during such a short-waiting time. This is in contrary to the situation in DDLT, where the long-waiting time can naturally select cases with indolent behavior.

- The growth factors and cytokines released during rapid regeneration of the partial grafts might contribute to tumor progression and recurrence.

- The extensive dissection and mobilization of the liver might increase the feasibility of tumor dissemination through the hepatic vein and increased potential for leaving residual tumor cells.

- The exaggerated vascular inflow associated with small size grafts elicits vast angiogenesis with subsequent carcinogenic effect.

- The less radical hepatectomy in LDLT with the native IVC left in place may constitute a suboptimal oncologic procedure [15, 55, 86–88].

A multi-center study was carried out on the database of China Liver Transplant Registry (CLTR) to highlight this issue. They explored the data of 6860 patients (6471 (DDLT) and 389 LDLT and concluded that both overall survival and recurrence-free survival were comparable between both approaches [89]. In an international consensus conference of liver transplantation (Zurich 2012), it had been stated that no convincing difference in outcome could be identified according to the type of graft, although a higher risk of recurrence was noted in fast-tracked patients. The experts advised an interval of observation for the biological behavior of the tumor to manifest. A period of 3 months had been suggested [12]. Many other groups reported similar recurrence rates after LDLT and DDLT and also similar long-term outcomes [14, 87].

However, others have found significantly higher rates of tumor recurrence after LDLT compared with DDLT for HCC. The Adult to Adult Living Donor Liver transplantation (A2ALL) study reported a significantly higher 3-year tumor recurrence rate after LDLT [15, 88, 90, 91]. One should consider that many studies that reported better outcome of DDLT than LDLT are conducted in the west and some of them were flawed by small sample sizes and the possibility of selection bias since DDLT was applied mostly on cases within Milan criteria only and those beyond Milan criteria are relegated to LDLT [92].

A systematic review and meta-analysis addressed this question (Is the regenerating liver of LDLT a fertile environment for HCC recurrence?). Though no randomized controlled trials were included, they came to a similar conclusion; disease-free survival (DFS) is worse after LDLT compared with DDLT but there was no difference observed in overall survival (OS). In the same meta-analysis, there was a concern that the follow-up periods in the included studies are probably too brief to detect a major impact on survival resulting from differences in disease recurrence. The same study revealed that the overall survival after LDLT vs. DDLT was better —though not statistically significant—in studies from eastern centers compared with studies from western centers. This may reflect differences between these regions in patient selection or case-volumes effects on surgical outcomes [6]. In conclusion, to date there is no definite evidence supporting higher recurrence after LDLT than DDLT [55, 92].

10.3. Pre-LDLT liver biopsy, can the trend be changed?

Because the risk of tumor seeding may be 2–4% along the needle biopsy tract and thus increasing the risk of metastases, liver biopsy should be considered only when there is uncertainty as to the diagnosis. This might occur, for example, in the presence of an HCC arising in the noncirrhotic liver or contradictory clinical, laboratory, and radiological findings [81]. However, a biopsy has the potential problems of sampling error. For example, different nodules may have different grades within the index tumor. It has also been demonstrated that even in a single-needle biopsy, adjacent tumor cells can be of different degrees of differentiation. Nevertheless, if transplantation is planned for HCC beyond the standard criteria, tumor biopsy appears to be a logical approach if there is suspicion of diagnosis [28].

Dubay et al. [44] have provided their experience in the University of Toronto based solely on a liver biopsy before LT. They have no size or number restriction for LT. They concluded that a protocol using a biopsy to exclude poorly differentiated tumors achieved excellent survival rates (70% at 5 years) [44].

10.4. Can we exclude morphological selection criteria in the coming era?

Morphological criteria of HCC describe the appearance, while biological criteria describe the concealed behavior. Ultimately, the behavior of HCC is the final-deciding factor on patient outcome. As shown earlier, modification of morphological criteria is pursued in many studies with the incorporation of biological factors [13]. In a study from Korea, the recipient selection based on pure biological factors was proposed. The group showed that FDG PET positivity with a cutoff point of maximum systemic uptake value (SUV_{max}) of 1.1 combined with the AFP serum level at 400 ng/ml is able—alone—to predict patient outcome more precise than morphological criteria [35]. More studies are needed to explore nonmorphological selection processes.

11. Conclusions

LDLT is a robust treatment pathway for HCC. Indeed, it may be the only pathway in this era of organ shortage especially in some Asian countries. The employment and dynamic application of selection criteria of LDLT for HCC are the cornerstone to acquire the best outcome. The number and size of the tumor(s) are not the only factors to consider for patient selection but some other factors are also present. Most of transplantation centers are combining biological (AFP-tumor avidity in PET scan) and pathological (pretransplant biopsy) factors of the tumors to the morphological factors aiming at refined patient selection for the optimal outcome. In the current era of personalized medicine, treatment of HCC should be tailored according to each individual patient and tumor criteria. A sound oncological surgical procedure is the core of successful LDLT and has its direct impact on the final outcome.

Author details

Chih-Che Lin[1*], Ahmed Mohammed Abdel Aziz Elsarawy[2] and Chao-Long Chen[1]

*Address all correspondence to: immunologylin@gmail.com

1 Department of general surgery and liver transplant center, Chang Gung Memorial Hospital, Kaohsiung, Taiwan

2 Liver transplant center, Chang Gung Memorial Hospital, Kaohsiung, Taiwan

References

[1] Knox JJ, Cleary SP, Dawson LA. Localized and systemic approaches to treating hepatocellular carcinoma. J Clin Oncol. 2015;33(16):1835–44. Available from: http://jco.ascopubs.org/content/33/16/1835.long

[2] Bruix J, Gores GJ, Mazzaferro V. Hepatocellular carcinoma: clinical frontiers and perspectives. Gut. 2014;844–55.

[3] Sonnenday CJ. Recurrent hepatocellular carcinoma after living donor liver transplantation: a preventable problem or an acceptable risk? Ann Surg Oncol. United States; 2010;17:2262–3.

[4] de Villa VH, Lo C-M, Chen C-L. Ethics and rationale of living-donor liver transplantation in Asia. Transplant. 2003;75(3 Suppl):S2–5. Available from: http://www.ncbi.nlm.nih.gov/pubmed/12589129

[5] Chen C-L, Concejero AM. Liver transplantation for hepatocellular carcinoma in the world: the Taiwan experience. J Hepatobil Pancreat Sci. Japan. 2010;17(5):555–8.

[6] Grant RC, Sandhu L, Dixon PR, Greig PD, Grant DR, McGilvray ID. Living vs. deceased donor liver transplantation for hepatocellular carcinoma: a systematic review and meta-analysis. Clin Transplant. Denmark; 2013;27(1):140–7.

[7] Dufour JF, Greten TF, Raymond E, Roskams T, De T, Ducreux M, et al. EASL–EORTC clinical practice guidelines: management of hepatocellular carcinoma. J Hepatol. 2012;56(4):908–43. Available from: http://linkinghub.elsevier.com/retrieve/pii/S0168827811008737

[8] Torre LA, Bray F, Siegel RL, Ferlay J. Global cancer statistics. CA Cancer J Clin. 2015;65(2):87–108.

[9] Shirabe K, Taketomi A, Morita K, Soejima Y, Uchiyama H, Kayashima H, et al. Comparative evaluation of expanded criteria for patients with hepatocellular carcinoma beyond the Milan criteria undergoing living-related donor liver transplantation. Clin Transplant. Denmark; 2011;25(5):E491–8.

[10] Chen C-L, Kabiling CS, Concejero AM. Why does living donor liver transplantation flourish in Asia? Nat Rev Gastroenterol Hepatol. 2013;10(12):746–51. Available from: http://www.ncbi.nlm.nih.gov/pubmed/24100300

[11] Khalaf H, Marwan I, Al-Sebayel M, El-Meteini M, Hosny A, Abdel-Wahab M, et al. Status of liver transplantation in the Arab world. Transplantation. 2014;97(7):722–4. Available from: http://www.ncbi.nlm.nih.gov/pubmed/24603475

[12] Clavien P-A, Lesurtel M, Bossuyt PMM, Gores GJ, Langer B, Perrier A. Recommendations for liver transplantation for hepatocellular carcinoma: an international consensus conference report. Lancet Oncol. England; 2012;13(1):e11–22.

[13] Mazzaferro V, Chun YS, Poon RTP, Schwartz ME, Yao FY, Marsh JW, et al. Liver transplantation for hepatocellular carcinoma. Ann Surg Oncol. United States; 2008;15(4):1001–7.

[14] Bhangui P, Vibert E, Majno P, Salloum C, Andreani P, Zocrato J, et al. Intention-to-treat analysis of liver transplantation for hepatocellular carcinoma: living versus deceased donor transplantation. Hepatology. United States; 2011;53(5):1570–9.

[15] Ng KK, Lo CM. Liver transplantation in Asia: past, present and future. Ann Acad Med Singapore. Singapore; 2009;38(4):310–22.

[16] Chen C, Cheng Y, Yu C, Ou H, Tsang LL, Huang T, et al. Living donor liver transplantation: the Asian perspective. Transplantat. 2014;97 Suppl 8: S3.

[17] Barr ML, Belghiti J, Villamil FG, Pomfret EA, Sutherland DS, Gruessner RW, et al. A report of the vancouver forum on the care of the live organ donor: lung, liver, pancreas, and intestine data and medical guidelines. Transplantat. 2006;81(10):1373–85. Available from: http://content.wkhealth.com/linkback/openurl?sid=WKPTLP:landingpage&an=00007890-200605270-00004

[18] Nadalin S, Bockhorn M, Malagó M, Valentin-Gamazo C, Frilling A, Broelsch CE. Living donor liver transplantation. HPB (Oxford). 2006;8(1):10–21. Available from: http://www.pubmedcentral.nih.gov/articlerender.fcgi?artid=2131378&tool=pmcentrez&rendertype=abstract

[19] Mazzaferro V, Bhoori S, Sposito C, Bongini M, Langer M, Miceli R, et al. Milan criteria in liver transplantation for hepatocellular carcinoma: an evidence-based analysis of 15 years of experience. Liver Transpl. United States; 2011;17 Suppl 2:S44–57.

[20] Farkas S, Hackl C, Schlitt HJ. Overview of the indications and contraindications for liver transplantation. Cold Spring Harb Perspect Med. United States; 2014;4(5).

[21] Majno PE, Sarasin FP, Mentha G, Hadengue A. Primary liver resection and salvage transplantation or primary liver transplantation in patients with single, small hepatocellular carcinoma and preserved liver function: an outcome-oriented decision analysis. Hepatology. United States; 2000;31(4):899–906.

[22] Lee HS, Choi GH, Joo DJ, Kim MS, Choi JS. The clinical behavior of transplantable recurrent hepatocellular carcinoma after curative resection: implications for salvage liver. Transplantation. 2014;2717–24.

[23] Concejero A, Chen C-L, Wang C-C, Wang S-H, Lin C-C, Liu Y-W, et al. Living donor liver transplantation for hepatocellular carcinoma: a single-center experience in Taiwan. Transplantation. United States; 2008;85(3):398–406.

[24] Cherqui D, Laurent A, Alain. Liver resection for transplantable hepatocellular carcinoma. Ann Surg. 2009;250(5). 738–46.

[25] Chan K-M, Yu M-C, Chou H-S, Wu T-J, Lee C-F, Lee W-C. Significance of tumor necrosis for outcome of patients with hepatocellular carcinoma receiving locoregional therapy prior to liver transplantation. Ann Surg Oncol. United States; 2011;18(9):2638–46.

[26] Yoshizumi T, Harimoto N, Itoh S, Okabe H, Kimura K, Uchiyama H, et al. Living donor liver transplantation for hepatocellular carcinoma within milan criteria in the present era. Anticancer Res. Greece; 2016;36(1):439–45.

[27] Mazzaferro V, Regalia E, Doci R, Andreola S, Pulvirenti A, Bozzetti F, et al. Liver transplantation for the treatment of small hepatocellular carcinomas in patients with cirrhosis. N Engl J Med. United States; 1996;334(11):693–9.

[28] Chan SC, Fan ST. Selection of patients of hepatocellular carcinoma beyond the Milan criteria for liver transplantation. Hepatobiliary Surg Nutr. China (Republic: 1949); 2013;2(2):84–8.

[29] Toso C, Meeberg G, Hernandez-Alejandro R, Dufour J-F, Marotta P, Majno P, et al. Total tumor volume and alpha-fetoprotein for selection of transplant candidates with hepatocellular carcinoma: a prospective validation. Hepatology. United States; 2015;62(1):158–65.

[30] Majno P, Mazzaferro V. Living donor liver transplantation for hepatocellular carcinoma exceeding conventional criteria: questions, answers and demands for a common language. Vol. 12, Liver transplantation: official publication of the American Association for the Study of Liver Diseases and the International Liver Transplantation Society. United States; 2006. p. 896–8.

[31] Kornberg A, Freesmeyer M, Barthel E, Jandt K, Katenkamp K, Steenbeck J, et al. 18F-FDG-uptake of hepatocellular carcinoma on PET predicts microvascular tumor invasion in liver transplant patients. Am J Transplant. Denmark; 2009;9(3):592–600.

[32] Hirakawa M, Yoshimitsu K, Irie H, Tajima T, Nishie A, Asayama Y, et al. Performance of radiological methods in diagnosing hepatocellular carcinoma preoperatively in a recipient of living related liver transplantation: comparison with step section histopathology. Jpn J Radiol. Japan; 2011;29(2):129–37.

[33] Piardi T, Gheza F, Ellero B, Woehl-Jaegle ML, Ntourakis D, Cantu M, et al. Number and Tumor Size Are Not Sufficient Criteria to Select Patients for Liver Transplantation for Hepatocellular Carcinoma. Ann Surg Oncol. 2012;19(6):2020–6.

[34] Na GH, Kim DG, Han JH, Kim EY, Lee SH, Hong TH, et al. Inflammatory markers as selection criteria of hepatocellular carcinoma in living-donor liver transplantation. World J Gastroenterol. United States; 2014;20(21):6594–601.

[35] Hong G, Suh K-S, Suh S-W, Yoo T, Kim H, Park M-S, et al. Alpha-fetoprotein and (18)F-FDG positron emission tomography predict tumor recurrence better than Milan criteria in living donor liver transplantation. J Hepatol. Netherlands; 2016;64(4):852–9.

[36] Ito T, Takada Y, Ueda M, Haga H, Maetani Y, Oike F, et al. Expansion of selection criteria for patients with hepatocellular carcinoma in living donor liver transplantation. Liver Transpl. United States; 2007;13(12):1637–44.

[37] Yao FY, Ferrell L, Bass NM, Watson JJ, Bacchetti P, Venook A, et al. Liver transplantation for hepatocellular carcinoma: expansion of the tumor size limits does not adversely impact survival. Hepatology. United States; 2001;33(6):1394–403.

[38] Lee S-G, Hwang S, Moon D-B, Ahn C-S, Kim K-H, Sung K-B, et al. Expanded indication criteria of living donor liver transplantation for hepatocellular carcinoma at one large-volume center. Liver Transpl. United States; 2008;14(7):935–45.

[39] Zheng S-S, Xu X, Wu J, Chen J, Wang W-L, Zhang M, et al. Liver transplantation for hepatocellular carcinoma: Hangzhou experiences. Transplantation. United States; 2008;85(12):1726–32.

[40] Sugawara Y, Tamura S, Makuuchi M. Living donor liver transplantation for hepatocellular carcinoma: Tokyo University series. Dig Dis. Switzerland; 2007;25(4):310–2.

[41] Mazzaferro V, Llovet JM, Miceli R, Bhoori S, Schiavo M, Mariani L, et al. Predicting survival after liver transplantation in patients with hepatocellular carcinoma beyond the Milan criteria: a retrospective, exploratory analysis. Lancet Oncol. 2009;10(1):35–43. Available from: http://dx.doi.org/10.1016/S1470-2045(08)70284-5

[42] Taketomi A, Sanefuji K, Soejima Y, Yoshizumi T, Uhciyama H, Ikegami T, et al. Impact of des-gamma-carboxy prothrombin and tumor size on the recurrence of hepatocellular carcinoma after living donor liver transplantation. Transplantation. United States; 2009;87(4):531–7.

[43] Takada Y, Uemoto S. Liver transplantation for hepatocellular carcinoma: the Kyoto experience. J Hepatobiliary Pancreat Sci. Japan; 2010;17(5):527–32.

[44] DuBay D, Sandroussi C, Sandhu L, Cleary S, Guba M, Cattral MS, et al. Liver transplantation for advanced hepatocellular carcinoma using poor tumor differentiation on biopsy as an exclusion criterion. Ann Surg. United States; 2011;253(1):166–72.

[45] Yoshizumi T, Ikegami T, Toshima T, Harimoto N, Uchiyama H, Soejima Y, et al. Two-step selection criteria for living donor liver transplantation in patients with hepatocellular carcinoma. Transplant Proc. United States; 2013;45(9):3310–3.

[46] Yao FY, Xiao L, Bass NM, Kerlan R, Ascher NL, Roberts JP. Liver transplantation for hepatocellular carcinoma: validation of the UCSF-expanded criteria based on preoperative imaging. Am J Transplant. 2007;7(11):2587–96.

[47] Toso C, Asthana S, Bigam DL, Shapiro AMJ, Kneteman NM. Reassessing selection criteria prior to liver transplantation for hepatocellular carcinoma utilizing the scientific registry of transplant recipients database. Hepatology. 2009;49(3):832–8.

[48] Yang SH, Suh KS, Lee HW, Cho EH, Cho JY, Cho YB, et al. A revised scoring system utilizing serum alphafetoprotein levels to expand candidates for living donor transplantation in hepatocellular carcinoma. Surgery. 2007;141(5):598–609.

[49] Lu C-H, Chen C-L, Cheng Y-F, Huang T-L, Tsang LL-C, Ou H-Y, et al. Correlation between imaging and pathologic findings in explanted livers of hepatocellular carcinoma cases. Transplant Proc. United States; 2010;42(3):830–3.

[50] Wu Y-J, Lin C-C, Lin Y-H, Wang S-H, Lin T-L, Chen C-L, et al. Incidentally small pulmonary nodule in candidates for living donor liver transplantation. Ann Transplant. Poland; 2015;20:734–40.

[51] Hameed B, Mehta N, Sapisochin G, Roberts JP, Yao FY. Alpha-fetoprotein level> 1000 ng/mL as an exclusion criterion for liver transplantation in patients with hepatocellular carcinoma meeting the milan criteria. Liver Transpl. 2014;20(8):945–51.

[52] Chiu KW, Nakano T, Chen KD, Hsu LW, Lai CY, Huang CY, et al. Repeated-measures implication of hepatocellular carcinoma biomarkers in living donor liver transplantation. PLoS One. 2015;10(5):1–12. Available from: <Go to ISI>://WOS:000354916100020

[53] Hsu C-C, Chen C-L, Wang C-C, Lin C-C, Yong C-C, Wang S-H, et al. Combination of FDG-PET and UCSF criteria for predicting HCC recurrence after living donor liver transplantation. Transplantat. 2016 Sep;100(9):1925–32.

[54] Orci LA, Berney T, Majno PE, Lacotte S, Oldani G, Morel P, et al. Donor characteristics and risk of hepatocellular carcinoma recurrence after liver transplantation. Br J Surg. England; 2015;102(10):1250–7.

[55] Park G-C, Song G-W, Moon D-B, Lee S-G. A review of current status of living donor liver transplantation. Hepatobiliary Surg Nutr. China (Republic: 1949); 2016;5(2):107–17.

[56] Toso C, Mentha G, Kneteman NM, Majno P. The place of downstaging for hepatocellular carcinoma. J Hepatol. 2010;52(6):930–6. Available from: http://dx.doi.org/10.1016/j.jhep.2009.12.032

[57] Yu CY, Ou HY, Huang TL, Chen TY, Tsang LLC, Chen CL, et al. Hepatocellular carcinoma downstaging in liver transplantation. Transplant Proc. 2012;44(2):412–4.

[58] Na GH, Kim EY, Hong TH, You YK, Kim DG. Effects of loco regional treatments before living donor liver transplantation on overall survival and recurrence-free survival in South Korean patients with hepatocellular carcinoma. HPB (Oxford). England; 2016;18(1):98–106.

[59] Parikh ND, Waljee AK, Singal AG. Downstaging hepatocellular carcinoma: a systematic review and pooled analysis. Liver Transplant. 2015;21(9):1142–52. Available from: http://www.ncbi.nlm.nih.gov/pubmed/25981135 [cited 2015 Nov 17].

[60] Xu D-W, Wan P, Xia Q. Liver transplantation for hepatocellular carcinoma beyond the Milan criteria: a review. World J Gastroenterol. United States; 2016;22(12):3325–34.

[61] Majeed TA, Wai CT, Rajekar H, Lee KH, Wong SY, Leong SO, et al. Experience of the transplant team is an important factor for posttransplant survival in patients with hepatocellular carcinoma undergoing living-donor liver transplantation. Transplant Proc. United States; 2008;40(8):2507–9.

[62] Chen C-L, Concejero AM. Early post-operative complications in living donor liver transplantation: prevention, detection and management. HBPD INT. China; 2007;6(4): 345–7.

[63] Chen C-L, Concejero AM, Cheng Y-F. More than a quarter of a century of liver transplantation in Kaohsiung Chang Gung Memorial Hospital. Clin Transpl. United States; 2011;213–21.

[64] Jawan B, Wang C-H, Chen C-L, Huang C-J, Cheng K-W, Wu S-C, et al. Review of anesthesia in liver transplantation. Acta Anaesthesiol Taiwanica. Taiwan LLC; 2014;52(4):185–96. Available from: http://linkinghub.elsevier.com/retrieve/pii/S1875459714001088

[65] Nadalin, S., Bockhorn, M., Malagó, M., Valentin-Gamazo, C., Frilling, A., & Broelsch, C. E. (2006). Living donor liver transplantation. *HPB* :8(1), 10–21. http://doi.org/10.1080/13651820500465626.

[66] Abdeldayem HM, editor. Living Donor Liver Transplantation, Liver Transplantation - Technical Issues and Complications. InTech. 2012. Available from: http://www.intechopen.com/books/liver-transplantation-technical-issues-and-complications/living-donor-livertransplantation

[67] Ercolani G, Grazi GL, Ravaioli M, Grigioni WF, Cescon M, Gardini A, et al. The role of lymphadenectomy for liver tumors. Ann Surg. 2004;239(2):202–9.

[68] Sotiropoulos GC, Malago M, Molmenti EP, Losch C, Lang H, Frilling A, et al. Hilar lymph nodes sampling at the time of liver transplantation for hepatocellular carcinoma: to do or not to do? Meta-analysis to determine the impact of hilar lymph nodes metastases on tumor recurrence and survival in patients with hepatocellular carcin. Transpl Int. 2007;20(2):141–6. Available from: http://www.ncbi.nlm.nih.gov/pubmed/17239022\nhttp://onlinelibrary.wiley.com/doi/10.1111/j.1432-2277.2006.00412.x/abstract?systemMessage=Wiley+Online+Library+will+be+disrupted+on+7+July+from+10:00-12:00+BST+(05:00-07:00+EDT)+for+essential+maintenance

[69] Suh S-W, Lee J-M, You T, Choi YR, Yi N-J, Lee K-W, et al. Hepatic venous congestion in living donor grafts in liver transplantation: is there an effect on hepatocellular carcinoma recurrence? Liver Transplant Off Publ Am Assoc Study Liver Dis Int Liver Transplant Soc. United States; 2014;20(7):784–90.

[70] Matsuda H, Sadamori H, Shinoura S, Umeda Y, Yoshida R, Satoh D, et al. Aggressive combined resection of hepatic inferior vena cava, with replacement by a ringed expanded polytetrafluoroethylene graft, in living-donor liver transplantation for hepatocellular carcinoma beyond the Milan criteria. J Hepatobiliary Pancreat Sci. Japan; 2010;17(5):719–24.

[71] Pahari H, Li W-F, Lin T-S, Wang C-C, Yong C-C, Lin T-L, et al. Extensive adhesions in living donor liver transplantation: a retrospective analysis. World J Surg. 2015;40(2): 427–32. Available from: http://link.springer.com/10.1007/s00268-015-3219-x

[72] Memeo R, De'Angelis N, de Blasi V, Cherkaoui Z, Brunetti O, Longo V, et al. Innovative surgical approaches for hepatocellular carcinoma. World J Hepatol. United States; 2016;8(13):591–6.

[73] Lin T-S, Chiang Y-C, Chen C-L, Concejero AM, Cheng Y-F, Wang C-C, et al. Intimal dissection of the hepatic artery following transarterial embolization for hepatocellular carcinoma: an intraoperative problem in adult living donor liver transplantation. Liver Transplant Off Publ Am Assoc Study Liver Dis Int Liver Transplant Soc. United States; 2009;15(11):1553–6.

[74] Pomfret EA, Lodge JPA, Villamil FG, Siegler M. Should we use living donor grafts for patients with hepatocellular carcinoma? Ethical considerations. Liver Transplant Off Publ Am Assoc Study Liver Dis Int Liver Transplant Soc. United States; 2011;17 Suppl 2:S128–32.

[75] Mizuno S, Yokoi H, Shiraki K, Usui M, Sakurai H, Tabata M, et al. Prospective study on the outcome of patients with hepatocellular carcinoma registered for living donor liver transplantation: how long can they wait? Transplantat. United States; 2010;89(6): 650–4.

[76] Taefi a, Abrishami a, Eghtesad B, Sherman M. Surgical resection versus liver transplant for patients with hepatocellular carcinoma (Review). Cochrane Database Syst Rev. 2013;(6).

[77] Ho C, Lee P, Chen C, Ho M. Long-Term outcomes after resection versus transplantation for hepatocellular carcinoma within UCSF criteria. Ann Surg Oncol. 2012;19(3):826–33.

[78] Dai WC, Chan SC, Chok KSH, Cheung TT, Sharr WW, Chan ACY, et al. Good longterm survival after primary living donor liver transplantation for solitary hepatocellular carcinomas up to 8 cm in diameter. HPB (Oxford). England; 2014;16(8):749–57.

[79] Blumgart LH, Jarnagin WR, Belghiti J, Buchler MW, Chapman WC, M.I. D, et al., editors. Liver Transplantation: Indications and General Considerations. In: Blumgart's Surgery of the Liver, Biliary Tract, and Pancreas. 5th ed. Philadelphia: Elsevier; 2012.

[80] Silva MF, Sapisochin G, Strasser SI, Hewa-geeganage S, Chen J, Wigg AJ. Liver resection and transplantation offer similar 5-year survival for Child-Pugh-Turcotte A HCC-patients with a single nodule up to 5 cm: a multicenter, exploratory analysis. Eur J Surg Oncol. 2013;39(4):386–95. Available from: http://dx.doi.org/10.1016/j.ejso.2012.12.011

[81] Bruix J, Sherman M. Management of hepatocellular carcinoma: an update. Hepatol. United States; 2011;53(3):1020–2.

[82] Sapisochin G, Castells L, Dopazo C. Single HCC in cirrhotic patients: liver resection or liver transplantation?? Long-term outcome according to an intention-to-treat basis. Ann Surg Oncol. 2013;20(4):1194–202.

[83] Dhir M, Lyden ER, Smith LM, Are C. Comparison of outcomes of transplantation and resection in patients with early hepatocellular carcinoma: a meta-analysis. Hpb. 2012;14(9):635–45.

[84] Proneth A, Zeman F, Schlitt HJ, Schnitzbauer A. Is resection or transplantation the ideal treatment in patients with hepatocellular carcinoma in cirrhosis if both are possible? A systematic review and metaanalysis. Ann Surg Oncol. 2014;21(9):3096–107. Available from: http://www.ncbi.nlm.nih.gov/pubmed/24866437

[85] Kaido T, Morita S, Tanaka S, Ogawa K, Mori A, Hatano E, et al. Long-term outcomes of hepatic resection versus living donor liver transplantation for hepatocellular carcinoma: a propensity score-matching study. Dis Markers. United States; 2015;2015:425926.

[86] Dionigi R. One Liver for Two: Split and Living Donor Liver Transplantation for Adult and Pediatric Patients. In: Recent Advances in Liver Surgery. Austin, TX: Landes Bioscience; 2009.

[87] Di Sandro S, Slim AO, Giacomoni A, Lauterio A, Mangoni I, Aseni P, et al. Living donor liver transplantation for hepatocellular carcinoma: long-term results compared with deceased donor liver transplantation. Transplant Proc. United States; 2009;41(4):1283–5.

[88] Lee S-G, Moon D-B, Shin H, Kim K-H, Ahn C-S, Ha T-Y, et al. Living donor liver transplantation for hepatocellular carcinoma: current status in Korea. Transplant Proc. United States; 2012;44(2):520–2.

[89] Hu Z, Qian Z, Wu J, Zhou J, Zhang M, Zhou L, et al. Clinical outcomes and risk factors of hepatocellular carcinoma treated by liver transplantation: a multi-centre comparison of living donor and deceased donor transplantation. Clin Res Hepatol Gastroenterol. 2015; 2016 Jun;40(3):315–26

[90] Fisher RA, Kulik LM, Freise CE, Lok ASF, Shearon TH, Brown RSJ, et al. Hepatocellular carcinoma recurrence and death following living and deceased donor liver transplantation. Am J Transplant. Denmark; 2007;7(6):1601–8.

[91] Park M-S, Lee K-W, Suh S-W, You T, Choi Y, Kim H, et al. Living-donor liver transplantation associated with higher incidence of hepatocellular carcinoma recurrence than deceased-donor liver transplantation. Transplant J. 2014;97(1):71–7. Available from: http://content.wkhealth.com/linkback/openurl?sid=WKPTLP:landingpage&an=00007890-201401150-00012

[92] Ninomiya M, Shirabe K, Facciuto ME, Schwartz ME, Florman SS, Yoshizumi T, et al. Comparative study of living and deceased donor liver transplantation as a treatment for hepatocellular carcinoma. J Am Coll Surg. United States; 2015;220(3):297–304.e3.

7

Metabolic Risk Factors in Hepatocellular Carcinoma

Andra-Iulia Suceveanu, Laura Mazilu,
Andreea-Daniela Gheorghe, Anca Pantea Stoian,
Felix Voinea and Adrian-Paul Suceveanu

Abstract

Hepatocellular carcinoma (HCC) is the most frequent primary malignancy of the liver and it is one of the leading causes of cancer-related deaths worldwide. The global burden of hepatocellular carcinoma is growing nowadays. Most cases of hepatocellular carcinoma develop in the background of chronic hepatitis C and B and liver cirrhosis-well-known risk factor. But despite the reducing incidence of chronic hepatitis infections, an increase in the incidence of hepatocellular carcinoma was observed in the last decades. This could be explained by the increasing prevalence of obesity, type 2 diabetes mellitus, nonalcoholic fatty liver disease (NAFLD) and nonalcoholic steatohepatitis (NASH), which are becoming important risk factors in hepatocellular carcinoma. Regular surveillance, as performed for patients with viral hepatitis, is required for patients with metabolic risk factors.

Keywords: hepatocellular carcinoma, nonalcoholic fatty liver disease, nonalcoholic steatohepatitis

1. Introduction

Hepatocellular carcinoma (HCC) is one of the dominant histopathological types of liver cancer, accounting for almost 90% of primary liver cancers worldwide, it is the sixth most common cancer and it is the third cause of cancer-related deaths worldwide [1]. Despite the decreasing incidence of HCC related to viral hepatitis, an increase in the incidence of HCC was observed especially in Europe and America [2]. The global burden of hepatocellular carcinoma in 2012 was of 14 million cases and it is predicted to grow to 22 million over the next two decades.

The most common and known risk factor for HCC are viral infection, virus B or C, toxic factors - alcohol and aflatoxin and immune diseases like primary biliary cirrhosis. There is an increasing number of HCC developed on liver metabolic diseases, including NAFLD and NASH, based on epidemiological evidence that shows a relationship of these diseases with an incident of HCC, regardless of the common known risk factors like alcohol consumption or chronic viral hepatitis.

It is not surprising the growing interest in the last few years on the mechanisms underlying the transition from liver metabolic disorders to HCC that is involving these new metabolic risk factors that include inflammation, insulin resistance, lipid and bile acids metabolism and the gut microbiota. A better understanding of the impact of these factors on the liver microenvironment may have potential benefit on the management of liver disease [3].

Metabolic syndrome has been associated with an increased risk of HCC and each component of this syndrome may increase cancer risk and also a synergic effect has been described [4, 5]. Overweight and obesity are well recognized independent risk factors for HCC, visceral adiposity showing stronger association with HCC risk than general body weight [6, 7]. Studies demonstrated that obesity may also influence HCC prognosis, Body Mass Index (BMI) seems to be a predictor of microvascular invasion and poor prognosis, while visceral adiposity is associated with HCC recurrence after treatment [8, 9]. Type 2 diabetes mellitus has been recognized in various studies as an important independent risk factor for HCC regardless of alcohol consumption [10]. Hyperlipidemia and hypertension are two additional components of metabolic syndrome that have been studied as risk factors for HCC, and hypertension seems to be related to a higher risk of HCC, whereas the relation between HCC and hyperlipidemia remains controversial [4, 5]. Also, synergism between the new risk factors and traditional risk factors has to be considered, for example, a strong synergic effect of alcohol abuse and type 2 diabetes mellitus has been described, also diabetes and obesity have been reported to enhance the risk of HCC in patients with chronic hepatitis [11, 12].

Non alcoholic fatty liver disease (NAFLD) is one of the most common cause of chronic liver disease and include a large spectrum of chronic liver disorders ranging from simple hepatic steatosis with no evidence of hepatocellular injury to non-alcoholic steatohepatitis (NASH), advanced fibrosis, cirrhosis and liver failure and currently, all guidelines agree that NAFLD is associated with the increasing percentage of obesity, type 2 diabetes mellitus, hypertension and dyslipidemia in our population [13, 14]. Several studies have demonstrated a strong association between NAFLD and each components of metabolic syndrome and there is enough evidence to define NAFLD itself as a liver component of metabolic syndrome [15–19, 46].

The rising incidence of NAFLD/NASH worldwide led to an important rise in HCC incidence related to these chronic liver diseases [3]. Many studies have demonstrated over the years that NAFLD can lead to hepatic fibrosis and cirrhosis, increasing therefore the risk for developing HCC [20, 21]. Among these patients with Non alcoholic fatty liver disease or non-alcoholic steatohepatitis, studies show that the third cause of death is liver disease, and HCC represents the main cause of death in these patients [20–23]. The incidence rate for developing HCC in patients with NASH related hepatic cirrhosis is up to 27% in retrospective studies [24]. Increased incidence of HCC was also been reported in patients with NAFLD in the absence of hepatic cirrhosis, and several risk factors for HCC development have been identified [6, 25–29].

2. Natural history: Progression from hepatic steatosis to HCC

The term nonalcoholic fatty liver refers to a variety of liver disease that ranges from simple isolated hepatic steatosis, to non-alcoholic steatohepatitis with or without cirrhosis, and progression to HCC.

Although NAFLD diagnosis can be made by imaging (ultrasound or magnetic resonance), biopsy still remain the gold standard for diagnosis. Histology generally displays the accumulation of triglycerides in hepatocytes, usually in mixed macrovesicular or microvesicular droplets, in the absence of alcohol abuse, steatogenic medication or hereditary disorders [30].

The prevalence of NASH is difficult to determine because biopsy is required, with specific criteria such as steatosis, hepatocellular injury, mainly in the form of ballooning, and lobular inflammation, and once cirrhosis is present, NASH may be difficult to evaluate because often the fatty deposition disappear. Liver fibrosis may be present in non-cirrhotic NASH, initially in perisinusoidal acinar zone 3 [31]. Because of the need of histopathologic confirmation, NASH is most likely underdiagnosed and it may be misclassified as cryptogenic cirrhosis, which shares the same risk factors including diabetes and obesity [32, 33, 46]. Therefore, to estimate correctly the prevalence of NASH, a novel NASH category including obese patients with cryptogenic cirrhosis or with unknown HCC etiology has been proposed.

The prevalence of NAFLD and NASH is variable and it is depended on the method of diagnostic used to confirm the disease, and it is usually underreported because of the asymptomatic nature and can be underestimated and poorly treated.

NAFLD is present in more than 25% of adult population and about 10 to 20% of NAFLD patients may progress to NASH, which may progress to cirrhosis in 20–45% of cases, and cirrhosis is a well-known risk factor for HCC, and approximately 7% of patients with NASH-related cirrhosis may progress to HCC within 6 years [31].

Patients with nonalcoholic steatohepatitis are more susceptible to develop progressive advanced liver disease when compared to benign course of simple hepatic steatosis. In a study that included 420 patients with NAFLD/NASH, it was demonstrated a higher mortality in these patients when compared to the general population and also liver-related deaths occurred in 13% compared to 1% in general population, and 3% of patients with NAFLD developed hepatic cirrhosis. [34] Another study showed increased rates of hepatic cirrhosis in patients with non-alcoholic steatohepatitis (25%) compared to patients with fatty liver without non-alcoholic steatohepatitis (3%), and also showed an increased risk of liver disease related death in these patients (11% *vs* 2% in patients with fatty liver without NASH) [35].

Patients with compensated liver cirrhosis related to non-alcoholic steatohepatitis present with better survival outcomes compared to patients with HCV related cirrhosis, but in the presence of uncompensated liver cirrhosis poor prognosis was observed in both populations [36, 37], and currently, both, the American and European Associations for the Study of Liver Diseases, recommend screening for HCC in all patients with non-alcoholic steatohepatitis related cirrhosis [38].

Evidence from studies suggests that an important proportion of patients with NAFLD-associated HCC, do not have histologic evidence of liver cirrhosis. In one study from 1168 patients that underwent hepatic surgery for HCC, 6 out of 8 patients with NASH-related HCC did not had any histopathological evidence of liver cirrhosis and also the study suggested that the presence of hepatic cirrhosis in NASH-related HCC patients is lower compared to HCV-related HCC [29].

In another study that analyzed 128 patients with HCC recruited over a period of 12 years, it was reported that a significant number of patients with NASH developed HCC in the absence of fibrosis when compared to HCC of other etiology [39]. To explain this phenomenon in non-cirrhotic NAFLD patients, one proposed hypothesis is the malignant transformation of liver cell adenoma, and there are some published reports that have suggested that in the presence of metabolic syndrome features, liver cell adenoma may incur a malignant transformation [40, 41].

In the last years, many studies tried to establish the relationship between NAFLD and NASH, cryptogenic cirrhosis and HCC. The true prevalence of NASH and NASH-related HCC is probably underestimated due to the asymptomatic nature of the disease, and in up to 29% of HCC cases, the underlying etiology of liver disease remains unknown or are considered as cryptogenic cirrhosis [40]. Histopathological features that are suggestive for non-alcoholic steatohepatitis are more frequently observed in patients with HCC of unknown etiology than in patients with HCC related to chronic viral hepatitis or alcoholic etiology [32]. Even if the true prevalence of NAFLD/NASH-related HCC is not yet well defined, the increasing incidence of obesity and diabetes, suggests that the incidence NAFLD/NASH-related HCC will continue to grow in the next years, and there are already numerous studies that are investigated the relation between these diseases [46].

3. Metabolic risk factors, NAFLD and HCC

It is established that HCC and NAFLD share many risk factors and the development of HCC in NAFLD/NASH patients is probably multifactorial and involves low grade chronic systemic inflammatory response, excessive fat accumulation and insulin resistance [40, 46].

3.1. Obesity

There is more evidence that overweight and obesity and metabolic syndrome have reached a epidemic proportion over the last decades, and there are evident data that show that 80% of NAFLD patients are overweight or obese [42]. According to the World Health Organization, in 2008, more than 35% of adults worldwide are overweight, and of these, 13% are obese [29] and if overweight and obesity rates continue at their current ascending trend, it is estimated that more than 3.3 billion adults will become overweight or obese by year 2030 [43].

Overweight and obesity are leading risk factors for overall mortality, accounting for more than 3.4 million adult deaths every year, and are considered risk factors for 44% of the diabetes, 23% of the ischemic heart disease, and between 7 and 40% of certain cancer [42].

Body Mass Index is the most commonly used index in epidemiologic studies, but body fat topography, and especially central obesity, seems to be more important in pathophysiologic mechanisms that connect obesity to cancer. Central obesity, is the key feature in most metabolic syndrome definitions, and has also been directly correlated with insulin resistance [44, 46].

Obesity have been associated with disproportion between visceral and subcutaneous adipose tissue and with chronic inflammatory state due to adipokine imbalance that is defined as increased levels of leptin and decreased levels of adiponectin. Furthermore, obesity has been associated with other risk factors including insulin resistance, increased hepatic lipid storage and alteration of intestinal flora [46].

Adipokine imbalance as mentioned before occurs with simultaneous increased leptin and decreased adiponectin levels resulting in a pro-inflammatory and pro-oncogenic state. Both leptin and adiponectin are hallmarks of obesity, and have been extensively studied and both have been related to NAFLD and progression to liver cancer.

Leptin is secreted by adipose tissue and acts as a hormone and it is involved in the process of satiety. High levels of leptin and resistance to its action are observed in obese persons. Leptin has been demonstrated to be implicated in NAFLD progression, liver fibrosis, NASH and eventually in the carcinogenesis process of HCC through multiple molecular mechanisms. And these mechanisms are the activation of JAK2/STAT3, PI-3 K/Akt, ERK pathways and the inhibition of the TGFβ1-induced apoptotic pathway [24]. For example, the activation of Akt pathway was observed in about 40% of HCC patients. Leptin's role is to have growth factor-like activities on hepatic cells and HCC cells, and also have proinflammatory, profibrogenic and proangiogenic role on liver microenvironment and also it is implicated in the process of cell growth, angiogenesis and metastasis [31].

Adiponectin is the most abundant hormone of adipose tissue and has well known metabolic functions, having anti-inflammatory, antifibrotic, antiangiogenic, and antiproliferative activities on the liver microenvironment. Adiponectin exerts antifibrotic effects on hepatic cells through activation of the signaling AMPK axis and inhibition of TGFβ-mediated profibrogenic gene expression, and in addition, adiponectin may also induce apoptosis of hepatic cells. The anti-inflammatory activity of adiponectin is mostly related to inhibition of NFkB signaling axis [31]. A direct effect of adiponectin on HCC cells has also been described, induces apoptosis and inhibits HCC cell proliferation and migration. In addition, adiponectin prevents HCC development by activation of the AMPK signaling pathway and consequent modulation of mTOR and JNK/caspase 3 axis, resulting in growth cell inhibition and enhanced apoptosis [4]. A number of observations support the reduced adiponectin levels observed in obese patients and were associated to increased incidence of hepatic steatosis, fibrosis and accelerated progression to HCC [45].

3.2. Insulin resistance

Insulin resistance it is another important component of the metabolic syndrome, and along with obesity, is involved in the chronic inflammatory state directly linked to NAFLD. Insulin resistance is also related to oxidative stress, which has the most important role in carcinogenesis in the presence of NAFLD and NASH.

Epidemiologic studies show that diabetes is associated with an increased risk of developing HCC compared with non-diabetics patients, regardless of other HCC risk factors and also seems to be independent of obesity [47]. In a large study conducted on patients with and without diabetes, with a follow-up period of 10–15 years, NAFLD incidence was significantly higher among patients with diabetes and a significantly higher incidence of HCC among patients with diabetes was observed [7]. Meta-analysis published over the years, revealed a 2 to 3-fold greater risk of HCC in patients with diabetes compared with non-diabetic patients, and this significant association was reported independent of alcohol abuse or chronic viral hepatitis in studies that examined these factors [48, 49].

Epidemiologic data demonstrate that both obesity and type 2 diabetes mellitus have increases the risk for HCC, and NAFLD, which is present in up to 90% of obese persons and up to 70% of type 2 diabetes mellitus patients [24], appears to play an important role in HCC development. NAFLD is nowadays considered the most common risk factor for HCC, followed by type 2 diabetes and it is exceeding the incidence of chronic viral infections and alcoholic liver disease [48, 50]. These can be explained by effective measures to reduce HCV infection incidence, which was the major cause of HCC in the United States and in other developed countries, and also can be explained by the increasing prevalence of NAFLD in these areas [51].

The strong relationship between visceral obesity and insulin resistance (IR) is well known, but insulin resistance is not related only to adipose tissue, in fact, liver accumulation of fatty acid metabolites can induce hepatic insulin resistance. One of the main fatty acid metabolite involved in hepatic insulin resistance is diacylglycerol (DAG) and it has been proposed as a predictor for hepatic insulin resistance [52]. The consequent hyperinsulinemia downregulates s expression of IRS2 in the hepatic cells increasing hepatic insulin resistance and in addition, insulin stimulates lipogenesis through activation of SREBP-1c, inducing, in a vicious circle with further fat accumulation and insulin resistance [31]. The liver microenvironment may induce insulin resistance also in other tissues, in fact, an increase in liver fat content may be considered a very strong predictor of insulin resistance in skeletal muscles, hepatic and adipose tissue, regardless of adiposity. In conclusion, liver fat content may predict the development of metabolic syndrome or diabetes, and the underlying mechanism may be the altered gene expression and protein synthesis and secretion also observed in NAFLD [53]. It is known that hyperinsulinemia occurs as a response to insulin resistance, and that is considered a risk factor for liver fibrosis and HCC development by activation of hepatic stellate cells, by dysregulation in the proliferation-apoptosis balance in hepatic cells, and by stimulation of angiogenesis. The most studied mechanism involved in NAFLD-related HCC is the IGF signaling axis that has a growth factor-like activity on hepatic cells and also a pro-angiogenic activity on the hepatic vascular system. Dysregulation of the IGF signaling axis has an important role in hepatic carcinogenesis and it is represented by the low levels of IGF1 in serum and overexpression of IGF-II. Insulin receptors (IRS) bind to insulin or IGF and share the same pro-oncogenic pathways with IGF1 receptor (IGF1R), including the activation of P13K/Akt and MAPK [54, 55].

3.3. Lipotoxicity

Increased lipid accumulation in the liver arises from lipolysis within peripheral adipose tissue, dietary sources and de novo hepatic lipogenesis, and this increased lipid accumulation causes hepatic lipotoxicity resulting in the excessive production of saturated and monounsaturated free fatty acids (FFAs) [40, 46, 56]. These FFAs undergo β-oxidation leading to formation of reactive oxygen species that will further induce mitochondrial damage, endothelial reticulum stress, and gene transcription promoting inflammatory cell signaling pathways.

As a result of the hepatic insulin resistance an increase in the liver of free fatty acids (FFAs) is observed, mainly due to dysregulation of the lipolysis and lipogenesis balance, resulting lipotoxicity that will determine chronic damage to hepatic tissue [51]. But, lipotoxicity is not due only as consequence of the excessive accumulation of FFAs in the liver, and the modification of lipid composition is another contributor to lipotoxicity, and recent studies are aimed at searching for specific metabolic changes as potential signatures of development of HCC in patients with NAFLD [57]. For example, some studies show that, during natural history of progression from normal liver to NAFLD or NASH, the ratio of polyunsaturated fatty acids (PUFAs) is increased in NASH, and phosphatidylcholine (PC) levels are reduced in both NAFLD and NASH, and based on these observations, it has been suggested that the LPA signaling axis may be one of the mechanism that is connecting hepatic steatosis to HCC [58–61].

3.4. Microbiota: Intestinal flora dysregulation

The basis for the ongoing interest on the role of gut microbiota in progression of NAFLD was the observation of fatal NASH that occurred in patients undergoing jejunoileal bypass in bariatric surgery and the reversal after metronidazol therapy [62]. There are several evidences that demonstrate a high prevalence of small intestinal bacterial overgrowth in patients with NAFLD/NASH and that also demonstrate the role of microbiota modifications in the development of NAFLD and NASH [45]. Specific microflora changes may play an important role in progression of hepatic steatosis, especially in obese patients. In patients with NAFLD and NASH was observed a difference in microbiota composition compared with healthy population [63, 64]. The mechanisms implicated in the progression of gut microbiota-related NAFLD and NASH and HCC are: alteration of intestine permeability, persistent activation of innate immune system with consequent chronic inflammation, changes in bile acid metabolism [65].

Patients with NAFLD or NASH show increased levels of lipopolysaccharides (LPS), a known innate immune system activator, on serum confirming the inflammatory state associated with this conditions and alteration in gut permeability with disruption of intercellular tight junctions observed in patients with NAFLD can contribute directly to lipopolysaccharides action to the liver [65, 66].

All these findings were confirmed in human study wherein increased LPS-binding protein (LBP) levels were observed in obese patients with NAFLD and even more in obese patients with NASH, correlating with liver TNFα increased expression [67].

All these mechanisms show how changes in the microbiota, in combination with loss of innate immune sensors, may induce metabolic liver disorders.

Gut microbiota also influences bile acid metabolisms mainly through the stimulation of the bile-acid-activated nuclear receptor and also by interacting with farnesoid X receptor (FXR) which induce excretion of bile acids from the liver and production of antimicrobial peptides [65].

4. Conclusions

Although significant progress has been made in NAFLD/NASH related HCC, many issues still remain to be resolved. With the prevalence of HCV declining in the last years, the incidence of NAFLD/NASH is expected to account for a greater proportion of HCC incidence in the near future due to the growing epidemic of obesity, diabetes and metabolic syndrome, known as independent metabolic risk factors for development of HCC. The annual incidence rate of HCC developed in patients with NASH-related cirrhosis is not yet clearly established and recent evidence show that a significant number of patients with NAFLD or NASH progress to HCC in the absence of hepatic cirrhosis. NAFLD/NASH-related cirrhotic patients receive significantly less surveillance for HCC than those with HCV-related cirrhosis, in contrast to epidemiological data and this represents an important public health problem. Also dysbiosis play an important role in progression of liver disease via changes in bile acids metabolism and dysregulation of intestinal barrier.

In conclusion, metabolic syndrome comprising of obesity, type 2 diabetes, dyslipidemia, hypertension, is related with an increased risk for development of HCC. NAFLD considered the liver manifestation of metabolic syndrome is an important factor implicated in progression to HCC. Also alteration in gut microbiota seems to be connected with HCC occurrence but many questions still remain to be answered.

Acknowledgements

All authors contributed equally to this chapter.

Author details

Andra-Iulia Suceveanu[1]*, Laura Mazilu[2], Andreea-Daniela Gheorghe[2], Anca Pantea Stoian[3], Felix Voinea[4] and Adrian-Paul Suceveanu[5]

*Address all correspondence to: andrasuceveanu@yahoo.com

1 Faculty of Medicine, Department of Gastroenterology, Emergency Hospital of Constanta, Ovidius University, Constanta, Romania

2 Faculty of Medicine, Department of Oncology, Emergency Hospital of Constanta, Ovidius University, Constanta, Romania

3 University of Medicine and Farmacy, Carol Davila, Department of Diabetes, Nutrition and Metabolic Disease, Bucharest, Romania

4 Faculty of Medicine, Department of Urology, Emergency Hospital of Constanta, Ovidius University, Constanta, Romania

5 Faculty of Medicine, Department of Internal Medicine, Emergency Hospital of Constanta, Ovidius University, Constanta, Romania

References

[1] Ferlay J, Shin HR, Bray F, Forman D, Mathers C, Parkin DM. Estimates of worldwide burden of cancer in 2008: GLOBOCAN 2008. International Journal of Cancer. 2010;**127** 2893-2917. PMID: 21351269. DOI: 10.1002/ijc.25516

[2] Bertuccio P, Turati F, Carioli G, Rodriguez T, La Vecchia C, Malvezzi M, et al. Global trends and predictions in hepatocellular carcinoma mortality. Journal of Hepatology. 2017;**67**:302-309

[3] Agosti P, Sabbà C, Mazzocca A. Emerging metabolic risk factors in hepatocellular carcinoma and their influence on the liver microenvironment. Biochimica et Biophysica Acta. 2018 Feb;**1864**(2):607-617. DOI: 10.1016/j.bbadis.2017.11.026 Epub 2017 Nov 29

[4] Welzel TM, Graubard BI, Zeuzem S, El-Serag HB, Davila JA, McGlynn KA. Metabolic syndrome increases the risk of primary liver cancer in the United States: a study in the SEER-Medicare database. Hepatology. 2011 Aug;**54**(2):463-471. DOI: 10.1002/hep.24397

[5] Borena W, Strohmaier S, Lukanova A, Bjørge T, Lindkvist B, Hallmans G, Edlinger M, Stocks T, Nagel G, Manjer J, Engeland A, Selmer R, Häggström C, Tretli S, Concin H, Jonsson H, Stattin P, Ulmer H. Metabolic risk factors and primary liver cancer in a prospective study of

578, 700 adults. International Journal of Cancer. 2012 Jul 1;**131**(1):193-200. DOI: 10.1002/ijc.26338

[6] Karagozian R, Derdák Z, Baffy G. Obesity-associated mechanisms of hepatocarcinogenesis. Metabolism. 2014 May;**63**(5):607-617. DOI: 10.1016/j.metabol.2014.01.011

[7] Schlesinger S, Aleksandrova K, Pischon T, Fedirko V, Jenab M, Trepo E, et al. Abdominal obesity, weight gain during adulthood and risk of liver and biliary tract cancer in a European cohort. International Journal of Cancer. 2013 Feb 1;**132**(3):645-657. DOI: 10.1002/ijc.27645

[8] Siegel AB, Lim EA, Wang S, Brubaker W, Rodriguez RD, Goyal A, et al. Diabetes, body mass index, and outcomes in hepatocellular carcinoma patients undergoing liver transplantation. Transplantation. 2012 Sep 15;**94**(5):539-543

[9] Ohki T, Tateishi R, Shiina S, Goto E, Sato T, Nakagawa H, et al. Visceral fat accumulation is an independent risk factor for hepatocellular carcinoma recurrence after curative treatment in patients with suspected NASH. Gut. 2009 Jun;**58**(6):839-844. DOI: 10.1136/gut.2008.164053

[10] Raff EJ, Kakati D, Bloomer JR, Shoreibah M, Rasheed K, Singal AK. Diabetes mellitus predicts occurrence of cirrhosis and hepatocellular cancer in alcoholic liver and non-alcoholic fatty liver diseases. Journal of Clinical and Translational Hepatology. 2015 Mar; **3**(1):9-16. DOI: 10.14218/JCTH.2015.00001

[11] Balbi M, Donadon V, Ghersetti M, Grazioli S, Valentina GD, Gardenal R, et al. Alcohol and HCV chronic infection are risk cofactors of type 2 diabetes mellitus for hepatocellular carcinoma in Italy. International Journal of Environmental Research and Public Health. 2010 Apr;**7**(4):1366-1378. DOI: 10.3390/ijerph7041366

[12] Chen CL, Yang HI, Yang WS, Liu CJ, Chen PJ, You SL, et al. Metabolic factors and risk of hepatocellular carcinoma by chronic hepatitis B/C infection: A follow-up study in Taiwan. Gastroenterology. 2008 Jul;**135**(1):111-121. DOI: 10.1053/j.gastro.2008.03.073

[13] Chalasani N, Younossi Z, Lavine JE, Diehl AM, Brunt EM, Cusi K, Charlton M, Sanyal AJ. The diagnosis and management of nonalcoholic fatty liver disease: Practice guideline by the American Association for the Study of Liver Diseases, American College of Gastroenterology, and the American Gastroenterological Association. Hepatology. 2012;**55**:2005-2023. PMID: 22488764. DOI: 10.1002/hep.25762

[14] Nascimbeni F, Pais R, Bellentani S, Day CP, Ratziu V, Loria P, Lonardo A. From NAFLD in clinical practice to answers from guidelines. Journal of Hepatology. 2013;**59**:859-871. PMID: 23751754. DOI: 10.1016/j.jhep.2013.05.044

[15] Marchesini G, Brizi M, Morselli-Labate AM, Bianchi G, Bugianesi E, McCullough AJ, Forlani G, Melchionda N. Association of nonalcoholic fatty liver disease with insulin resistance. The American Journal of Medicine. 1999;**107**:450-455. PMID: 10569299

[16] Marchesini G, Brizi M, Bianchi G, Tomassetti S, Bugianesi E, Lenzi M, McCullough AJ, Natale S, Forlani G, Melchionda N. Nonalcoholic fatty liver disease: a feature of the metabolic syndrome. Diabetes. 2001;**50**:1844-1850. PMID: 11473047. DOI: 10.2337/diabetes.50.8.1844

[17] Hsiao PJ, Kuo KK, Shin SJ, Yang YH, Lin WY, Yang JF, Chiu CC, Chuang WL, Tsai TR, Yu ML. Significant correlations between severe fatty liver and risk factors for metabolic syndrome. Journal of Gastroenterology and Hepatology. 2007;**22**:2118-2123. PMID: 18031368. DOI: 10.1111/j.1440-1746.2006.04698.x

[18] Jimba S, Nakagami T, Takahashi M, Wakamatsu T, Hirota Y, Iwamoto Y, Wasada T. Prevalence of non-alcoholic fatty liver disease and its association with impaired glucose metabolism in Japanese adults. Diabetic Medicine. 2005;**22**:1141-1145. PMID: 16108839. DOI: 10.1111/j.1464-5491.2005.01582.x

[19] Tarantino G, Finelli C. What about non-alcoholic fatty liver disease as a new criterion to define metabolic syndrome? World Journal of Gastroenterology. 2013 Jun 14;**19**(22):3375-3384. DOI: 10.3748/wjg.v19.i22.3375

[20] Adams LA, Lymp JF, St Sauver J, Sanderson SO, Lindor KD, Feldstein A, Angulo P. The natural history of nonalcoholic fatty liver disease: A population-based cohort study. Gastroenterology. 2005;**129**:113-121 PMID: 16012941

[21] Jansen PL. Non-alcoholic steatohepatitis. European Journal of Gastroenterology & Hepatology. 2004;**16**:1079-1085. PMID: 15489564

[22] Nagaoki Y, Hyogo H, Aikata H, Tanaka M, Naeshiro N, Nakahara T, et al. Recent trend of clinical features in patients with hepatocellular carcinoma. Hepatology Research. 2012;**42**: 368-375. PMID: 22151896. DOI: 10.1111/j.1872-034X.2011.00929.x

[23] Yatsuji S, Hashimoto E, Tobari M, Taniai M, Tokushige K, Shiratori K. Clinical features and outcomes of cirrhosis due to nonalcoholic steatohepatitis compared with cirrhosis caused by chronic hepatitis C. Journal of Gastroenterology and Hepatology. 2009;**24**:248-254. PMID: 19032450. DOI: 10.1111/j.1440-1746.2008.05640.x

[24] White DL, Kanwal F, El-Serag HB. Association between nonalcoholic fatty liver disease and risk for hepatocellular cancer, based on systematic review. Clinical Gastroenterology and Hepatology. 2012;**10**:1342-1359.e2. PMID: 23041539. DOI: 10.1016/j.cgh.2012.10.001

[25] Marrero JA, Fontana RJ, Su GL, Conjeevaram HS, Emick DM, Lok AS. NAFLD may be a common underlying liver disease in patients with hepatocellular carcinoma in the United States. Hepatology. 2002;**36**:1349-1354. PMID: 12447858. DOI: 10.1053/jhep.2002.36939

[26] Guzman G, Brunt EM, Petrovic LM, Chejfec G, Layden TJ, Cotler SJ. Does nonalcoholic fatty liver disease predispose patients to hepatocellular carcinoma in the absence of cirrhosis? Archives of Pathology & Laboratory Medicine. 2008;**132**:1761-1766. PMID: 1897 6012. DOI: 10.1043/1543-2165-132.11.1761

[27] Reddy SK, Steel JL, Chen HW, DeMateo DJ, Cardinal J, et al. Outcomes of curative treatment for hepatocellular cancer in nonalcoholic steatohepatitis versus hepatitis C and alcoholic liver disease. Hepatology. 2012;**55**:1809-1819. PMID: 22183968. DOI: 10.1002/hep.25536

[28] Starley BQ, Calcagno CJ, Harrison SA. Nonalcoholic fatty liver disease and hepatocellular carcinoma: A weighty connection. Hepatology. 2010;**51**:1820-1832. PMID: 20432259. DOI: 10.1002/ hep.23594

[29] Kawada N, Imanaka K, Kawaguchi T, Tamai C, Ishihara R, et al. Hepatocellular carcinoma arising from non-cirrhotic nonalcoholic steatohepatitis. Journal of Gastroenterology. 2009; **44**:1190-1194. PMID: 19672551. DOI: 10.1007/s00535-009-0112-0

[30] Ong JP, Younossi ZM. Epidemiology and natural history of NAFLD and NASH. Clinics in Liver Disease. 2007;**11**:1-16, vii. PMID:17544968. DOI: 10.1016/j.cld.2007.02.009

[31] Hardy T, Oakley F, Anstee QM, Day CP. Nonalcoholic fatty liver disease: Pathogenesis and disease spectrum. Annual Review of Pathology. 2016 May 23;**11**:451-496. DOI: 10.1146/annurev-pathol-012615-044224

[32] Bugianesi E, Leone N, Vanni E, Marchesini G, Brunello F, et al. Expanding the natural history of nonalcoholic steatohepatitis: from cryptogenic cirrhosis to hepatocellular carcinoma. Gastroenterology. 2002 Jul;**123**(1):134-140

[33] Regimbeau JM, Colombat M, Mognol P, Durand F, Abdalla E, et al. Obesity and diabetes as a risk factor for hepatocellular carcinoma. Liver Transplantation. 2004 Feb;**10**(2 Suppl 1): S69-S73

[34] Rafiq N, Bai C, Fang Y, Srishord M, McCullough A, Gramlich T, Younossi ZM. Long-term follow-up of patients with nonalcoholic fatty liver. Clinical Gastroenterology and Hepatology. 2009;**7**:234-238. PMID: 19049831. DOI: 10.1016/j.cgh.2008.11.005

[35] Matteoni CA, Younossi ZM, Gramlich T, Boparai N, Liu YC, McCullough AJ. Nonalcoholic fatty liver disease: A spectrum of clinical and pathological severity. Gastroenterology. 1999;**116**:1413-1419. PMID: 10348825

[36] Hui JM, Kench JG, Chitturi S, Sud A, Farrell GC, Byth K, Hall P, Khan M, George J. Long-term outcomes of cirrhosis in nonalcoholic steatohepatitis compared with hepatitis C. Hepatology. 2003;**38**:420-427. PMID: 12883486. DOI: 10.1053/jhep.2003.50320

[37] Sanyal AJ, Banas C, Sargeant C, Luketic VA, Sterling RK, Stravitz RT, et al. Similarities and differences in outcomes of cirrhosis due to nonalcoholic steatohepatitis and hepatitis C. Hepatology. 2006;**43**:682-689. PMID: 16502396. DOI: 10.1002/hep.21103

[38] Bruix J, Sherman M. Management of hepatocellular carcinoma: An update. Hepatology. 2011;**53**:1020-1022. PMID: 21374666. DOI: 10.1002/hep.24199

[39] Paradis V, Zalinski S, Chelbi E, Guedj N, Degos F, Vilgrain V, Bedossa P, Belghiti J. Hepatocellular carcinomas in patients with metabolic syndrome often develop without

significant liver fibrosis: A pathological analysis. Hepatology. 2009;**49**:851-859. PMID: 19115377. DOI: 10.1002/hep.22734

[40] Margini C, Dufour JF. The story of HCC in NAFLD: From epidemiology, across pathogenesis, to prevention and treatment. Liver International. 2016;**36**:317-324. PMID: 26601627. DOI: 10.1111/liv.13031

[41] Farges O, Ferreira N, Dokmak S, Belghiti J, Bedossa P, Paradis V. Changing trends in malignant transformation of hepatocellular adenoma. Gut. 2011;**60**:85-89. PMID: 21148580. DOI: 10.1136/gut.2010.222109

[42] World Health Organisation (WHO): Overweight and Obesity Factsheet. Available from: http://www.who.int/mediacentre/factsheets/fs311/en/

[43] Kelly T, Yang W, Chen CS, Reynolds K, He J. Global burden of obesity in 2005 and projections to 2030. International Journal of Obesity. 2008;**32**:1431-1437. PMID: 18607383. DOI: 10.1038/ijo.2008.102

[44] Alberti KG, Zimmet PZ. Definition, diagnosis and classification of diabetes mellitus and its complications. Part 1: Diagnosis and classification of diabetes mellitus provisional report of a WHO consultation. Diabetic Medicine. 1998;**15**:539-553. PMID: 9686693. DOI: 10.1002/(SICI)1096-9136(199807)15

[45] Jiang CM, Pu CW, Hou YH, Chen Z, Alanazy M, Hebbard L. Non alcoholic steatohepatitis a precursor for hepatocellular carcinoma development. World Journal of Gastroenterology. 2014 Nov 28;**20**(44):16464-16473. DOI:10.3748/ wjg.v20.i44.16464

[46] Cholankeril G, Patel R, Khurana S, Sanjaya K. Satapathy, Hepatocellular carcinoma in non-alcoholic steatohepatitis: Current knowledge and implications for management. World Journal of Hepatology. 2017 Apr 18;**9**(11):533-543. Published online 2017 Apr 18. DOI: 10.4254/wjh.v9.i11.533

[47] Hung CH, Wang JH, Hu TH, Chen CH, Chang KC, Yen YH, Kuo YH, Tsai MC, Lu SN, Lee CM. Insulin resistance is associated with hepatocellular carcinoma in chronic hepatitis C infection. World Journal of Gastroenterology. 2010;**16**:2265-2271. PMID: 20458764. DOI: 10.3748/wjg.v16.i18.2265

[48] El-Serag HB, Hampel H, Javadi F. The association between diabetes and hepatocellular carcinoma: a systematic review of epidemiologic evidence. Clinical Gastroenterology and Hepatology. 2006;**4**:369-380. PMID: 16527702. DOI: 10.1016/j.cgh.2005.12.007

[49] Wang P, Kang D, Cao W, Wang Y, Liu Z. Diabetes mellitus and risk of hepatocellular carcinoma: A systematic review and metaanalysis. Diabetes/Metabolism Research and Reviews. 2012;**28**:109-122. PMID: 21898753. DOI: 10.1002/dmrr.1291

[50] Ertle J, Dechêne A, Sowa JP, Penndorf V, Herzer K, Kaiser G, et al. Non-alcoholic fatty liver disease progresses to hepatocellular carcinoma in the absence of apparent cirrhosis. International Journal of Cancer. 2011;**128**:2436-2443. PMID: 21128245. DOI: 10.1002/ijc.25797

[51] Baffy G, Brunt EM, Caldwell SH. Hepatocellular carcinoma in non-alcoholic fatty liver disease: an emerging menace. Journal of Hepatology. 2012;**56**:1384-1391. PMID: 22326465. DOI: 10.1016/ j.jhep.2011.10.027

[52] Kumashiro N, Erion DM, Zhang D, Kahn M, Beddow SA, Chu X, et al. Cellular mechanism of insulin resistance in nonalcoholic fatty liver disease. Proceedings of the National Academy of Sciences of the United States of America. 2011 Sep 27;**108**(39):16381-16385. DOI: 10.1073/pnas.1113359108

[53] Meex RCR, Watt MJ. Hepatokines: linking nonalcoholic fatty liver disease and insulin resistance. Nature Reviews. Endocrinology. 2017 Sep;**13**(9):509-520. DOI: 10.1038/nrendo.2017.56

[54] Siddique A, Kowdley KV. Insulin resistance and other metabolic risk factors in the pathogenesis of hepatocellular carcinoma. Clinics in Liver Disease. 2011 May;**15**(2):281-296 vii-x. DOI: 10.1016/j.cld.2011.03.007

[55] Chun YS, Huang M, Rink L, Von Mehren M. Expression levels of insulin-like growth factors and receptors in hepatocellular carcinoma: A retrospective study. World Journal of Surgical Oncology. 2014 Jul 22;**12**:231. DOI: 10.1186/1477-7819-12-231

[56] Hirsova P, Ibrabim SH, Gores GJ, Malhi H. Lipotoxic lethal and sublethal stress signaling in hepatocytes: relevance to NASH pathogenesis. Journal of Lipid Research. 2016;**57**:1758-1770. PMID: 27049024. DOI: 10.1194/jlr.R066357

[57] Beyoğlu D, Idle JR. The metabolomic window into hepatobiliary disease. Journal of Hepatology. 2013 Oct;**59**(4):842-858. DOI:10.1016/j.jhep.2013.05. 030

[58] Puri P, Baillie RA, Wiest MM, Mirshahi F, Choudhury J, et al. A lipidomic analysis of nonalcoholic fatty liver disease. Hepatology. 2007 Oct;**46**(4):1081-1090

[59] Lopane C, Agosti P, Gigante I, Sabbà C, Mazzocca A. Implications of the lysophosphatidic acid signaling axis in liver cancer. Biochimica et Biophysica Acta. 2017 Aug;**1868**(1):277-282. DOI: 10.1016/j.bbcan.2017.06.002

[60] Lade A, Noon LA, Friedman SL. Contributions of metabolic dysregulation and inflammation to nonalcoholic steatohepatitis, hepatic fibrosis, and cancer. Current Opinion in Oncology. 2014 Jan;**26**(1):100-107. DOI: 10.1097/CCO.0000000000000042

[61] Shi H, Kokoeva MV, Inouye K, Tzameli I, Yin H, Flier JS. TLR4 links innate immunity and fatty acid-induced insulin resistance. The Journal of Clinical Investigation. 2006 Nov;**116** (11):3015-3025

[62] Drenick EJ, Fisler J, Johnson D. Hepatic steatosis after intestinal bypass–prevention and reversal by metronidazole, irrespective of protein-calorie malnutrition. Gastroenterology. 1982 Mar;**82**(3):535-548

[63] Mouzaki M, Comelli EM, Arendt BM, Bonengel J, Fung SK, Fischer SE, McGilvray ID, Allard JP. Intestinal microbiota in patients with nonalcoholic fatty liver disease. Hepatology. 2013 Jul;**58**(1):120-127. DOI: 10.1002/hep.26319

[64] Zhu JL, Baker SS, Gill C, Liu W, Alkhouri R, Baker RD, Gill SR. Characterization of gut microbiomes in nonalcoholic steatohepatitis (NASH) patients: A connection between endogenous alcohol and NASH. Hepatology. 2013 Feb;**57**(2):601-609. DOI: 10.1002/hep.26093

[65] Aron-Wisnewsky J, Gaborit B, Dutour A, Clement K. Gut microbiota and nonalcoholic fatty liver disease: New insights. Clinical Microbiology and Infection. 2013 Apr;**19**(4):338-348. DOI: 10.1111/1469-0691.12140

[66] Cani PD, Bibiloni R, Knauf C, Waget A, Neyrinck AM, Delzenne NM, Burcelin R. Changes in gut microbiota control metabolic endotoxemia-induced inflammation in high-fat diet-induced obesity and diabetes in mice. Diabetes. 2008 Jun;**57**(6):1470-1481. DOI: 10.2337/db07-1403

[67] Ruiz AG, Casafont F, Crespo J, Cayón A, Mayorga M, Estebanez A, et al. Lipopolysaccharide-binding protein plasma levels and liver TNF-alpha gene expression in obese patients: evidence for the potential role of endotoxin in the pathogenesis of non-alcoholic steatohepatitis. Obesity Surgery. 2007 Oct;**17**(10):1374-1380

8

CBX4 Expression and AFB1-Related Liver Cancer Prognosis

Qun-Ying Su, Jun Lu, Xiao-Ying Huang, Jin-Guang Yao, Xue-Min Wu, Bing-Chen Huang, Chao Wang, Qiang Xia and Xi-Dai Long

Abstract

Background: Previous studies have shown that chromobox 4 (CBX4) expression may involve in the progression of liver cancer, however, it is unclear whether it affects the prognosis of hepatocellular carcinoma (HCC) related to aflatoxin B1 (AFB1).

Methods: A retrospective study was conducted in the high AFB1 exposure areas and a total of 428 patients with HCC were included in the final survival analyses. AFB1 exposure levels and CBX4 expression in the tumor tissues were tested using enzyme-linked immunosorbent assay and immunohistochemistry, respectively. The effects of AFB1 and CBX4 on HCC outcome were elucidated by Kaplan–Meier survival method and Cox regression model.

Results: We found that the levels of AFB1 exposure and CBX4 expression in tumor tissues were significantly associated with some clinicopathological features such as microvessel density and tumor stage. Furthermore, both AFB1 and CBX4 significantly modified overall survival and tumor reoccurrence-free survival status of HCC. Additionally, some evidence of CBX4-AFB1 interaction affecting HCC prognosis was observed, with an interactive value of 1.98 for overall survival and 1.94 for tumor reoccurrence-free survival, respectively.

Conclusion: These results suggest that CBX4 expression might be a useful marker for AFB1-related HCC prognosis.

Keywords: CBX4, AFB1, HCC, prognosis

1. Introduction

Aflatoxin B1 (AFB1) is a type of secondary metabolite of *Aspergillus parasiticus* and *Aspergillus flavus*, and frequently contaminates a series of staple foods, such as ground nuts, and maize [1–3]. Once this type foods contaminated by AFB1 entered into human bodies, it is metabolized into its epoxides consisting of AFB1–8,9-exo-epoxide (AFBEX) and AFB1–8,9-endo-epoxide (AFBEN) by cytochrome P450 (CYP) metabolic system [3]. These products of AFB1, especially AFBEX, are characterized by high reaction, genic toxicity, and carcinogenicity [3]. Evidence from molecular epidemiology and animal models has shown that AFB1 is an important carcinogen inducing hepatocellular carcinoma (HCC) [4–10]. Mechanically, the carcinogenesis of AFB1-related HCC mainly involves in the formation of DNA damage (including AFB1-DNA adducts, DNA single-strand breaks, DNA double-strands breaks, and gene mutations), the inactivation of such tumor suppressor gene as TP53, and the activation of cancer genes such as Ras [3, 11–15]. Although some advance in the pathogenesis of AFB1-related HCC has obtained in the past decades [16–18], it is still far for us to elucidate more detailed mechanisms.

The chromobox 4 (Cbx4) (GenBank accession NO. 8535) consists of six exons and spans about 6.26 kb on chromosome 17q25.3. This gene encodes a 560-amino acid protein which is the important component of polycomb repressive complex 1 (PRC1) [19–22]. Functionally, CBX4 involves in PRC1-regulated transcription repression and post-translation modification [19–22]. Recently, increasing evidence has exhibited that the dysregulation of this gene may affect the carcinogenic process of some tumors such as HCC, colorectal cancer, breast cancer, and so on, and may be a significant prognostic biomarker [19, 21, 23–29]. However, it is not clear whether CBX4 modify the prognosis of AFB1-related HCC. Here, we conducted a hospital-based retrospective study to investigate whether the CBX4 expression in the cancerous tissues is associated with the outcome of HCC related to AFB1 expression in the Guangxi Region, a high AFB1 exposure area.

2. Materials and methods

2.1. Study population

Between January 2009 and December 2012, 428 consecutive patients with histopathologically confirmed hepatocarcinoma were recruited at the Divisions of Oncology and Pathology, the affiliated Hospitals of Guangxi Medical University and Youjiang Medical University for Nationalities. During the recruitment phase, only 5 cases refused to participate in the study (response rate 98.8%). All cases were from high AFB1 exposure areas, including Nanning, Bose, Tiandong, and Tianyang. After informed consent was obtained, surgically removed tumor samples were collected to analyze the amounts of AFB1-DNA adducts and CBX4 protein in the cancerous tissues. Additionally, all corresponding clinicopathological and survival following-up data were also collected in the hospitals as previously described methods [30-32]. In this study, the status of hepatitis B virus (HBV) and hepatitis C virus (HCV) infection was evaluated using serum hepatitis B surface antigen (HBsAg) and anti-HCV, respectively; whereas the grade and stage of tumor was elucidated using the Edmondson and Steiner (ES) grading system and the Barcelona Clinic Liver Cancer (BCLC) staging system, respectively. For survival analyses, the last follow-up day was set on December 31, 2017. The study protocol was carried out according to the approved guidelines by the Institutional Ethics Committee from the Affiliated Hospitals of Youjiang Medical University for Nationalities and Guangxi Medical University.

2.2. Microvessel density (MVD) assay

MVD in the cancerous tissues was assessed using the immunohistochemistry staining of CD31 as our previously descripted [30]. In this study, positive status of MVD was defined as microvessel counts more than 50 per ×200 magnifications.

2.3. AFB1 exposure data

AFB1 exposure levels were evaluated using the amounts of AFB1-DNA adducts in the cancerous tissues as our previously descripted [31, 32]. The amounts of AFB1-DNA adduct were tested using the competitive enzyme-linked immunosorbent assay. In this study, a value than less 1.00 μmol/mol DNA was considered as negative status for AFB1 exposure.

2.4. CBX4 expression assays

The level of CBX4 protein expression in cancerous tissues was elucidated using our previously published immunohistochemistry method [33, 34]. Briefly, the amounts of CBX4 protein were tested using anti-CBX4 antibody and calculated using immunoreactive score system (IRS). In the present study, positive CBX4 protein in cancerous tissues was define as IRS > 4.

2.5. Statistical analysis

Logistic regression model with enter method for variables (including all known clinicopathological features) was used for statistical comparison between groups. The odd ratios (ODs) and corresponding 95% confidence intervals (CIs) were calculated in this model for evaluating the association between clinicopathological features of HCCs and either AFB1 exposure or CBX4 expression. Kaplan–Meier survival method with log-rank test was used for statistical comparisons between different levels of AFB1 expression and CBX4 expression. Multivariate Cox regression model (with retread method based on likelihood ratio test) analyses were performed to calculate the risk strength of independent variates and prognostic values. In this study, all analyses were finished using the SPSS soft version 18.0 (SPSS Inc. Chicago, IL), and a *P*-value less than 0.05 was defined as statistical significance.

3. Results

3.1. The clinicopathological and survival features of HCC cases

Table 1 gave the clinicopathological characteristics of all cases, and a total of 428 patients with HCC were included in the final analyses. All cases were followed-up more than 5 years to obtain median survival time. During the follow-up period, 261 patients with

Variables	n	%
Total	428	100.0
Age, years		
Mean ± SE	47.9 ± 10.1	—
Range	30–75	—
Sex		
Man	290	68.9
Female	138	32.8
Ethnicity		
Han	229	54.4
Zhuang	199	47.3
HBV status		
HBsAg (−)	113	26.8
HBsAg (+)	315	74.8
HCV status		
anti-HCV (−)	378	89.8
anti-HCV (+)	50	11.9
Smoking status		
No	315	74.8
Yes	113	26.8
Drinking status		
No	304	72.2
Yes	124	29.5
AFP (ng/mL)		
≤ 20	154	36.6
> 20	274	65.1
Liver cirrhosis		
No	104	24.7
Yes	324	77.0
BCLC stage		
A	167	39.7
B	121	28.7
C	140	33.3
Tumor size		
≤ 3 cm	211	50.1
> 3 cm	217	51.5
MVD		
Negative	192	45.6

Variables	n	%
Positive	236	56.1
ES grade		
Low	226	53.7
High	202	48.0

Abbreviations: AFP, α-fetoprotein; BCLC, the Barcelona Clinic Liver Cancer staging system; ES, Edmondson and Steiner grading system; HBsAg, hepatitis B surface antigen; HBV, hepatitis B virus; HCV, hepatitis C virus; MVD, microvessel density.

Table 1. The clinic-pathological features of cases with hepatocellular carcinoma.

HCC featured cancer recurrences with 30.00 (22.20–37.80) months of median recurrence-free survival time (MRT), and 270 died with 45.00 (38.98–51.02) months of median overall survival time (MST).

3.2. The effects of AFB1 exposure on the clinicopathological features and the prognosis of HCC cases

In this study, the status of AFB1 exposure was elucidated using the amount of AFB1-DNA adducts in the cancerous tissues. Results from competitive ELISA exhibited the patients with HCC featured a 2.82 ± 1.60 μmol/mol DNA of AFB1 exposure level. To investigate the effects of AFB1 exposure on the clinicopathological features of HCC cases, we defined the amount of AFB1-DNA adducts ≤1.00 μmol/mol DNA as negative AFB1 exposure according to our previous published results [31, 32]. Our results showed that these patients with positive AFB1 status (AFB1-DNA adducts: > 1.00 μmol/mol DNA) had higher BCLC stage (adjusted OR = 2.09 and adjusted 95% CI = 1.04–4.24), bigger tumor size (adjusted OR = 69.06 and adjusted 95% CI = 33.62–141.86), and higher MVD (adjusted OR = 2.56 and adjusted 95% CI = 1.36–4.81) compared with those without positive AFB1 status (OR = 1) (**Table 2**). Additionally, we also found that the levels of AFB1 exposure were significantly associated with the age of patients with hepatocarcinoma (adjusted OR = 1.80, adjusted 95% CI = 1.22–2.66, and $P = 3.07\times10^{-3}$). However, AFB1 exposure was not correlated with other clinicopathological features of HCCs (**Table 2**).

Next, we investigated the effects of AFB1 exposure on the HCC prognosis using Kaplan–Meier survival model (**Figure 1A**). Results exhibited that HCC cases with negative AFB1 status (AFB1-DNA adducts: ≤ 1.00 μmol/mol DNA) featured longer median overall survival time (MST) [69.00 (55.41–82.59) months] and median tumor reoccurrence-free survival time (MRT) [70.00 (44.93–95.07) months] compared with those with positive AFB1 status [20.00 (13.04–26.96) months for MST and 13.00 (9.54–16.46) months for MRT, respectively].

3.3. The effects of CBX4 expression on the clinicopathological features and the prognosis of HCC cases

In the present, the levels of CBX4 protein in the cancerous tissues were amounted using immunohistochemistry technique with IRS counting system and the median IRS value was 5.58 for

	AFB1 (–)		AFB1 (+)			
Variables	n	%	n	%	OR (95% CI)	P_{trend}
Total	244	100.0	184	100.0	—	—
Age (years)						
≤ 48	148	60.7	86	46.7	Reference	
> 48	96	39.3	98	53.3	1.80 (1.22–2.66)	3.07×10^{-3}
Sex						
Man	160	65.6	130	70.7	Reference	
Female	84	34.4	54	29.3	1.13 (0.59–2.13)	0.72
Ethnicity						
Han	124	50.8	105	57.1	Reference	
Zhuang	120	49.2	79	42.9	0.99 (0.55–1.78)	0.98
HBsAg						
Negative	65	26.6	48	26.1	Reference	
Positive	179	73.4	136	73.9	1.19 (0.60–2.34)	0.61
anti-HCV						
Negative	217	88.9	161	87.5	Reference	
Positive	27	11.1	23	12.5	1.25 (0.51–3.09)	0.62
Smoking status						
No	181	74.2	134	72.8	Reference	
Yes	63	25.8	50	27.2	0.48 (0.12–1.85)	0.28
Drinking status						
No	174	71.3	130	70.7	Reference	
Yes	70	28.7	54	29.3	2.61 (0.69–9.89)	0.27
AFP (ng/mL)						
≤ 20	82	33.6	72	39.1	Reference	
> 20	162	66.4	112	60.9	1.00 (0.55–1.82)	0.99
Liver cirrhosis						
No	58	23.8	46	25.0	Reference	
Yes	186	76.2	138	75.0	0.84 (0.42–1.69)	0.63
BCLC stage						
A	113	46.3	54	29.3	Reference	
B	69	28.3	52	28.3	1.27 (0.61–2.61)	0.52
C	62	25.4	78	42.4	2.09 (1.04–4.24)	0.04
Tumor size						
≤ 3 cm	197	80.7	14	7.6	Reference	

	AFB1 (−)		AFB1 (+)			
Variables	n	%	n	%	OR (95% CI)	P_{trend}
> 3 cm	47	19.3	170	92.4	69.06 (33.62–141.86)	9.36×10^{-31}
MVD						
Negative	118	48.4	74	40.2	Reference	
Positive	126	51.6	110	59.8	2.56 (1.36–4.81)	3.46×10^{-3}
ES grade						
Low	129	52.9	97	52.7	Reference	
High	115	47.1	87	47.3	1.52 (0.64–2.07)	0.64

Abbreviations: AFP, α-fetoprotein; BCLC, the Barcelona Clinic Liver Cancer staging system; ES, Edmondson and Steiner grading system; HBsAg, hepatitis B surface antigen; HBV, hepatitis B virus; HCV, hepatitis C virus; MVD, microvessel density.

Table 2. The association between AFB1 exposure and clinic-pathological features of hepatocellular carcinoma cases.

all cases with hepatocarcinoma. According to the results from the CBX4 expression in cancerous tissues based on a large sample, IRS > 4 was regarded as positive CBX4 status. **Table 3** summarized the association between CBX4 expression in the cancerous tissues and the clinicopathological features, and results from multivariable logistic regression models proved that the levels of CBX4 expression were significantly related to increasing risk of liver cirrhosis (OR = 1.75 and 95% CI = 1.07–2.88), higher tumor stage (OR = 2.02 and 95% CI = 1.23–3.33), and increasing MVD (OR = 2.66 and 95% CI = 1.74–4.07). However, CBX4 expression levels did not affect other clinicopathological features such as tumor size, grade, AFP, and so on.

Results from Kaplan–Meier survival analyses further displayed that HCC patients with positive status of CBX4 protein expression had short MST [22.00 (18.00–26.00) months] and MRT [16.00 (10.88–21.12) months] compared with those with negative-status CBX4 protein [69.00 (52.75–85.25) months for MST and 48.00 (23.69–72.31) months for MRT, respectively] (**Figure 1B**). Taken together, CBX4 expression in the cancerous might be an important biomarker for HCC prognosis.

3.4. The joint effects of AFB1 exposure and CBX4 expression on HCC prognosis

Given that both AFB1 exposure and CBX4 expression modified HCC outcome, we questioned whether CBX4 expression interacted with AFB1 expression, and whether this interaction affected the prognosis of hepatocarcinoma. First, we analyzed the joint effects of AFB1 exposure and CBX4 expression on the prognosis of patients with HCC using Kaplan–Meier survival model (**Figure 2**). In this model, the combination of AFB1 exposure and CBX4 expression was divided into four groups: cases with negative-AFB1 and negative-CBX4 status (AC-1), cases with negative-AFB1 and positive-CBX4 status (AC-2), cases with positive-AFB1 and negative-CBX4 status (AC-3), and cases with positive-AFB1 and positive-CBX4 status (AC-4). We found MST and MRT gradually decreased from AC-1 to AC-4 (89.00–11.00 months for MST and more than 125.00–7.00 months for MRT, respectively) (**Figure 2A** and **B**).

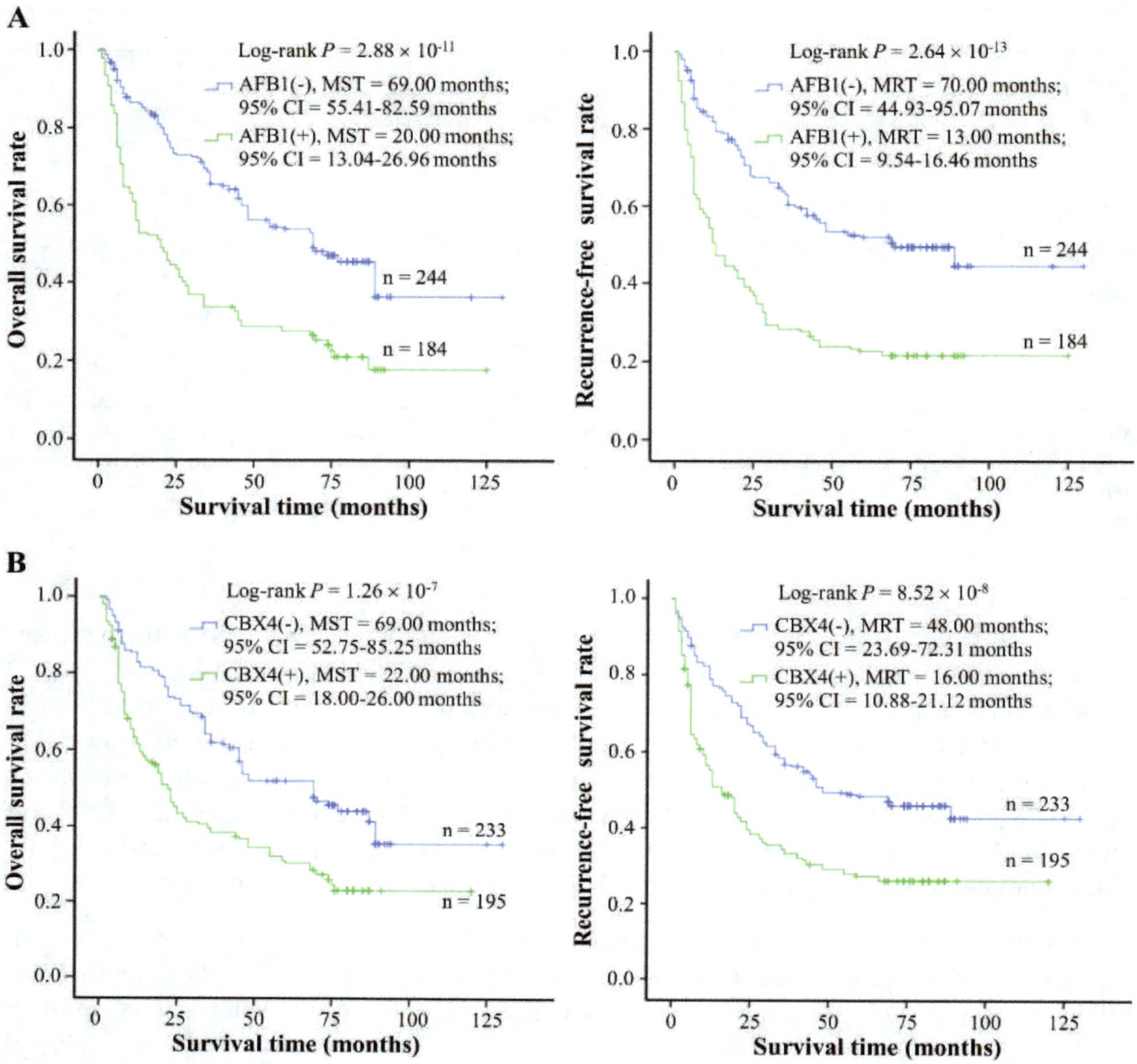

Figure 1. Both AFB1 exposure and CBX4 expression significantly correlating with hepatocellular carcinoma. AFB1 exposure levels were elucidated using the amount of AFB1-DNA adducts in the cancerous tissues. The CBX4 expression in cancerous tissues from 428 patients with hepatocellular carcinoma was tested using immunohistochemistry technique based on immunoreactive score system (IRS). To analyze, the levels of CBX4 expression were divided into two groups: Negative group (IRS ≤ 4) and positive group (IRS > 4). AFB1 exposure (A) and CBX4 expression (B) are associated with overall survival (left) and tumor recurrence-free survival (right) of hepatocellular carcinoma. Cumulative hazard function was plotted by Kaplan–Meier's methodology, and *P* value was calculated with two-sided log-rank tests. ***Abbreviations:*** CBX4, chromobox 4; MST, median overall survival time; MRT, median tumor recurrence-free survival time; CI, confidence interval.

We next finished multivariable Cox regression analyses based on the retread method with likelihood ratio test (including significant variables and all kinds of possible interactive variables) (**Table 4**), and found both AFB1 exposure and CBX4 expression in the cancerous tissues were independent prognostic factors. Furthermore, we also observed that AFB1 exposure significantly and multiplicatively interacted with CBX4 protein expression (interactive values, 1.98 for overall survival and 1.94 for tumor reoccurrence-free survival, respectively).

	CBX4 (–)		CBX4 (+)			
Variables	n	%	n	%	OR (95% CI)	P_{trend}
Total	233	100.0	195	100.0	—	—
Age (years)						
≤ 48	136	58.4	98	50.3	Reference	
> 48	97	41.6	97	49.7	1.35 (0.89–2.05)	0.67
Sex						
Man	160	68.7	130	66.7	Reference	
Female	73	31.3	65	33.3	1.14 (0.73–1.78)	0.57
Ethnicity						
Han	121	51.9	108	55.4	Reference	
Zhuang	112	48.1	87	44.6	0.96 (0.63–1.46)	0.85
HBsAg						
Negative	65	27.9	48	24.6	Reference	
Positive	168	72.1	148	75.9	1.17 (0.73–1.89)	0.51
anti-HCV						
Negative	209	89.7	169	86.7	Reference	
Positive	24	10.3	26	13.3	1.43 (0.74–2.75)	0.29
Smoking status						
No	176	75.5	139	71.3	Reference	
Yes	57	24.5	56	28.7	1.04 (0.37–2.93)	0.94
Drinking status						
No	172	73.8	132	67.7	Reference	
Yes	61	26.2	63	32.3	1.40 (0.51–3.83)	0.51
AFP (ng/mL)						
≤ 20	84	36.1	70	35.9	Reference	
> 20	149	63.9	125	64.1	1.11 (0.72–1.70)	0.64
Liver cirrhosis						
No	69	29.6	35	17.9	Reference	
Yes	164	70.4	160	82.1	1.75 (1.07–2.88)	0.03
BCLC stage						
A	112	48.1	55	28.2	Reference	
B	58	24.9	63	32.3	1.94 (1.16–3.24)	0.01
C	63	27.0	77	39.5	2.02 (1.23–3.33)	5.79×10^{-3}
Tumor size						
≤ 3 cm	121	51.9	90	46.2	Reference	
> 3 cm	112	48.1	105	53.8	1.24 (0.81–1.88)	0.33

	CBX4 (–)		CBX4 (+)			
MVD						
Negative	131	56.2	61	31.3	Reference	
Positive	102	43.8	134	68.7	2.66 (1.74–4.07)	6.65×10^{-6}
ES grade						
Low	132	56.7	94	48.2	Reference	
High	101	43.3	101	51.8	1.39 (0.92–2.11)	0.12

Abbreviations: AFP, α-fetoprotein; BCLC, the Barcelona Clinic Liver Cancer staging system; CBX4, chromobox 4; ES, Edmondson and Steiner grading system; HBsAg, hepatitis B surface antigen; HBV, hepatitis B virus; HCV, hepatitis C virus; MVD, microvessel density.

Table 3. The correlation between CBX4 expression and clinical pathological features of hepatocellular carcinoma.

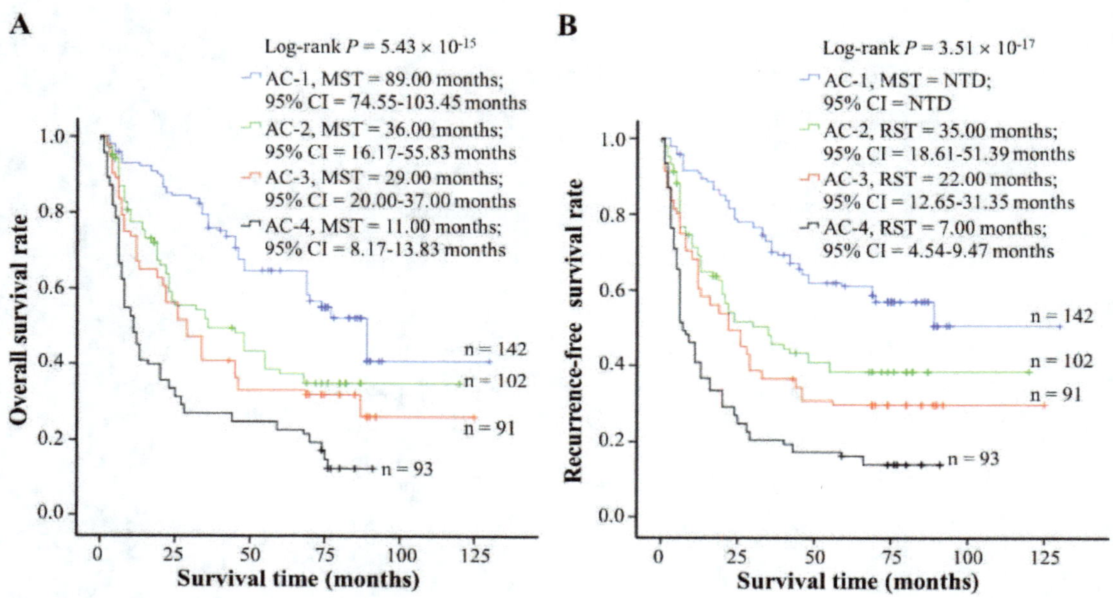

Figure 2. Survival analysis of CBX4 expression binding AFB1 exposure levels. The combination of CBX4 expression and AFB1 exposure was divided into 4 strata: Cases with negative-AFB1 and negative-CBX4 status (AC-1), cases with negative-AFB1 and positive-CBX4 status (AC-2), cases with positive-AFB1 and negative-CBX4 status (AC-3), and cases with positive-AFB1 and positive-CBX4 status (AC-4). This kind of joint analyses showed that interactive effects on the overall survival (A) and tumor recurrence-free survival (B) of patients with hepatocarcinoma. Cumulative hazard function was plotted by Kaplan–Meier's methodology, and *P* value was calculated with two-sided log-rank tests. ***Abbreviations:*** CBX4, chromobox 4; MST, median overall survival time; MRT, median tumor recurrence-free survival time; CI, confidence interval.

4. Discussion

In Guangxi Zhuang Autonomous Region, HCC is the most malignant disease. In the past decades, the annual incidence and death rate (AIR and ADR) of hepatocarcinoma in this area has been reported to remarkably increase (up to about 100–200 per 10,000 for AIR about 50 per 10,000 for ADR) [1]. Lots of epidemiological studies have shown that AFB1 exposure is

	OS		RFS	
Variables	HR (95%CI)	Ptrend	HR (95%CI)	Ptrend
AFB1	2.09 (1.64–2.65)	2.34×10^{-9}	2.29 (1.79–2.93)	3.82×10^{-11}
CBX4	1.76 (1.38–2.24)	4.66×10^{-6}	1.80 (1.41–2.30)	3.12×10^{-6}
AFB1 × CBX4	1.98 (1.61–2.59)	9.43×10^{-7}	1.94 (1.58–2.54)	8.17×10^{-5}

HR and corresponding 95% CI was calculated using multivariable Cox regression model (with retread method based on likelihood ratio test). ***Abbreviations:*** AFB1, aflatoxin B1; CBX4, chromobox 4; OS, overall survival; RFS, tumor reoccurrence-free survival; HR, hazard ratio; CI, confidence interval.

Table 4. The effects of AFB1 and CBX4 expression on the prognosis of cases with hepatocellular carcinoma.

the most important cause for this high AIR and ADR [1]. AFB1 is a known I-type chemical carcinogen produced by *Aspergillus parasiticus* and *Aspergillus flavus*, and has been proved to involve in the carcinogenesis and progression of HCC [4–10]. This carcinogenicity of AFB1 mainly results from its metabolic product binding to DNA and inducing DNA damage. Among DNA damage types induced by AFB1, AFB1-DNA adducts are very important, because of its non-enzymatic, time-dependent, and apparent persistent characteristics in the genomic DNA strands [3, 35]. Our previous studies have exhibited that AFB1-DNA adducts, especially from liver tissues, are highly associated not only with increasing HCC risk, but with the poor prognosis of HCC [2, 31, 36–39]. Here, our data displayed that increasing levels of AFB1 exposure significantly correlated with higher tumor stage, increasing tumor size, and higher MVD; furthermore, AFB1 was also poor prognostic marker for HCC. Taken together, these data suggest that AFB1 may involve in the startup and progression of HCC.

Because several previous studies have exhibited that CBX4 can progress tumorigenesis via several signal pathways, including CBX4/HIF-1α/VEGF pathway [20, 25, 26, 34], CBX4/HDAC3/Runx2 pathway [21], CBX4/P63 pathway [22], CBX4/miR-195 pathway [40], CBX4/CtIP pathway [41], and CBX4/P53 pathway [42, 43], here we investigated the effects of CXB4 expression on HCC outcome. We not only found that increasing CBX4 expression in the cancerous tissues is a poor prognostic biomarker for HCC, but this increasing expression is associated with clinicopathological features such as tumor size, tumor stage, and angiogenesis. Supporting our findings, several recent reports further prove that CBX4 can govern the several biofunctions of HCC, including proliferation, invasion and metastasis, angiogenesis, and metastasis [20, 25, 26, 34, 40, 44].

Noticeably, some evidence of the joint effects of CBX4 and AFB1 on HCC outcome was observed in the prognostic analyses based on the gene-environmental joint effects. Our results showed that CBX4 expression significantly and multiplicatively interacted with AFB1 exposure levels, and that this multiplicative interaction remarkably increased the death risk and tumor reoccurrence risk of patients with HCC. Recently, two studies from high AFB1 exposure areas have also reported that the dysregulation of CBX4 in the cancerous tissues from patients with hepatocarcinoma increases MVD, promotes angiogenesis, and increases sensitivity of HCC cells on anti-cancer drugs [33, 34]. Altogether, these results are indicative of the angiogenesis induced by CBX4 involving in the progression of AFB1-related HCC.

In summary, our present study proposes that CBX4 expression in the cancerous tissues can act as a valuable biomarker for AFB1-related HCC. However, several limitations confine the value of this study. First, because of the hospital-based retrospective design, selective bias may take place. Second, because liver damage itself affects AFB1 metabolite and may increase the amount of AFB1-DNA adducts, the prognostic and interactive values of AFB1 and CBX4 may be underestimated. Finally, we did not do functional and mechanical analyses. Therefore, detailed functional analyses deserve further evaluation on the basis of the foresighted design and the combination of AFB1 and CBX4.

Conflicts of interest and source of funding

The authors declare no competing financial interests. This study was supported in part by the National Natural Science Foundation of China (Nos. 81,760,502, 81,572,353, 81,372,639, 81,472,243, 81,660,495, and 81,460,423), the Innovation Program of Guangxi Municipal Education Department (Nos. 201204LX674 and 201204LX324), Innovation Program of Guangxi Health Department (No. Z2013781), the Natural Science Foundation of Guangxi (Nos. 2017GXNSFAA198002, 2017GXNSFGA198002, 2016GXNSFDA380003, 2015GXNSFAA139223, 2013GXNSFAA019251, 2014GXNSFDA118021, and 2014GXNSFAA118144), Research Program of Guangxi "Zhouyue Scholar" (No. 2017–2038), Research Program of Guangxi Specially invited Expert (No. 2017-6th), Research Program of Guangxi Clinic Research Center of Hepatobiliary Diseases (No.AD17129025), and Open Research Program from Molecular Immunity Study Room Involving in Acute & Severe Diseases in Guangxi Colleges and Universities (Nos. kfkt20160062 and kfkt20160063).

Abbreviations

AFB1	aflatoxin B1
AFBEX	AFB1–8,9-exo-epoxide
AFBEN	AFB1–8,9-endo-epoxide
BCLC	The Barcelona Clinic Liver Cancer
CBX4	chromobox 4
CI	confidence interval
CYP	cytochrome P450
ES	The Edmondson and Steiner
HBV	hepatitis B virus
HCC	hepatocellular carcinoma
HCV	hepatitis C virus

HBsAg	hepatitis B surface antigen
IRS	immunoreactive score system
MRT	median tumor reoccurrence-free survival time
MST	median overall survival time
MVD	microvessel density
OD	odd ratio.

Author details

Qun-Ying Su[1], Jun Lu[2], Xiao-Ying Huang[1], Jin-Guang Yao[1], Xue-Min Wu[1], Bing-Chen Huang[1], Chao Wang[3], Qiang Xia[2] and Xi-Dai Long[1,2,4*]

*Address all correspondence to: sjtulongxd@263.net

1 Department of Pathology, The Affiliated Hospital of Youjiang Medical University for Nationalities, Baise, China

2 Department of Liver Surgery, Renji Hospital, School of Medicine, Shanghai Jiao Tong University, Shanghai, China

3 Department of Digestive Medicine, The Affiliated Hospital of Youjiang Medical University for Nationalities, Baise, China

4 Guangxi Clinic Research Center of Hepatobiliary Diseases, Baise, China

References

[1] Wu XM, Xi ZF, Lu J, Wang XZ, Zhang TQ, Huang XY, Yao JG, Wang C, Wei ZH, Luo CY, Huang BC, Xu QQ, Yang WP, Xia Q, Long XD. Genetic single nucleotide polymorphisms (GSNPs) in the DNA repair genes and hepatocellular carcinoma related to aflatoxin B1 among Guangxiese population. In: Parine NR, editor. Genetic Polymorphisms. Vol. 1. Rijeka, Croatia: InTech; 2017. pp. 97-119. DOI: 10.5772/intechopen.69530

[2] Long XD, Yao JD, Yang Q, Huang CH, Liao P, Nong LG, Tang YJ, Huang XY, Wang C, Wu XM, Huang BC, Ban FZ, Zeng LX, Ma Y, Zhai B, Zhang JQ, Xue F, Lu CX, Xia Q. Polymorphisms of DNA repair genes and toxicological effects of aflatoxin B1 exposure. In: Faulkner AG, editor. Aflatoxins: Food Sources, Occurrence and Toxicological Effects. 1st ed. New York: Nova Science Publishers; 2014. pp. 125-156. DOI: 978-1-63117-298-4

[3] Kew MC. Aflatoxins as a cause of hepatocellular carcinoma. Journal of Gastrointestinal and Liver Diseases. 2013;**22**:305-310

[4] Rushing BR, Selim MI. Adduction to arginine detoxifies aflatoxin B1 by eliminating genotoxicity and altering in vitro toxicokinetic profiles. Oncotarget. 2018;**9**:4559-4570. DOI: 10.18632/oncotarget.23382

[5] Xiang X, Qin HG, You XM, Wang YY, Qi LN, Ma L, Xiang BD, Zhong JH, Li LQ. Expression of P62 in hepatocellular carcinoma involving hepatitis B virus infection and aflatoxin B1 exposure. Cancer Medicine. 2017;**6**:2357-2369. DOI: 10.1002/cam4.1176

[6] Weng MW, Lee HW, Choi B, Wang HT, Hu Y, Mehta M, Desai D, Amin S, Zheng Y, Tang MS. AFB1 hepatocarcinogenesis is via lipid peroxidation that inhibits DNA repair, sensitizes mutation susceptibility and induces aldehyde-DNA adducts at p53 mutational hotspot codon 249. Oncotarget. 2017;**8**:18213-18226. DOI: 10.18632/oncotarget.15313

[7] Narkwa PW, Blackbourn DJ, Mutocheluh M. Aflatoxin B1 inhibits the type 1 interferon response pathway via STAT1 suggesting another mechanism of hepatocellular carcinoma. Infectious Agents and Cancer. 2017;**12**:17. DOI: 10.1186/s13027-017-0127-8

[8] Maurya BK, Trigun SK. Fisetin attenuates AKT associated growth promoting events in AflatoxinB1 induced hepatocellular carcinoma. Anti-Cancer Agents in Medicinal Chemistry. 2017. DOI: 10.2174/1871520618666171229223335. E-pub Ahead of Print

[9] Huang MN, Yu W, Teoh WW, Ardin M, Jusakul A, Ng AWT, Boot A, Abedi-Ardekani B, Villar S, Myint SS, Othman R, Poon SL, Heguy A, Olivier M, Hollstein M, Tan P, Teh BT, Sabapathy K, Zavadil J, Rozen SG. Genome-scale mutational signatures of aflatoxin in cells, mice, and human tumors. Genome Research. 2017;**27**:1475-1486. DOI: 10.1101/gr.220038.116

[10] Chu YJ, Yang HI, Wu HC, Liu J, Wang LY, Lu SN, Lee MH, Jen CL, You SL, Santella RM, Chen CJ. Aflatoxin B1 exposure increases the risk of cirrhosis and hepatocellular carcinoma in chronic hepatitis B virus carriers. International Journal of Cancer. 2017;**141**:711-720. DOI: 10.1002/ijc.30782

[11] Chawanthayatham S, Valentine CC, 3rd, Fedeles BI, Fox EJ, Loeb LA, Levine SS, Slocum SL, Wogan GN, Croy RG, Essigmann JM. Mutational spectra of aflatoxin B1 in vivo establish biomarkers of exposure for human hepatocellular carcinoma. Proceedings of the National Academy of Sciences of the United States of America. 2017;**114**:E3101-E3109. DOI: 10.1073/pnas.1700759114

[12] Umesha S, Manukumar HM, Chandrasekhar B, Shivakumara P, Shiva Kumar J, Raghava S, Avinash P, Shirin M, Bharathi TR, Rajini SB, Nandhini M, Vinaya Rani GG, Shobha M, Prakash HS. Aflatoxins and food pathogens: Impact of biologically active aflatoxins and their control strategies. Journal of the Science of Food and Agriculture. 2017;**97**:1698-1707. DOI: 10.1002/jsfa.8144

[13] Sarma UP, Bhetaria PJ, Devi P, Varma A. Aflatoxins: Implications on health. Indian Journal of Clinical Biochemistry. 2017;**32**:124-133. DOI: 10.1007/s12291-017-0649-2

[14] Kowalska A, Walkiewicz K, Koziel P, Muc-Wierzgon M. Aflatoxins: Characteristics and impact on human health. Postępy Higieny i Medycyny Doświadczalnej (Online). 2017;**71**:315-327. DOI: 10.5604/01.3001.0010.3816

[15] Woloshuk CP, Shim WB. Aflatoxins, fumonisins, and trichothecenes: A convergence of knowledge. FEMS Microbiology Reviews. 2013;**37**:94-109. DOI: 10.1111/1574-6976.12009

[16] Khlangwiset P, Shephard GS, Wu F. Aflatoxins and growth impairment: A review. Critical Reviews in Toxicology. 2011;**41**:740-755. DOI: 10.3109/10408444.2011.575766

[17] Wu Q, Jezkova A, Yuan Z, Pavlikova L, Dohnal V, Kuca K. Biological degradation of aflatoxins. Drug Metabolism Reviews. 2009;**41**:1-7. DOI: 10.1080/03602530802563850

[18] Villar S, Ortiz-Cuaran S, Abedi-Ardekani B, Gouas D, Nogueira da Costa A, Plymoth A, Khuhaprema T, Kalalak A, Sangrajrang S, Friesen MD, Groopman JD, Hainaut P. Aflatoxin-induced TP53 R249S mutation in hepatocellular carcinoma in Thailand: Association with tumors developing in the absence of liver cirrhosis. PLoS One. 2012; **7**:e37707. DOI: 10.1371/journal.pone.0037707

[19] Zeng JS, Zhang ZD, Pei L, Bai ZZ, Yang Y, Yang H, Tian QH. CBX4 exhibits oncogenic activities in breast cancer via Notch1 signaling. The International Journal of Biochemistry & Cell Biology. 2018;**95**:1-8. DOI: 10.1016/j.biocel.2017.12.006

[20] Yang J, Cheng D, Zhu B, Zhou S, Ying T, Yang Q. Chromobox homolog 4 is positively correlated to tumor growth, survival and activation of HIF-1alpha signaling in human osteosarcoma under normoxic condition. Journal of Cancer. 2016;**7**:427-435. DOI: 10.7150/jca.13749

[21] Wang X, Li L, Wu Y, Zhang R, Zhang M, Liao D, Wang G, Qin G, Xu RH, Kang T. CBX4 suppresses metastasis via recruitment of HDAC3 to the Runx2 promoter in colorectal carcinoma. Cancer Research. 2016;**76**:7277-7289. DOI: 10.1158/0008-5472.CAN-16-2100

[22] Cohen I, Ezhkova E. Cbx4: A new guardian of p63's domain of epidermal control. The Journal of Cell Biology. 2016;**212**:9-11. DOI: 10.1083/jcb.201512032

[23] Liang YK, Lin HY, Chen CF, Zeng. Prognostic values of distinct CBX family members in breast cancer. Oncotarget. 2017;**8**:92375-92387. DOI: 10.18632/oncotarget.21325

[24] Lin FM, Kumar S, Ren J, Karami S, Bahnassy S, Li Y, Zheng X, Wang J, Bawa-Khalfe T. SUMOylation of HP1alpha supports association with ncRNA to define responsiveness of breast cancer cells to chemotherapy. Oncotarget. 2016;**7**:30336-30349. DOI: 10.18632/oncotarget.8733

[25] Mei Z, Jiao H, Wang W, Li J, Chen G, Xu Y. Polycomb chromobox 4 enhances migration and pulmonary metastasis of hepatocellular carcinoma cell line MHCC97L. Science China. Life Sciences. 2014;**57**:610-617. DOI: 10.1007/s11427-014-4663-9

[26] Li J, Xu Y, Jiao H, Wang W, Mei Z, Chen G. Sumoylation of hypoxia inducible factor-1alpha and its significance in cancer. Science China. Life Sciences. 2014;**57**:657-664. DOI: 10.1007/s11427-014-4685-3

[27] Oh Y, Chung KC. Small ubiquitin-like modifier (SUMO) modification of zinc finger protein 131 potentiates its negative effect on estrogen signaling. The Journal of Biological Chemistry. 2012;**287**:17517-17529. DOI: 10.1074/jbc.M111.336354

[28] Ismail IH, Gagne JP, Caron MC, McDonald D, Xu Z, Masson JY, Poirier GG, Hendzel MJ. CBX4-mediated SUMO modification regulates BMI1 recruitment at sites of DNA damage. Nucleic Acids Research. 2012;**40**:5497-5510. DOI: 10.1093/nar/gks222

[29] Vandamme J, Volkel P, Rosnoblet C, Le Faou P, Angrand PO. Interaction proteomics analysis of polycomb proteins defines distinct PRC1 complexes in mammalian cells. Molecular & Cellular Proteomics. 2011;**10**:M110-M002642. DOI: 10.1074/mcp.M110.002642

[30] Liu YX, Long XD, Xi ZF, Ma Y, Huang XY, Yao JG, Wang C, Xing TY, Xia Q. MicroRNA-24 modulates aflatoxin B1-related hepatocellular carcinoma prognosis and tumorigenesis. BioMed Research International. 2014;**2014**:482926. DOI: 10.1155/2014/482926

[31] Long XD, Yao JG, Zeng Z, Ma Y, Huang XY, Wei ZH, Liu M, Zhang JJ, Xue F, Zhai B, Xia Q. Polymorphisms in the coding region of X-ray repair complementing group 4 and aflatoxin B1-related hepatocellular carcinoma. Hepatology. 2013;**58**:171-181. DOI: 10.1002/hep.26311

[32] Long XD, Ma Y, Huang HD, Yao JG, Qu de Y, Lu YL. Polymorphism of XRCC1 and the frequency of mutation in codon 249 of the p53 gene in hepatocellular carcinoma among Guangxi population, china. Molecular Carcinogenesis. 2008;**47**:295-300. DOI: 10.1002/mc.20384

[33] Jiao HK, Xu Y, Li J, Wang W, Mei Z, Long XD, Chen GQ. Prognostic significance of Cbx4 expression and its beneficial effect for transarterial chemoembolization in hepatocellular carcinoma. Cell Death & Disease. 2015;**6**:e1689. DOI: 10.1038/cddis.2015.57

[34] Li J, Xu Y, Long XD, Wang W, Jiao HK, Mei Z, Yin QQ, Ma LN, Zhou AW, Wang LS, Yao M, Xia Q, Chen GQ. Cbx4 governs HIF-1alpha to potentiate angiogenesis of hepatocellular carcinoma by its SUMO E3 ligase activity. Cancer Cell. 2014;**25**:118-131. DOI: 10.1016/j.ccr.2013.12.008

[35] Kensler TW, Roebuck BD, Wogan GN, Groopman JD. Aflatoxin: A 50-year odyssey of mechanistic and translational toxicology. Toxicological Sciences. 2011;**120**(Suppl 1):S28-S48. DOI: 10.1093/toxsci/kfq283

[36] Yao JG, Huang XY, Long XD. Interaction of DNA repair gene polymorphisms and aflatoxin B1 in the risk of hepatocellular carcinoma. International Journal of Clinical and Experimental Pathology. 2014;**7**:6231-6244. DOI: 10.2016/1936-2625.25337275

[37] Long XD, Zhao D, Wang C, Huang XY, Yao JG, Ma Y, Wei ZH, Liu M, Zeng LX, Mo XQ, Zhang JJ, Xue F, Zhai B, Xia Q. Genetic polymorphisms in DNA repair genes XRCC4 and XRCC5 and aflatoxin B1-related hepatocellular carcinoma. Epidemiology. 2013;**24**:671-681. DOI: 10.1097/EDE.0b013e31829d2744

[38] Long XD, Yao JG, Zeng Z, Huang CH, Huang ZS, Huang YZ, Ban FZ, Huang XY, Yao LM, Fan LD, Fu GH. DNA repair capacity-related to genetic polymorphisms of DNA repair genes and aflatoxin B1-related hepatocellular carcinoma among Chinese population. In: Kruman I, editor. DNA Repair. Rijeka, Croatia: InTech; 2011. pp. 505-524. DOI: 10.5772/20792

[39] Long XD, Ma Y, Zhou YF, Ma AM, Fu GH. Polymorphism in xeroderma pigmentosum complementation group C codon 939 and aflatoxin B1-related hepatocellular carcinoma in the Guangxi population. Hepatology. 2010;**52**:1301-1309. DOI: 10.1002/hep.23807

[40] Zheng C, Li J, Wang Q, Liu W, Zhou J, Liu R, Zeng Q, Peng X, Huang C, Cao P, Cao K. microRNA-195 functions as a tumor suppressor by inhibiting CBX4 in hepatocellular carcinoma. Oncology Reports. 2015;**33**:1115-1122. DOI: 10.3892/or.2015.3734

[41] Soria-Bretones I, Cepeda-Garcia C, Checa-Rodriguez C, Heyer V, Reina-San-Martin B, Soutoglou E, Huertas P. DNA end resection requires constitutive sumoylation of CtIP by CBX4. Nature Communications. 2017;**8**:113. DOI: 10.1038/s41467-017-00183-6

[42] Peuget S, Bonacci T, Soubeyran P, Iovanna J, Dusetti NJ. Oxidative stress-induced p53 activity is enhanced by a redox-sensitive TP53INP1 SUMOylation. Cell Death and Differentiation. 2014;**21**:1107-1118. DOI: 10.1038/cdd.2014.28

[43] Pelisch F, Pozzi B, Risso G, Munoz MJ, Srebrow A. DNA damage-induced heterogeneous nuclear ribonucleoprotein K sumoylation regulates p53 transcriptional activation. The Journal of Biological Chemistry. 2012;**287**:30789-30799. DOI: 10.1074/jbc.M112.390120

[44] Wang B, Tang J, Liao D, Wang G, Zhang M, Sang Y, Cao J, Wu Y, Zhang R, Li S, Ding W, Zhang G, Kang T. Chromobox homolog 4 is correlated with prognosis and tumor cell growth in hepatocellular carcinoma. Annals of Surgical Oncology. 2013;**20**(Suppl 3): S684-S692. DOI: 10.1245/s10434-013-3171-7

9

What Chinese Medicine can do for Liver Cancer?

Feiyu Chen, Ning Wang and Yibin Feng

Abstract

Liver cancer is an international problem, especially in Asian countries. It is because that most liver cancers are already late stage when they are diagnosed, and also most liver cancers have various previous chronic liver diseases induced by alcoholic, virus, and steatosis, etc. In recent years, laboratory and clinical studies focusing on liver cancer by Chinese medicine has been extensively studied. What Chinese medicine treatment formalities can be used in liver cancer? How Chinese medicine can be employed in treatment of liver cancer? What Chinese medicine can contribute to liver cancer? To answer these questions in this chapter, we will review and discuss treatment of liver cancer from Chinese medicine's perspective with scientific evidences as following three parts: (1) Chinese medicine as the source of discovering new treatment for liver cancer, (2) Chinese medicine as a complementary treatment of liver cancer, and (3) to discuss future research and application of Chinese medicine in liver cancer treatment.

Keywords: Chinese medicine, liver cancer, source of drug discovery, complementary medicine, clinical application

1. Introduction

Liver cancer is one of the most common malignancies with high morbidity and mortality all over the world. Despite the number of new cases of liver cancer appears to be plateauing, large population size of liver cancer patients, especially in China, still greatly contributes to the global cancer deaths [1]. Hepatocellular carcinoma (HCC) is the most commonly observed histological subgroup of primary liver cancer, accounting for 70–90% of the cases. With a global status quo that 746,000 deaths only in 2012 and 10.1 new cases diagnosed within every 10,000 people, HCC ranks the sixth lethal malignancy and the third leading cause of cancer-related deaths [2].

Over the past decades, the clinical approaches to treat liver cancer have considerably evolved. Patients can benefit from partial hepatectomy, radiotherapy, systemic or local chemotherapy, liver transplantation, and radiofrequency ablative surgery. Nevertheless, numerous adverse events and dismal outcomes still seriously affect the life quality of patients. On the background of shortcomings, developing improved preventive and therapeutic strategy is urgently necessary.

Considering its low toxicity and high activity, Chinese medicine has been deemed as one of the prominent complementary and alternative approaches in tumor therapy. As unique biomedical and pharmaceutical resources, Chinese medicine owns the ability of providing better treatment for liver cancer, either alone or in integrative way [3]. According to Hong Kong Liver Cancer staging system in a population-based investigation, for patients with Va/Vb (tumor status being early, intermediate or locally advanced), the most frequent treatment was Chinese medicine [4]. Another cohort study in Taiwan reported that Chinese medicine users exhibited significant lower risk to suffer HCC, which supported the application of Chinese medicine into the clinical practice of liver cancer treatment [5]. A recent meta-analysis showed that add-on therapy with Chinese medicine regimens in HCC could reduce side effects, activate tumor responses, and improve overall survival. Moreover, cancer subjects were reported to be more inclined to integrating Chinese medicine regimens with conventional therapies rather than conventional treatment only [6]. In this regard, Chinese medicine has been considered as a potential curative choice of method for controlling the proliferation of liver cancer, and thus improving the quality of life and prolonging overall survival of the patients.

Historically, the medical foundation of Chinese medicine can be traced back to 5000 years ago. With contributions and dedications of Chinese medical people in modern and old times, Chinese medicine has been gradually evolved and accepted by the mainstream society. In particular, accompanying the tide of Chinese immigration and cultural communication, Chinese medicine has been approved worldwide and employed in clinical practice in at least 183 countries [7]. Even though many regions have the regulations imposing restrictions to ensure that Chinese medicine is beneficial to liver cancer patients instead of being harmful to public health, the evidence-based guideline has not been covered every field [8, 9].

However, due to its effective curative outcomes in real life, the usage of Chinese medicine in various forms of single compounds, extracted fractions, and composite formulae has attracted a great deal of attentions over the past few decades. Chinese medicine may be capable of retarding liver cancer progression with its multitargets and coordinated intervention actions, either in combination with conventional therapies or radiation alone. Here, we retrospectively reviewed and analyzed the functional roles of Chinese medicine in the treatment of liver cancer.

2. Chinese medicine as the source of discovering new treatment for liver cancer

As mentioned above, currently there are various therapies for liver neoplasm. However, the overall survival rate of patients still remains unsatisfactory on account of high invasiveness and metastasis, chemotherapeutic resistance, and so on. Chinese medicine, in various forms including composite formulae, extracted fractions, monomers, and their derivatives, has been pursued as ideal and novel sources for therapeutic agent development for cancer.

2.1. Single compounds from Chinese medicine for the treatment of liver cancer

Berberine is a natural product in many Chinese medicinal herbs, especially *Coptidis rhizoma,* which has been extensively studied and reported to show the antitumor action mostly by modulation of a number of different signal transductions. Currently, scholars have explored the antitumor action of berberine in liver cancer by various different strategies. For instance, in our laboratory, we found that berberine-induced cell death and tumor growth inhibition in xenograft model were demonstrated and mechanism was revealed that miR-23a might play a mediated role in berberine-suppressing HCC growth [10]. Also, cyclin D1 overexpression is mainly responsible for tumor expansion, metastasis as well as angiogenesis. Berberine was found to repress the expression of cyclin D1 via proteasomal degradation in HCC [11]. In addition, our group identified that berberine exerted antimigratory and anti-invasive abilities in HCC cells involving the upregulation of PAI-1 and downregulation of uPA [12]. On the other hand, our group described for the first time that berberine could trigger autophagic cell death, in which the compound was shown to activate Beclin-1 and suppress mTOR [13]. Actually, lung metastases in liver cancer are also a serious problem for patients, and we identified that the anti-invasive and antiproliferative actions of berberine in liver cancer was at least in part involved in the downregulation of Id-1, revealing a new anti-invasive mechanism [14]. Hence, berberine is predicted as a new and potent natural molecule targeting liver cancer.

Flavonoids commonly exist in Chinese medicine and could be isolated from many different kinds of herbal medicine. In recent years, the precise molecular mechanism underlying the obvious antiliver tumor effect of flavonoids has been studied. For example, hydroxysafflor yellow A (HSYA), a kind of flavonoid extracted from *Carthamus tinctorius* L. owns the ability of antitumor. It was demonstrated that HSYA could result in angiogenesis inhibition of HCC by blocking signaling pathways of ERK/MAPK and NF-κB in comparison with negative control group. More interestingly, spleen and thymus indexes have been demonstrated to be improved, suggesting improvement on the immune system by HSYA [15]. Oroxin B (OB) is one of the flavonoids isolated from *Oroxylum indicum* (L.) Vent. Li et al. investigated the antitumor effects of OB on HCC cell line SMMC-772 and studied the underlying mechanisms by which OB markedly inhibited expansion and induced apoptosis of the HCC cells. The antitumor activity of OB probably involved the inhibition of COX-2/VEGF and PTEN/PI3K/AKT signaling pathways, providing evidence for OB being used as a new therapeutic agent for liver cancer [16]. Another flavonoid, namely luteolin, showed antineoplastic activity in a number of cancer cells. In SMMC-7721 HCC cells, luteolin induced apoptosis partially via modulation of autophagy, indicating luteolin serving as a regulator of autophagy in treating liver cancer [17].

Brucein D (BD) is an active constituent derived from *Brucea javanica* fruit, which has been employed as an antitumor recipe in Chinese medical practice. It was revealed that BD exerted observable apoptotic induction in HCC in vitro and in vivo, which was attributed to the reduced expression of miR-95 [18].

Matrine, a chemical component came from the roots of sophora species, mainly *Sophora flavescens* Ait (SF), has been used clinically to treat diseases such as liver fibrosis. The hepato-specific *miR-122a* has been found decreased in HCC cell lines [19]. Zhou et al. reported that in HepG2 cells, matrine could cause cell arrest alteration as well as apoptosis induction with recovering expression of miR-122a [20]. Actually, matrine is the prominent bioactive compound in one adjuvant treatment of liver cancer, namely Fufang Kushen injection, which was approved by Chinese FDA in 1995. Matrine has been deemed as the favorable lead source for drug discovery owing to its changeable structure and stable safety profile. Researchers designed and synthesized a group of matrine derivatives, which improved the antitumor activities of matrine in several human cancer cell lines. Among four tested cell lines, HCC cell line Bel-7402 responded more sensitively to compounds than the other three cell lines. Matrine and its derivatives induced G1 cell cycle blockage as well as migration inhibition in HCC cells [21]. Another matrine derivative named WM622 showed remarkable inhibitory effect on HCC both in vivo and in vitro. Further study showed the apoptotic induction, cell cycle blocking in G0/G1 phase and the inhibition of PI3K/AKT signaling were involved in the antiliver cancer effect of WM622 [22].

Longikaurin A (LK-A) is a naturally occurring compound of ent-kaurane obtained from *I. aternifolius*. Researchers explored LK-A administration in liver of tumor-bearing mice models and discovered that LK-A could induce cell cycle arrest at G2/M phase with downregulation of Skp2 and subsequently resulted in induction of ROS/JNK/c-Jun apoptotic pathway in HCC cells [23].

The antitumor of two known pennogenyl saponins, which are derived from *R. paridis axialis*, was investigated in orthotopic nude-mouse model. The data indicated that these two monomers dose dependently suppressed the HCC progression through activating both caspase-independent and caspase-dependent apoptotic pathways. Furthermore, possible mechanism probably involved the modulation of mitogen-related protein kinase pathway as well as the suppression of PI3K/Akt signaling [24].

Isoquercitrin was found to strongly repress liver tumor cells via retarding the G1 phase cell cycle and promoting cancer cells apoptosis. In nude mice, the proliferation of transplanted tumors was suppressed after treatment with isoquercitrin. Further study showed that the underlying mechanism might be closely involved in the MAPK and PKC signaling pathways [25].

Zhang et al. investigated the effect of astragaloside IV (AS-IV) and curcumin on tumor expansion and angiogenesis in nude mice bearing xenografts of HCC. Combining AS-IV and curcumin revealed significant synergistic repressive efficacy against both angiogenic and thrombosis-related factors, which might be mediated by downregulation of *miR-221* as well as upregulation of *miR-122*. This current study indicated future clinical potential of combination therapy with AS-IV and curcumin for treatment of liver cancer [26].

Ursolic acid (UA), a naturally occurring pentacyclic triterpenoid carboxylic acid found among Chinese herbal medicine, has been reported to be a potent component for cancer prevention, including liver cancer. Yie et al. explored the probable mechanisms underlying the antiliver cancer action of UA. Taken together, the results demonstrated that UA inhibited proliferation and induced apoptosis of HCC cells via AMPKα-mediated suppression of Sp1, followed by suppressing DNMT1 expression. The investigation revealed a potential novel mechanism by which UA controlled proliferation of HCC cells, suggesting the critical effect of DNMT1 in HCC chemoprevention and treatment [27].

Bilobol is a Chinese medical ingredient. Xu et al. identified that bilobol administration could suppress expansion of HepG2 cells, which pretreated with lipopolysaccharide (LPS) to induce inflammation. Bilobol appeared to exhibit antitumor effect via inhibiting the RhoA/ROCK signal transduction during the anti-inflammatory response [28].

Fucoidan, a sulfated polysaccharide isolated from brown algae, has been applied as an anti-cancer drug for hundreds of years in Chinese medicine. The results from Zhu et al. revealed that fucoidan had the capacity of antitumor partially through inhibiting the proliferation of HCC cells, although it is unable to repress the angiogenesis induced by HCC [29]. In another study, fucoidan displayed the antimetastatic efficacy on HCC cell lines via upregulating p42/44 MAPK-dependent NDRG-1/CAP43 pathway. Also, fucoidan was found to protect against bile acid-induced hepatocyte apoptosis. This ability suggested fucoidan presented a potent therapeutic agent for HCC treatment [30].

Telekin is a eudesmane-type sesquiterpene lactone extracted from the natural plant *Carpesium divaricatum*, which presents strong antiproliferative activity in cancer cells. Zheng et al. found that telekin promoted HCC cells apoptosis by activating the mitochondria-mediated apoptotic pathway [31].

Gigantol is a phenolic substance derived from the genus Dendrobium. Chen et al. investigated gigantol efficacy on liver cancer cells and the results suggested gigantol inhibited cells expansion and induced apoptosis in HepG2 cells through PI3K/Akt/NF-kappaB signal transduction [32].

The endoplasmic reticulum (ER) stress and unfolded protein response (UPR) play critical roles in the modulation of cell fate. The two factors even could become potent targets and provide support for the development of antineoplastic agents. Celastrol, one of the triterpene compounds derived from herbal medicine, exerts antitumor effects on various malignancies. Ren et al. demonstrated that for HCC cells, exposure to celastrol led to the sensitivity of the intrinsic apoptotic pathway, at least partly through ER stress and the UPR. Moreover, celastrol was found to repress H22 tumor growth in murine syngeneic model studies by inducing ER stress and apoptosis. These data suggested that targeting ER-stress/UPR was an efficient way for celastrol becoming a potent drug for HCC therapy [33]. Cytisine, a quinolizidine alkaloid, also a major bioactive constituent purified from the *Sophora alopecuroides* L. It was reported to exhibit inhibitory effects in treating liver cancer by inducing the ER stress-mediated apoptotic pathway through activating CHOP, JNK, and caspase-4 signaling pathways in liver cancer cells. This phenomenon suggested a novel target compound potentially to treat liver cancer [34].

RA-XII, a naturally occurring compound originated from Chinese herbal medicine Rubia yunnanensis, possesses activities of anti-inflammatory and antitumor. Song et al. revealed that RA-XII accelerated apoptosis and repressed protective autophagy via signaling pathway AMPK/mTOR/P70S6K in HepG2 cells, suggesting RA-XII, a cyclopeptide, provides the therapeutic support for potentially being an autophagy inhibitor drug in the therapy of hepatic tumor [35].

There are many bioactive compounds from Chinese medicine, which are also one part of daily diet. For example, *Bullacta exarata* is widely used as a part of normal diet in Asia, and also it is an agent with liver- and kidney-nourishing functions. One polysaccharide conjugate BEPS-IA was extracted from *B. exarata*. Liao et al. reported that BEPS-IA exerted a potent inhibition in HepG2 cells growth in a concentration-dependent manner via inducing apoptosis and blocking cell cycle. Furthermore, it was corroborated that this effect was involved in downregulation of Bcl-2, upregulation of p53, p21 and Bax, suggesting that BEPS-IA may be a new dietary drug for HCC obtained from herbals and shed light on getting a deeper understanding on the action mechanisms [36]. Diosgenin is a major bioactive component of Dioscoreaceae plants including yam, which is commonly prescribed in Chinese medicine, and a common vegetable all over the world. Diosgenin remarkably repressed the proliferation of several HCC cell lines in a dosage-dependent manner. Deeper investigation reported the apoptosis and cell cycle G2/M arrest were involved in the inactivation of Akt, activation of the caspase cascades, and upregulation of p21 and p27 expression. These results suggested that diosgenin may serve potentially as a novel antiliver cancer dietary supplement [37]. *Armillaria mellea* (*A. mellea*) is a honey mushroom, which is currently often consumed worldwide as a dietary supplement. Armillarikin was purified from *A. mellea*, which is an important component of Chinese medicine "Tianma." Chen et al. investigated the cytotoxicity of armillarikin against HCC cell lines such as Huh7, HA22T, and HepG2 cells. Armillarikin treatment induced apoptosis that was mediated by ROS and accompanied by the collapse of mitochondrial and activation of caspase-8 and -3 in cancer cells, suggesting the potential of armillarikin serving as an potent antihepatoma drug [38]. Corosolic acid analogue (CAA) is a triterpenoid saponin isolated from *Actinidia valvata* Dunn (Actinidiaceae), a kind of well-known fruit. The study investigated the antiproliferation and inducing apoptosis effects of CAA in three hepatoma cell lines. The data showed for the first time that CAA inhibited expansion of liver cancer cell lines and induced G1 phase arrest. Moreover, proapoptotic effect of CAA was mediated by the activation of TNF-α, caspases, and mitochondrial pathway [39].

1,6,7-trihydroxyxanthone (THA) is an active small molecule purified from *Goodyera oblongifolia*. The compound was discovered to strongly inhibit cancer cell proliferation and induced apoptosis in hepatoma carcinoma cells partially mediated by the repression of Bmi-1 and activation of miR-218 [40].

An active ingredient cordycepin was extracted from "Dong Chong Xia Cao." It has been implicated in regulating multiple physiological actions especially antitumor effects. Yao et al. revealed that cordycepin might contribute to tumor progression, EMT, migration, and invasion inhibition in HCC by suppression of signaling pathways E-cadherin and integrin/FAK. Hence, cordycepin is a supplementary candidate or therapeutic agent for preventing liver tumor expansion [41].

Norcantharidin (NCTD), a small-molecule antitumor drug originated from small animal *blister beetle*, has been currently applied as a potent antineoplastic agent for several kinds of cancers including HCC. The expression of FAM46C, which has been firstly reported as a tumor suppressor for multiple myeloma, was demonstrated to enhance with NCTD administration. FAM46C, a tumor inhibitor for HCC, was important for proapoptotic effects and antiproliferation of NCTD

[42]. Another study investigated the mechanism of NCTD-induced apoptosis in HepG2 cells, which indicated that NCTD could reverse the methylation state of RASSF1A gene and recover its expression, providing the theoretical information for further development in clinical application [43]. Also, Zhang et al. found in multiple HCC cell lines that NCTD could induce transcriptional repression of Mcl-1 and significantly enhance ABT-737-triggered cell viability inhibition and apoptosis [44].

Bufalin is the major bioactive constituent of the Chinese medicine Chansu, which is presently employed in clinical practice for cancer therapy. A number of groups have investigated the therapy efficacy of bufalin on hepatoma, either in vivo or in vitro, to explore the therapeutic potential of the drug. Qiu et al. reported that bufalin exhibited considerable antitumor activities in liver cancer cell lines HCCLM3 and HepG2 and the underlying mechanism might be related to the repression of signaling pathway AKT/GSK3β/β-catenin/E-cadherin [45]. Tsai et al. demonstrated that bufalin led to autophagic cell death and G2/M cell cycle phase arrest in SK-HEP-1 HCC cells via activating AKT/mTOR signal transduction pathway [46]. Another group reported that bufalin exerted remarkable antiproliferative activity and apoptosis induction in Huh-7 and HepG-2 cancer cells. Further study supported the prosurvival role of bufalin-induced autophagy when the autophagy pathway was retarded with specific chemical inhibitors, indicating a promising therapeutic approach for HCC therapy combining bufalin with a specific autophagy inhibitor [47].

In searching for active antihepatoma ingredients from *toad venom*, which is a frequent prescription applied in HCC treatment, Zhang et al. discovered that arenobufagin, a bufadienolide derived from toad venom, had prominent anticancer capacity against HepG2 cells and the corresponding multidrug-resistant cells, namely HepG2/ADM. They illuminated the molecular mechanisms of arenobufagin, which involved crosstalk between autophagy and apoptosis through PI3K/Akt/mTOR pathway suppression. Consequently, these findings contributed to the development of arenobufagin into a chemotherapeutic agent in liver cancer treatment [48]. Another compound, namely hellebrigenin, which was also isolated from *Venenum bufonis*, was found to significantly repress HepG2 cell viability and colony formation. Further exploration revealed the cytotoxicity of hellebrigenin in HepG2 cells and underscored the antihepatoma activity of hellebrigenin as an active component of *Venenum bufonis*. Hellebrigenin induced DNA damage, triggered cell cycle arrest, and subsequently initiated mitochondrial apoptosis. Moreover, Akt was found to take a role in cell cycle and apoptosis modulation induced by hellebrigenin. The findings showed the potential of hellebrigenin used as a chemotherapeutic drug for future HCC clinical application [49].

2.2. Functional roles of Chinese medicine extracts and fractions in liver cancer

Asparagus is not only consumed in daily diet but also employed as an agent in Chinese medicine for multiple types of malignancies therapy. An extract from asparagus, asparagus polysaccharide, has been confirmed to be the major bioactive constituent of asparagus in the respect of antitumor as well as immunity-enhancing activities. In clinical practice, it has been used in a number of malignancies treatment [50]. Weng et al. applied tumor-bearing rat model to systemically evaluate the toxicity and antitumor activity of asparagus polysaccharide and asparagus gel-like material. The results showed a certain tumor inhibitory effect of them via promoting cell apoptosis and suppressing tumor angiogenesis when given as transarterial chemoembolization (TACE) therapy. Meanwhile, it exerted the antihepatoma activity with lower toxic effects as well as reduced kidney and liver functional damage, highlighting its chemotherapeutic potential in clinical application for future liver cancer TACE therapy [51].

Ganoderma lucidum polysaccharides (GLPS) have been exploited as folk Chinese medicine for their properties of immunomodulation and tumor prevention [52]. Li et al. measured the efficacy of GLPS on liver cancer cells in hepatoma-bearing mice model and effectively suppressed the tumor growth. The possible molecular mechanism may be related with an augment of the ratio of regulatory T cell (Treg) to effector T cell (Teff), which is caused by the augment of miR-125b, a predicative marker of poor prognosis and aggressiveness of liver cancer [53].

In China, *Trametes robiniophila Murr* (Huaier) has recently been used as Chinese medicine in China. It has a great clinical effect as adjuvant therapies in the treatment of HCC. Shan et al. investigated the functions of Huaier on HCC cells and confirmed that HCC growth could be restrained by Huaier through downregulation of yes-associated protein 1 (YAP1) [54].

Ampelopsis sinica root (ASR) is a well-known hepatoprotective Chinese medicine. Wang et al. explored whether ethyl acetate extract from ASRE had the antihepatoma activity both in vitro and in vivo. The findings showed that ASRE had prominent antihepatoma activity, which possibly involved the decreased regulation of inflammatory cytokines such as cyclooxygenase-2, 5-lipoxygenase and FLAP, augment of p53 protein expression and the ratio of bax/bcl-2, caspase-3 activation, as well as survivin repression. Moreover, ASR was found to be nontoxic on normal cells, suggesting that it may serve as a potential therapeutic agent for HCC treatment [55].

An extract of *Stellerachamaejasme* L. (ESC) had been confirmed as a potential antitumor extract of Chinese medicine. Liu et al. tested that the suppressive effects of ESC on propagation and epithelial mesenchymal transition (EMT) in liver cancer cells were associated with miR-107. The findings indicated ESC retarded HCC expansion and metastasis by regulating the expression of microRNAs and their according target genes [56].

Cnidium monnieri (L.) Cusson (CME) is a frequently used Chinese herbal medicine that treats gynecological diseases and carbuncles. A recent study showed the cell cycle alteration and apoptosis of HepG2 (wildtype p53) and Hep3B (p53null) by ethanol extract of CME, suggesting that CME induced G1 arrest and apoptosis via the Akt/GSK3β signaling pathway [57].

Astragalus membranaceus and Salvia miltiorrhiza are medical plants that have been applied for thousands of years in the treatment of liver diseases. According to previous researches, it has showed that these two herbs and their extracts own the ability to inhibit the development liver cancer. Rui et al. investigated that the compound astragalus and salvia miltiorrhiza extract (CASE) could repress diethylinitrosamine-induced hepatoma in rat model via the inhibition of fibrosis and PAI-1 mRNA transcription, indicating the possibility of being development as antihepatoma agents in preventing and treating human liver cancer [58].

Salvia chinensis Benth has been traditionally exploited for several centuries since old times to treat malignant diseases including HCC. In a study, total flavonoids isolated from *Salvia chinensis* Benth were shown to own the capability of inducing HCC cell apoptosis both in vitro and in vivo, which appeared to be implicated in the suppression of NF-κB activity [59]. *Coptidis rhizoma* has been used in clinical practice for tumor treatment in Chinese medicine, and recent experiments in our laboratory have supported its employment in tumor treatment. Zhu et al. examined the anticancer efficacy of *Coptidis rhizoma* aqueous extract (CRAE) on HCC cells and found the alterations of miR-21 and miR-23a after treatment with CRAE. The results suggested that CRAE targeted the miRNAs in hepatoma cells [60]. Wang et al. found that CRAE could remarkably downregulate Rho/ROCK signal transduction, then finally interfere MHCC97-L cell migration [61]. As we know, angiogenesis is an important factor, which is beneficial for tumor expansion. Tan et al. confirmed that antiangiogenic effect of CRAE on HCC was partially dependent to an eEF2-driven pathway [62]. All these findings supported the potential application of CRAE in HCC therapy.

Prunella vulgaris (PV) is a small tree that has been employed clinically for thousands of years in Asia to treat herpetic keratitis. According to previous researches, it has showed PV could repress TPA-induced activation of MMP-9 and suppress hepatoma cells migration and invasion. Data suggested that by modulating multiple signaling pathways, PV modified the metastatic microenvironment of HCC. PV thus may provide useful information for systemic therapies of HCC [63].

Ethyl acetate extract (EAE) of *Euphorbia helioscopia* L. played a critical role in repressing tumor cell proliferation, apoptosis, invasion, and metastasis in vitro. Meanwhile, Cheng et al. found that change of expression of cyclin D1, Bcl-2, Bax, MMP-9 by EAE may be associated with inhibition of tumor growth, induction apoptosis, and suppression of tumor metastasis and invasion in HCC xenografts [64].

Some Chinese medicine scholars have indicated that endogenous wind-evil acted as a critical role in tumor metastasis. On the basis of this, the agent of dispelling wind-evil could serve as a suppressor for cancer metastasis and poor prognosis. Yan et al. observed that scorpion-medicated serum could restrain proliferation, induce apoptosis, as well as inhibit the capacity of migration and invasion in vitro. Further experiments in HCC tumor-bearing metastasis mice models showed that water decoction of scorpion blocked tumor growth and metastasis. More importantly, these results suggested that scorpion, as an important wind calming drug, could inhibit the metastasis and invasion of liver cancer cells especially through epithelial-mesenchymal transition (EMT) reversal, thereby providing a possible potential approach to preventing HCC metastasis [65].

Actinidia chinensis Planch root extract (acRoots) has been shown to inhibit cell proliferation in numerous cancer cells. Hou et al. used acRoots to treat HCC cells and observed the distinct effects of acRoots on cell proliferation, cell cycle arrest, and apoptosis. Furthermore, the mechanism underlying these activities was attributed to LAMB3-mediated proliferation suppression and S-phase cell cycle arrest in HepG2 cells [66]. He et al. studied the mechanism in the extent of metabolic alterations. The data showed that acRoots could remarkably inhibit cholesterol metabolism through a PCSK9-mediated signaling pathway, which in turn limited the nutrients production that was essential for the proliferation of cancer cells [67].

Ethanol extract of root of *Prunus persica,* which is an important ingredient in Chinese medicine prescription, exhibited antitumor effect in liver cancer. Scholars recently reported that *Prunus persica* could repress cell growth in a time and dose-dependent fashion, causing sustained M/G2 phase arrest as well as notably suppressing the migration of HepG2 cells and the expression of extracellular matrix metalloproteases, MMP3 and MMP9 [68].

Realgar (As_4S_4), one of the most useful mineral drugs in Chinese medicine, has been employed in clinical therapy as a potential agent for cancer therapy. However, due to its low solubility and subsequent poor bioavailability, it is difficult to achieve the effective blood medicine dose unless with high dosage of realgar and long period of treatment. A recent study explored realgar transforming solution (RTS) and found the strong antihepatoma activity of RTS via inducing ROS [69].

2.3. The role of Chinese medicine composite formulae in regressing liver cancer

Huang-lian-jie-du-tang (HLJDT) is oriental medicinal formulation known to possess anti-inflammatory activity. The prescription has been well documented for thousands of years and used for liver protection in Asian community [70]. Recent researches have postulated HLJDT as a regimen for cancer treatment, particularly hepatoma. Hsu et al. found that HLJDT might have an effect on human liver cancer cell lines, Hep G2 and PLC/PRF/5. The results showed that HLJDT significantly triggered cell cycle arrest and contributed to the mitochondrial apoptotic pathway by reducing the level and activity of NF-κB, which suggested that HLJDT might be a promising chemotherapeutic agent without causing cytotoxicity to normal cellular environment [71]. Wang et al. examined the suppressive efficacy of HLJDT on the liver cancer expansion and found that involvement of eEF2 inhibition might be the key mechanism mediating the inhibitory effect of the formula [72].

Yiguanjian (YGJ), a classic liver-YIN tonifying herbal formula, was established by ancient Chinese medicine practitioner Wei Zhixian in the Qing Dynasty (AD 1722–1772). Researchers optimized the prescription of YGJ on the basis of modern principles in clinical practice of Chinese medicine and then evaluated the antitumor activity of modified YGJ (MYGJ) on Bel-7402 human liver cancer cells. These data showed that MYGJ could interfere proliferation suspension and induce anoikis in cancer cells. The mechanisms underlying the actions of MYGJ might involve in inhibiting the phosphorylation and expression of p38 MAPK, and subsequent regulating intrinsic and extrinsic pathways of apoptosis [73].

Pien Tze Huang (PZH) is an extensively employed prescription in the treatment of multiple malignancies and has possible therapeutic effects in clinical therapy for HCC. Qi et al. aimed to elucidate the efficacy of PZH on the proliferation and apoptosis of liver cancer cell lines and demonstrated PZH could effectively inhibit cancer cell proliferation and induce apoptosis in Bel-7402 HCC cells by upregulating miR-16, which has been verified as tumor suppressor, suggesting a novel potential therapeutic for HCC patients [74].

Sini-San (SNS) has been employed for the treatment of various types of liver disease. This formulation comprises four prescriptions of Chinese herbal medicine and was first described in "Shanghan Lun (Treatise on Cold Damage Disorders or the Treatise on Cold Injury)," established by one of the most famous ancient Chinese physicians, Zhang Zhongjing (150–219 AD). SNS has shown significant inhibition on tumor growth in HepG2 xenograft model. Lin et al. elucidated the molecular mechanism by which SNS exerted an antimigratory and anti-invasive effect on HBx-activated liver cancer cells. These results showed that SNS suppressed invasiveness and metastasis in HCC cells via multiple signal transduction pathways including downregulating PI3K/Akt, decreasing MAPK and IκB signaling, inhibiting NF-κB and AP-1 activity, and reducing MMP-9 expression. Thus, SNS might be helpful to interfere the invasion and metastasis of HCC [75].

Songyou Yin (SYY), a composite formula, showed efficacy to repress tumor proliferation, metastasis, and recurrence. An interesting study explored that SYY combining with moderate swimming has potent effect on retraining tumor growth and metastasis mainly via enhancing immune function [76].

Niu-Huang-Shen (NHS) has been accepted and used in China for a long time with its various effects such as antipyretic, anti-inflammatory, and vasodilatation effects. It was showed that NHS inhibited cell cycle arrest, induced cell apoptosis, and then repressed cell proliferation and invasion, probably through the significant suppression of Yes-associated protein (YAP) expression. NHS may have the therapeutic potential for treating HCC more effectively [77].

Shuihonghuazi formula (SHHZF) has been employed for early stage of liver cancer in clinical therapy for a long time; a study was designed to investigate potent effects of SHHZF on hepatoma and its metabolomic profiles. The results elucidated that SHHZF exerted inhibitory effects against liver cancer by adjusting the activities of PE N-methyl transferase, lysophospholipase D, methylenetetrahydrofolate reductase, and lysophospholipase [78].

3. Chinese medicine as a complementary treatment of liver cancer

Chinese medicine is appreciated for its 5000-year-old history and still holds a prominent position in primary health care in China. Chinese medicine could complement Western medicine by using modern techniques; thus, increasing interests in Chinese medicine has been observed over the Western world. In Chinese medicine, a wide range of ingredients have been proven to achieve various effects in cancer therapy, including alleviating the toxicity to human body, retraining tumor metastasis and recurrence, enhancing chemo- or radio-therapeutic effects, and subsequent improving the general status of patients and extending their survival time.

Long-term food restriction and diarrhea may be an adverse factor for liver cancer. Jian-pi-jie-du decoction (JPJD) could improve the quality of life of hepatoma subjects, in particular, the symptoms of diarrhea and decreased food intake. A research indicated JPJD could improve the condition of tumor-bearing rats, which were pretreated with diarrhea and food restriction by increasing ABCC2 expressional level and downregulating the OATP1B2 in liver normal tissues while downregulating ABCC2 as well as upregulating OATP1B2 in cancer tissues [79].

In terms of radioprotective and radiosensitizing functions of Chinese medicine, a series of concerning studies have been conducted. Numerous Chinese medicine agents have been confirmed to strengthen the therapeutic gain of radiotherapy by the way of serving as radioprotectors for healthy cells or as radiosensitizers for cancer cells [80, 81]. Botanical agents are comprised of multiple phytochemical compounds that may work synergistically or even individually, not only exhibiting favorable therapeutic effects, but also with safety profiles and lower toxicity [82].

Ganoderma lucidum polysaccharide (GLP) is well known for its various pharmacologic properties including antitumor effects [52]. A study recently demonstrated that GLP treatment may augment growth inhibition and apoptotic death of HepG2 cells, which induced by radiation, and revealed the regulatory role of Akt signaling pathway for GLP-mediated radiosensitivity in HCC cells exposed to radiation [83].

Kou et al. investigated the radiosensitizing effects of ultrafiltration extract of Radix Angelicae Sinensis-Radix Hedysari (RAS-RH) in human hepatoma cells. The results reported that the RAS-RH significantly enhanced the radiosensitivity of H22 cells of 12C6+ heavy ion radiation. Further study explored the underlying mechanism of radiosensitization, which is to increase caspase-dependent apoptosis via reducing surviving expressional level, suggesting a promising potent radiosensitizer [84].

Zhang et al. demonstrated that a flavonoid dihydromyricetin (DHM) exerted anticancer activity against hepatoma cells as well as xenotransplanted tumors in nude mice by activating the p53-dependent apoptosis pathway. And best of all, DHM was indicated to play a prominent role when administered in combination with cisplatin [85]. In this case, DHM could be an ideal anticancer drug with minimal side effects because it can alleviate cytotoxicity caused by cisplatin in normal liver cells.

Some studies investigated the adjunctive role of bufalin in reversal chemoresistance in the treatment of liver cancer. The Akt activation triggered by sorafenib is regarded to be responsible for this resistant phenomenon. Zhai et al. investigated that bufalin had the ability of reversing both inherent and acquired resistance to sorafenib via the IRE1 pathway in an ER-stress-dependent manner. These data warranted further studies to examine the utility of bufalin in combination with sorafenib as a first- or second-line treatment after sorafenib alone gains failure in advanced liver cancer [86]. Fluorouracil (5-FU) is a type of anticancer chemotherapeutics, which has been used for 40 years in clinical practice. A research confirmed the reversal effect of bufalin on drug resistance in a moderate multidrug resistance cell line Bel-7402/5-FU. They found Bufalin could block the cell cycle at G_0/G_1 phase, induce apoptosis through an increase of Bax/Bcl-xL ratio, inhibit the drug efflux pump activity via downregulation of MRP1, and reduce the expression of thymidylate synthase in vitro. All these data revealed that in Bel-7402/5-FU cells, the combination of bufalin with cytotoxic drugs could considerably reverse the MDR through multiple pathways including cell cycle arrest, apoptosis induction, etc., indicating an effective strategy for the chemotherapy of HCC [87].

Xu et al. investigated the efficacy of drug combination of luteolin and 5-FU on the proliferation of HepG2 and Bel-7402 cells. The data showed that luteolin synergized 5-FU at different dose ratios and then exerted the antitumor effects against HCC cells. Potential mechanism for synergistic effects may be associated with apoptosis and 5-FU metabolism, as evidenced by the increased bax/bcl-2 ratios, upregulated p53 expressions, and induced PARP cleavage [88].

ADCX, a natural cycloartane triterpenoid isolated from *Cimicifugae* rhizome, impaired autophagic degradation by inhibiting lysosomal cathepsin B expression in multidrug resistant cell line, namely HepG2/ADM, which consequently lead to apoptosis, suggesting that an active constituent from Cimicifugae rhizome could overcome multidrug resistance in hepatoma cells by the role of persistent Akt activation in inhibition of autophagic degradation [89].

Arsenic trioxide (As_2O_3) with high doses is employed to treat solid tumors and acute promyelocytic leukemia, which mostly induce toxic side effects to healthy cells. Andrographolide is a kind of Chinese medicine that exhibits various effects against diseases such as anti-inflammatory, antivirus, antitumor, and so on. Duan et al. demonstrated that andrographolide enhanced As_2O_3-induced apoptosis in a caspase-3-dependent manner via downregulation of EphB4 in HCC cells. These findings suggested that lower concentrations of As_2O_3 in combination with andrographolide could be used as chemotherapy for HCC with the potential to minimize the adverse events from As_2O_3 treatment alone [90].

The aqueous extract of *Solanum nigrum* (AE-SN) is an important constituent in some Chinese medicine formulae used in the treatment of cancer. Wang et al. explored the antitumor effect of AE-SN in combination with a normal chemotherapeutic drug, namely doxorubicin or cisplatin, in HCC cell lines Hep3B and HepJ5. The results indicated the integrated treatment with AE-SN-potentiated doxorubicin and cisplatin-induced cytotoxicity through the cleavage of caspase-7 and accumulation of microtubule-associated protein-1 light chain-3 A/1B II (LC-3 A/B II), which were involved in autophagic and apoptotic cell death, respectively. Thereby, this combinatorial strategy of AE-SN and cisplatin or doxorubicin may be exploited to be a candidate regimen to treat HCC patients [91].

A recent research was performed to explore the combination effect of Huaier aqueous extract and chemotherapeutic agent cisplatin or rapamycin. The findings showed that Huaier had the capacity of activating mTOR signaling, which contributed to the enhanced cancer cells sensitivity to chemotherapeutics in response to Huaier administration. Huaier, thus, can potentially be used in integrated chemotherapy with rapamycin or cisplatin for liver cancer therapy [92].

Cinobufacini, a mixture of a number of components in Chinese medicine, has been used extensively for HCC therapy with strong apoptosis-inducing activity. Xia et al. used a combination of doxorubicin with cinobufacini to achieve tumor-suppression efficiency and found the combination group had a more considerable apoptotic effect by affecting proteins and RNA of apoptosis-related elements, such as Bcl-2, Bax, Bid, and cytochrome C. Consequently, cinobufacini in combination with chemotherapeutic agents might be a new strategy to improve the treatment effect for HCC patients [93].

Shufeng Jiedu Capsule (SFJDC) has been widely used due to its various pharmacological actions such as anti-inflammation, antibacterial, antiviral, and antitumor. Recently, scholars used combination of SFJDC with doxorubicin to treat liver cancer cells and further explored the underlying mechanisms of SFJDC as well as its constituents in vitro. The data showed that the combination group induced more considerable apoptosis and invasion and migration suppression than control group by targeting NF-κB, Akt/mTOR, and mitochondrial signaling pathways [94].

Dahuang zhechong pill (DHZCP) is one of the most famous prescriptions from an ancient Chinese medical classic "Jin Kui Yao Lue (Essential Prescriptions from the Golden Cabinet)." DHZCP is officially recorded in the Chinese Pharmacopeia and is commonly used for clinical practice of hepatoma. Wu et al. found that inhibitory growth of doxorubicin-resistant HCC subcutaneous xenografts in nude mice was achieved by DHZCP, and apoptosis promotion was accelerated by doxorubicin. The reversal of doxorubicin resistance by DHZCP was related with energy metabolism decline and regulation of proapoptotic proteins expression [95].

4. Discussion

Accumulating researches have demonstrated that Chinese medicine is a promising substitute for therapy of liver cancer. Furthermore, increasing scholars starts to pay attention to clinical studies of Chinese medicine. For example, gambogic acid (GA), a naturally occurring compound from ancient China, has been demonstrated efficient antineoplastic activity in a number of malignancies. More importantly, it has entered phase II clinical trials. A team ?found GA might lead to oxidative stress and subsequently induce apoptosis in hepatoma cells through interacting with TrxR1. Thus, targeting TrxR1 by GA disclosed a previously unrecognized mechanism underlying the biological action of GA and provides useful information for further development of GA as a potential agent for cancer therapy [96]. On the other hand, the theory of "Jianpi Huayu Therapy" (JPHY) was rooted from "Jin Kui Yao Lue." According to the selection criteria, Zhong et al. recruited a total of 120 patients in a randomized trial, aiming to compare the curative outcome and safety profile of surgery in combination with "Jianpi Huayu Therapy" HCC treatment to surgery alone. The patients in treatment group received the basic prescription based on JPHY. The results showed that hepatectomy combined with JPHY was more effective with reducing postoperative metastasis and recurrence and prolonged overall survival of HCC patients [97]. JQ1, one of the bromodomain and extra-terminal domain (BET) inhibitors, has been emerged as a novel agent candidate for cancer treatment in clinical research. Nevertheless, a number of solid cancers are resistant to BET inhibitors. The results from a group showed that oridonin synergistically increased JQ1 capacity of inhibiting HCC cell survival, and considerably enhanced JQ1-caused apoptosis in HCC cells and in HCC cancer stem-like cells. Furthermore, they demonstrated that oridonin distinctly augmented the sensitivity of JQ1 via downregulation of the level of multiple antiapoptotic proteins, including Bcl-2, Mcl-1, and x-linked inhibitor of apoptosis, suggesting that the combination treatment of JQ1 and oridonin could be further pursued for clinical application and it was expected to provide a rational for HCC tumor prevention [98].

Collectively, the aforementioned findings showed the potential efficacy of Chinese medicine on numerous types of cancer, either alone or in combination with conventional treatment of method such as surgery, chemotherapy, or radiation. In particular, as stated above, when integrated with chemotherapy or radiotherapy, Chinese medicine may serve as complementary drugs strongly enhancing the positive effects or reducing the negative events induced by radiochemotherapy. However, in comparison with a great deal of laboratory researches, clinical trials still remain poor, which limits the wide application of Chinese medicine throughout the world.

5. Conclusion

Chinese medicine is increasingly emerging as a novel curative choice for liver cancer. This retrospective review systemically introduced and evaluated the functional roles of Chinese medicine in treating liver cancer. Chinese medicine has potentially exerted efficient anticancer properties. For example, liver cancer progression can be repressed by active constituents derived from Chinese medicine through multiple pathways. The specific network with regard to the potential therapeutic targets for liver cancer treatment was constructed (**Figure 1**). The detailed relationships between biological factors and refined extracts could be directly visualized in **Figure 1**. Moreover, composite formulae as promising curative are increasingly indispensable in current clinical practice. As summarized in **Table 1**, formulae potentially employed in practice were studied in laboratory and the regulatory mechanisms for the treatment of liver cancer have been showed clearly. Also, Chinese medicine may serve as adjuvant agents in surgery as well as in combination with conventional radio- and chemotherapy, to decrease the adverse events or enhance the treatment outcome. Taken all together, Chinese medicine possesses the potential in liver cancer treatment, and rational application in clinical therapy needs to be warranted in the future.

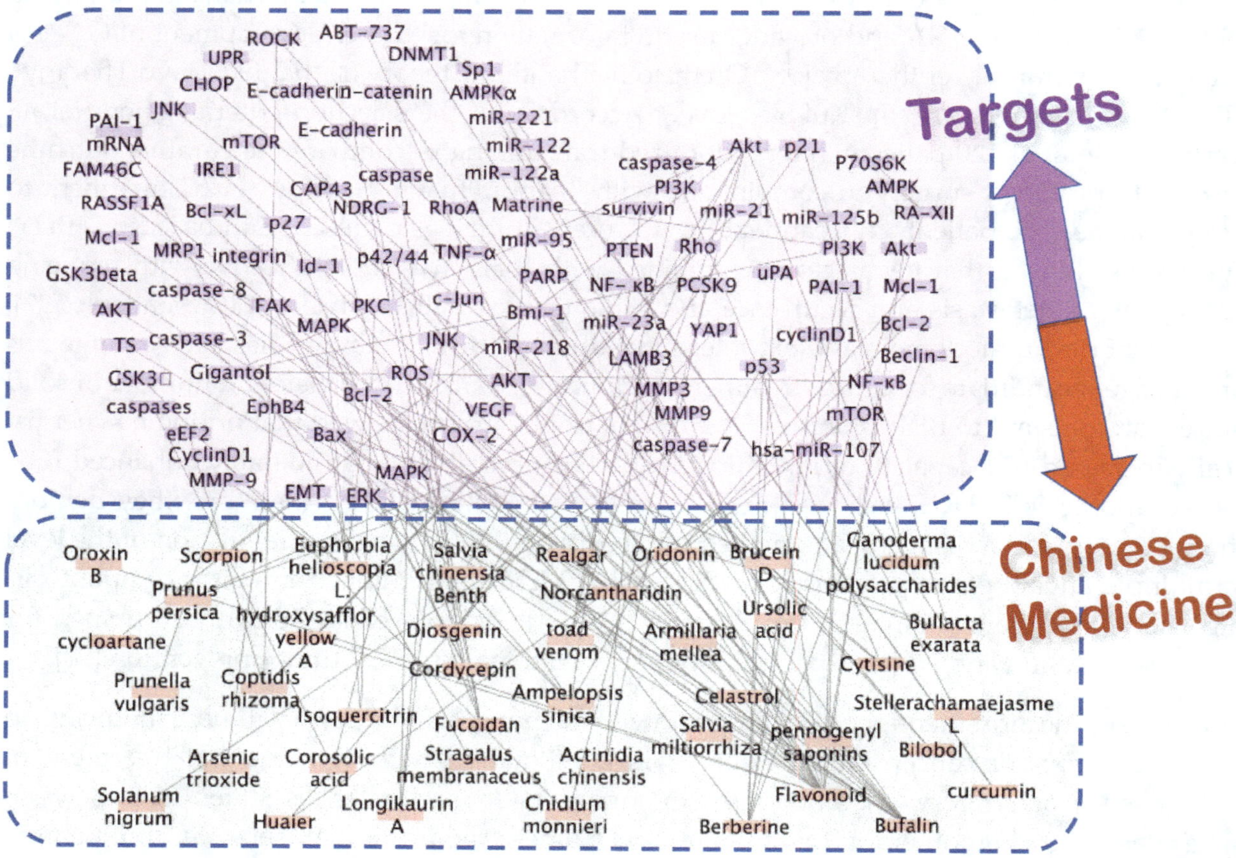

Figure 1. Target identification of Chinese medicine-derived compounds and extracts for liver cancer. Literature mining in PubMed with "Chinese Medicine" integrated with "liver cancer" was performed. All filtered data during the last 5 years were imported into a professional software Cytoscape for the establishment of the analysis of network pharmacology. The top five influential molecules including Akt, Bax, Bcl-2, mTOR, and PI3K could be figured out.

Name	Functions	Ref.
Huang-lian-jie-du-tang	Cell cycle arrest, induce mitochondrial apoptotic pathway, inhibit HCC cell proliferation, suppress growth and angiogenesis in xenografted murine model	[71, 72]
Yiguanjian	Interfere proliferation suspension and induce anoikis in cancer cells	[73]
Pien Tze Huang	Inhibit cancer cell proliferation and induce apoptosis	[74]
Sini-San	Suppressed invasiveness and metastasis in HCC cells	[75]
Songyou Yin	Repress tumor proliferation, metastasis, and recurrence	[76]
Niu-Huang-Shen	Cell cycle arrest, induce cell apoptosis, and cell invasion	[77]
Shuihonghuazi formula	Increase the uptake and utilization of linoleic acid and oleic acid, increase arachidonic acid-like substance content, and enhance organism immunity of liver cancer rats	[78]
Jian-pi-jie-du decoction	Improve the condition of tumor-bearing rats with the symptoms of diarrhea and decreased food intake	[79]
Cinobufacini	Combination of doxorubicin with cinobufacini to achieve a more considerable apoptotic effect	[93]
Shufeng Jiedu Capsule	Combination of SFJDC with doxorubicin induced more considerable apoptosis and invasion and migration suppression	[94]
Dahuang zhechong pill	Inhibit growth of doxorubicin-resistant HCC subcutaneous xenografts in nude mice and accelerate apoptosis promotion integration with doxorubicin	[95]

A comprehensive screening among literature searched with "Chinese Medicine" combined with "liver cancer" was performed. Potential composite formulae for therapeutic of liver cancer were screened out and corresponding possible action mechanisms were summarized.

Table 1. Summary on Chinese medicine composite formulae potentially used for liver cancer treatment.

Acknowledgements

The study was financially supported by grants from the research council of the University of Hong Kong (project codes: 104004092, 104004460, 104004746), the Research Grants Committee (RGC) of Hong Kong, HKSAR (project codes: 764708, 766211, 17152116), Wong's Donation on Modern Oncology of Chinese Medicine (project code: 200006276), and Gala Family Trust (project code: 200007008).

Author details

Feiyu Chen, Ning Wang and Yibin Feng*

*Address all correspondence to: yfeng@hku.hk

School of Chinese Medicine, Li Ka Shing Faculty of Medicine, The University of Hong Kong, China

References

[1] Chen WQ et al. Cancer statistics in China, 2015. CA: A Cancer Journal for Clinicians. 2016; **66**(2):115-132

[2] Forner A, Reig M, Bruix J. Hepatocellular carcinoma. Lancet. 2018;**391**(10127):1301-1314

[3] Ting CT et al. Preventive and therapeutic role of traditional Chinese herbal medicine in hepatocellular carcinoma. Journal of the Chinese Medical Association. 2015;**78**(3):139-144

[4] Zhong JH et al. Tumor stage and primary treatment of hepatocellular carcinoma at a large tertiary hospital in China: A real-world study. Oncotarget. 2017;**8**(11):18296-18302

[5] Tsai TY et al. Associations between prescribed Chinese herbal medicine and risk of hepatocellular carcinoma in patients with chronic hepatitis B: A nationwide population-based cohort study. BMJ Open. 2017;**7**(1):e014571

[6] Yang Z et al. Add-on therapy with traditional chinese medicine improves outcomes and reduces adverse events in hepatocellular carcinoma: A meta-analysis of randomized controlled trials. Evidence-based Complementary and Alternative Medicine. 2017;**2017**:3428253

[7] Cao BQ. Current status and future prospects of acupuncture and traditional Chinese medicine in Canada. Chinese Journal of Integrative Medicine. 2015;**21**(3):166-172

[8] Ling CQ et al. Clinical practice guidelines for the treatment of primary liver cancer with integrative traditional Chinese and Western medicine. Journal of Integrative Medicine. 2018;**16**(4):236-248

[9] Fan TP et al. Future development of global regulations of Chinese herbal products. Journal of Ethnopharmacology. 2012;**140**(3):568-586

[10] Wang N et al. Berberine-induced tumor suppressor p53 up-regulation gets involved in the regulatory network of MIR-23a in hepatocellular carcinoma. Biochimica et Biophysica Acta. 2014;**1839**(9):849-857

[11] Wang N et al. Berberine suppresses cyclin D1 expression through proteasomal degradation in human hepatoma cells. International Journal of Molecular Sciences. 2016;**17**(11):1899

[12] Wang X et al. Up-regulation of PAI-1 and down-regulation of uPA are involved in suppression of invasiveness and motility of hepatocellular carcinoma cells by a natural compound berberine. International Journal of Molecular Sciences. 2016;**17**(4):577

[13] Wang N et al. Berberine induces autophagic cell death and mitochondrial apoptosis in liver cancer cells: The cellular mechanism. Journal of Cellular Biochemistry. 2010;**111**(6): 1426-1436

[14] Tsang CM et al. Berberine suppresses Id-1 expression and inhibits the growth and development of lung metastases in hepatocellular carcinoma. Biochimica et Biophysica Acta. 2015;**1852**(3):541-551

[15] Yang F et al. Hydroxysafflor yellow A inhibits angiogenesis of hepatocellular carcinoma via blocking ERK/MAPK and NF-kappaB signaling pathway in H22 tumor-bearing mice. European Journal of Pharmacology. 2015;**754**:105-114

[16] Li NN et al. Evidence for the involvement of COX-2/VEGF and PTEN/Pl3K/AKT pathway the mechanism of Oroxin B treated liver cancer. Pharmacognosy Magazine. 2018;**14**(54): 207-213

[17] Cao Z et al. Luteolin promotes cell apoptosis by inducing autophagy in hepatocellular carcinoma. Cellular Physiology and Biochemistry. 2017;**43**(5):1803-1812

[18] Xiao Z et al. Role of microRNA-95 in the anticancer activity of Brucein D in hepatocellular carcinoma. European Journal of Pharmacology. 2014;**728**:141-150

[19] Gramantieri L et al. Cyclin G1 is a target of miR-122a, a microRNA frequently down-regulated in human hepatocellular carcinoma. Cancer Research. 2007;**67**(13):6092-6099

[20] Zhou W et al. TCM matrine inducescell arrest and apoptosis with recovery expression of the hepato-specific miR122a in human hepatocellular carcinomaHep G2cell line. International Journal of Clinical and Experimental Medicine. 2015;**8**(6):9004-9012

[21] Wu L et al. Synthesis and biological evaluation of matrine derivatives as anti-hepatocellular cancer agents. Bioorganic & Medicinal Chemistry Letters. 2016;**26**(17):4267-4271

[22] Sun X et al. A novel matrine derivative WM622 inhibits hepatocellular carcinoma by inhibiting PI3K/AKT signaling pathways. Molecular and Cellular Biochemistry. 2018;(8):1-8

[23] Liao YJ et al. Longikaurin A, a natural ent-kaurane, induces G2/M phase arrest via downregulation of Skp2 and apoptosis induction through ROS/JNK/c-Jun pathway in hepatocellular carcinoma cells. Cell Death & Disease. 2014;**5**(3):1136

[24] Chen YS et al. Growth inhibition by pennogenyl saponins from Rhizoma paridis on hepatoma xenografts in nude mice. Steroids. 2014;**83**:39-44

[25] Huang G et al. Isoquercitrin inhibits the progression of liver cancer in vivo and in vitro via the MAPK signalling pathway. Oncology Reports. 2014;**31**(5):2377-2384

[26] Zhang S et al. Synergistic inhibitory effect of traditional chinese medicine astragaloside IV and curcumin on tumor growth and angiogenesis in an orthotopic nude-mouse model of human hepatocellular carcinoma. Anticancer Research. 2017;**37**(2):465-473

[27] Yie Y et al. Ursolic acid inhibited growth of hepatocellular carcinoma HepG2 cells through AMPKalpha-mediated reduction of DNA methyltransferase 1. Molecular and Cellular Biochemistry. 2015;**402**(1-2):63-74

[28] Xu J et al. Bilobol inhibits the lipopolysaccharide-induced expression and distribution of RhoA in HepG2 human hepatocellular carcinoma cells. Oncology Letters. 2015;**10**(2):962-966

[29] Zhu C et al. Fucoidan inhibits the growth of hepatocellular carcinoma independent of angiogenesis. Evidence-based Complementary and Alternative Medicine. 2013;**2013**: 692549

[30] Cho Y et al. Fucoidan protects hepatocytes from apoptosis and inhibits invasion of hepatocellular carcinoma by up-regulating p42/44 MAPK-dependent NDRG-1/CAP43. Acta Pharmaceutica Sinica B. 2015;**5**(6):544-553

[31] Zheng B et al. Telekin induces apoptosis associated with the mitochondria-mediated pathway in human hepatocellular carcinoma cells. Biological & Pharmaceutical Bulletin. 2013;**36**(7):1118-1125

[32] Chen H et al. Gigantol attenuates the proliferation of human liver cancer HepG2 cells through the PI3K/Akt/NF-kappaB signaling pathway. Oncology Reports. 2017;**37**(2):865-870

[33] Ren B et al. Celastrol induces apoptosis in hepatocellular carcinoma cells via targeting ER-stress/UPR. Oncotarget. 2017;**8**(54):93039-93050

[34] Yu L et al. Cytisine induces endoplasmic reticulum stress caused by calcium overload in HepG2 cells. Oncology Reports. 2018;**39**(3):1475-1484

[35] Song L et al. Natural cyclopeptide RA-XII, a new autophagy inhibitor, suppresses protective autophagy for enhancing apoptosis through AMPK/mTOR/P70S6K pathways in HepG2 cells. Molecules. 2017;**22**(11):1934

[36] Liao N et al. A novel polysaccharide conjugate from bullacta exarata induces G1-phase arrest and apoptosis in human hepatocellular carcinoma HepG2 cells. Molecules. 2017;**22**(3):384

[37] Li Y et al. Diosgenin induces G2/M cell cycle arrest and apoptosis in human hepatocellular carcinoma cells. Oncology Reports. 2015;**33**(2):693-698

[38] Chen YJ, Chen CC, Huang HL. Induction of apoptosis by Armillaria mellea constituent armillarikin in human hepatocellular carcinoma. OncoTargets and Therapy. 2016;**9**:4773-4783

[39] Qu L et al. Corosolic acid analogue, a natural triterpenoid saponin, induces apoptosis on human hepatocarcinoma cells through mitochondrial pathway in vitro. Pharmaceutical Biology. 2016;**54**(8):1445-1457

[40] Fu WM et al. MiR-218-targeting-Bmi-1 mediates the suppressive effect of 1,6,7-trihydroxyxanthone on liver cancer cells. Apoptosis. 2015;**20**(1):75-82

[41] Yao WL et al. Cordycepin suppresses integrin/FAK signaling and epithelial-mesenchymal transition in hepatocellular carcinoma. Anti-Cancer Agents in Medicinal Chemistry. 2014; **14**(1):29-34

[42] Zhang QY et al. FAM46C is critical for the anti-proliferation and pro-apoptotic effects of norcantharidin in hepatocellular carcinoma cells. Scientific Reports. 2017;**7**(1):396

[43] Wang Y et al. Regulation of demethylation and re-expression of RASSF1A gene in hepatocellular carcinoma cell lines treated with NCTD in vitro. Journal of Cancer Research and Therapeutics. 2015;**11**(4):818-822

[44] Zhang S et al. Norcantharidin enhances ABT-737-induced apoptosis in hepatocellular carcinoma cells by transcriptional repression of Mcl-1. Cellular Signalling. 2012;**24**(9): 1803-1809

[45] Qiu DZ et al. Bufalin, a component in Chansu, inhibits proliferation and invasion of hepatocellular carcinoma cells. BMC Complementary and Alternative Medicine. 2013;**13**:185

[46] Tsai SC et al. Bufalin increases sensitivity to AKT/mTOR-induced autophagic cell death in SK-HEP-1 human hepatocellular carcinoma cells. International Journal of Oncology. 2012; **41**(4):1431-1442

[47] Hu F et al. Blocking autophagy enhances the apoptosis effect of bufalin on human hepatocellular carcinoma cells through endoplasmic reticulum stress and JNK activation. Apoptosis. 2014;**19**(1):210-223

[48] Zhang DM et al. Arenobufagin, a natural bufadienolide from toad venom, induces apoptosis and autophagy in human hepatocellular carcinoma cells through inhibition of PI3K/Akt/mTOR pathway. Carcinogenesis. 2013;**34**(6):1331-1342

[49] Deng LJ et al. Hellebrigenin induces cell cycle arrest and apoptosis in human hepatocellular carcinoma HepG2 cells through inhibition of Akt. Chemico-Biological Interactions. 2014;**219**:184-194

[50] Xiang JF et al. Anticancer effects of deproteinized asparagus polysaccharide on hepatocellular carcinoma in vitro and in vivo. Tumor Biology. 2014;**35**(4):3517-3524

[51] Weng LL et al. Asparagus polysaccharide and gum with hepatic artery embolization induces tumor growth and inhibits angiogenesis in an orthotopic hepatocellular carcinoma model. Asian Pacific Journal of Cancer Prevention. 2014;**15**(24):10949-10955

[52] Guo L et al. Characterization and immunostimulatory activity of a polysaccharide from the spores of *Ganoderma lucidum*. International Immunopharmacology. 2009;**9**(10):1175-1182

[53] Li A et al. *Ganoderma lucidum* polysaccharide extract inhibits hepatocellular carcinoma growth by downregulating regulatory T cells accumulation and function by inducing microRNA-125b. Journal of Translational Medicine. 2015;**13**:100

[54] Shan L et al. Huaier restrains proliferative and migratory potential of hepatocellular carcinoma cells partially through decreased Yes-associated protein 1. Journal of Cancer. 2017;**8**(19):4087-4097

[55] Wang JZ et al. Anti-hepatoma activities of ethyl acetate extract from *Ampelopsis sinica* root. Oncology Reports. 2017;**37**(4):2227-2236

[56] Liu X et al. Extract of Stellerachamaejasme L(ESC) inhibits growth and metastasis of human hepatocellular carcinoma via regulating microRNA expression. BMC Complementary and Alternative Medicine. 2018;**18**(1):99

[57] Lim EG et al. Ethanol extract from *Cnidium monnieri* (L.) Cusson induces cell cycle arrest and apoptosis via regulation of the p53independent pathway in HepG2 and Hep3B hepatocellular carcinoma cells. Molecular Medicine Reports. 2018;**17**(2):2572-2580

[58] Rui W et al. Compound Astragalus and Salvia miltiorrhiza extract suppresses hepatocellular carcinoma progression by inhibiting fibrosis and PAI-1 mRNA transcription. Journal of Ethnopharmacology. 2014;**151**(1):198-209

[59] Xiang M et al. Chemical composition of total flavonoids from Salvia chinensia Benth and their pro-apoptotic effect on hepatocellular carcinoma cells: Potential roles of suppressing cellular NF-kappaB signaling. Food and Chemical Toxicology. 2013;**62**:420-426

[60] Zhu M et al. Up-regulation of microRNAs, miR21 and miR23a in human liver cancer cells treated with Coptidis rhizoma aqueous extract. Experimental and Therapeutic Medicine. 2011;**2**(1):27-32

[61] Wang N et al. F-actin reorganization and inactivation of Rho signaling pathway involved in the inhibitory effect of Coptidis rhizoma on hepatoma cell migration. Integrative Cancer Therapies. 2010;**9**(4):354-364

[62] Tan HY et al. Suppression of vascular endothelial growth factor via inactivation of eukaryotic elongation factor 2 by alkaloids in Coptidis rhizome in hepatocellular carcinoma. Integrative Cancer Therapies. 2014;**13**(5):425-434

[63] Su YC et al. Modulation of the tumor metastatic microenvironment and multiple signal pathways by *Prunella vulgaris* in human hepatocellular carcinoma. The American Journal of Chinese Medicine. 2016;**44**(4):835-849

[64] Cheng J et al. Hepatocellular carcinoma growth is inhibited by *Euphorbia helioscopia* L. extract in nude mice xenografts. BioMed Research International. 2015;**2015**:601015

[65] Yan YQ et al. Scorpion inhibits epithelial-mesenchymal transition and metastasis of hepatocellular carcinoma. Experimental Biology and Medicine (Maywood, N.J.). 2018;**243**(7): 645-654

[66] Hou J, Wang L, Wu D. The root of *Actinidia chinensis* inhibits hepatocellular carcinomas cells through LAMB3. Cell Biology and Toxicology. 2018;**34**(4):321-332

[67] He M et al. *Actinidia chinensis* Planch root extract inhibits cholesterol metabolism in hepatocellular carcinoma through upregulation of PCSK9. Oncotarget. 2017;**8**(26):42136-42148

[68] Shen H et al. Ethanol extract of root of *Prunus persica* inhibited the growth of liver cancer cell HepG2 by inducing cell cycle arrest and migration suppression. Evidence-based Complementary and Alternative Medicine. 2017;**2017**:8231936

[69] Song P et al. Realgar transforming solution displays anticancer potential against human hepatocellular carcinoma HepG2 cells by inducing ROS. International Journal of Oncology. 2017;**50**(2):660-670

[70] Lin SC et al. Protective and therapeutic effects of Huanglian-Jie-Du-Tang on hepatotoxin-induced liver injuries. American Journal of Chinese Medicine. 1996;**24**(3-4):219-229

[71] Hsu YL et al. Huang-lian-jie-du-tang, a traditional Chinese medicine prescription, induces cell-cycle arrest and apoptosis in human liver cancer cells in vitro and in vivo. Journal of Gastroenterology and Hepatology. 2008;**23**(7 Pt 2):e290-e299

[72] Wang N et al. Inhibition of eukaryotic elongation factor-2 confers to tumor suppression by a herbal formulation Huanglian-Jiedu decoction in human hepatocellular carcinoma. Journal of Ethnopharmacology. 2015;**164**:309-318

[73] Hu B et al. Modified Yi Guan Jian, a Chinese herbal formula, induces anoikis in Bel-7402 human hepatocarcinoma cells in vitro. Oncology Reports. 2011;**26**(6):1465-1470

[74] Qi F et al. Pien Tze Huang inhibits the growth of hepatocellular carcinoma cells by upregulating miR-16 expression. Oncology Letters. 2017;**14**(6):8132-8137

[75] Lin HJ et al. The Chinese medicine Sini-San inhibits HBx-induced migration and invasiveness of human hepatocellular carcinoma cells. BMC Complementary and Alternative Medicine. 2015;**15**:348

[76] Zhang QB et al. Herbal compound Songyou Yin and moderate swimming suppress growth and metastasis of liver cancer by enhancing immune function. Integrative Cancer Therapies. 2016;**15**(3):368-375

[77] Peng Y et al. Niu-Huang-Shen suppresses hepatocellular carcinoma cell growth and metastasis by regulating Yap1 expression. Experimental and Therapeutic Medicine. 2017; **14**(6):5459-5463

[78] Bao Y et al. Metabolomic study of the intervention effects of Shuihonghuazi Formula, a Traditional Chinese Medicinal formulae, on hepatocellular carcinoma (HCC) rats using performance HPLC/ESI-TOF-MS. Journal of Ethnopharmacology. 2017;**198**:468-478

[79] Sun B et al. The Chinese Herb Jianpijiedu contributes to the regulation of OATP1B2 and ABCC2 in a rat model of orthotopic transplantation liver cancer pretreated with food restriction and diarrhea. BioMed Research International. 2015;**2015**:752850

[80] Fujii Y et al. Recipient-mediated effect of a traditional chinese herbal medicine, Ren-Shen-Yang-Rong-Tang (Japanese Name, Ninjin-Youei-to), on hematopoietic recovery following lethal irradiation and syngeneic bone-marrow transplantation. International Journal of Immunopharmacology. 1994;**16**(8):615-622

[81] Ohnishi Y et al. Effects of Juzen-Taiho-Toh (Tj-48), a traditional oriental medicine, on hematopoietic recovery from radiation-injury in mice. Experimental Hematology. 1990; **18**(1):18-22

[82] Jia LL et al. The synergistic effects of traditional Chinese herbs and radiotherapy for cancer treatment (review). Oncology Letters. 2013;**5**(5):1439-1447

[83] Yu Y et al. *Ganoderma lucidum* polysaccharide enhances radiosensitivity of hepatocellular carcinoma cell line HepG2 through Akt signaling pathway. Experimental and Therapeutic Medicine. 2017;**14**(6):5903-5907

[84] Kou W et al. Radix Angelicae Sinensis and Radix Hedysari enhance radiosensitivity of 12C6+ radiation in human liver cancer cells by modulating apoptosis protein. Saudi Medical Journal. 2014;**35**(9):945-952

[85] Zhang Q et al. Dihydromyricetin promotes hepatocellular carcinoma regression via a p53 activation-dependent mechanism. Scientific Reports. 2014;**4**:4628

[86] Zhai B et al. Bufalin reverses resistance to sorafenib by inhibiting Akt activation in hepatocellular carcinoma: The role of endoplasmic reticulum stress. PLoS One. 2015;**10**(9): e0138485

[87] Gu W et al. Reversal effect of bufalin on multidrug resistance in human hepatocellular carcinoma BEL-7402/5-FU cells. Oncology Reports. 2014;**31**(1):216-222

[88] Xu H et al. Luteolin synergizes the antitumor effects of 5-fluorouracil against human hepatocellular carcinoma cells through apoptosis induction and metabolism. Life Sciences. 2016;**144**:138-147

[89] Sun H et al. The cycloartane triterpenoid ADCX impairs autophagic degradation through Akt overactivation and promotes apoptotic cell death in multidrug-resistant HepG2/ADM cells. Biochemical Pharmacology. 2017;**146**:87-100

[90] Duan X et al. The antitumor effect of arsenic trioxide on hepatocellular carcinoma is enhanced by andrographolide. Oncotarget. 2017;**8**(53):90905-90915

[91] Wang CK et al. Integrated treatment of aqueous extract of *Solanum nigrum*-potentiated cisplatin- and doxorubicin-induced cytotoxicity in human hepatocellular carcinoma cells. Evidence-based Complementary and Alternative Medicine. 2015;**2015**:675270

[92] Hu Z et al. Huaier aqueous extract sensitizes cells to rapamycin and cisplatin through activating mTOR signaling. Journal of Ethnopharmacology. 2016;**186**:143-150

[93] Xia J et al. Combination of cinobufacini and doxorubicin increases apoptosis of hepatocellular carcinoma cells through the Fas- and mitochondria-mediated pathways. The American Journal of Chinese Medicine. 2017;**45**(7):1537-1556

[94] Xia J et al. Shufeng Jiedu Capsule and its active ingredients induce apoptosis, inhibit migration and invasion, and enhances doxorubicin therapeutic efficacy in hepatocellular carcinoma. Biomedicine & Pharmacotherapy. 2018;**99**:921-930

[95] Wu L et al. Effects of Dahuang zhechong pill on doxorubicin-resistant SMMC-7721 xenografts in mice. Journal of Ethnopharmacology. 2018;**222**:71-78

[96] Duan D et al. Gambogic acid induces apoptosis in hepatocellular carcinoma SMMC-7721 cells by targeting cytosolic thioredoxin reductase. Free Radical Biology & Medicine. 2014; **69**:15-25

[97] Zhong C et al. Clinical study of hepatectomy combined with Jianpi Huayu Therapy for hepatocellular carcinoma. Asian Pacific Journal of Cancer Prevention. 2014;**15**(14):5951-5957

[98] Zhang HP et al. Oridonin synergistically enhances JQ1-triggered apoptosis in hepatocellular cancer cells through mitochondrial pathway. Oncotarget. 2017;**8**(63):106833-106843

10

Interaction of Mitochondrial and Epigenetic Regulation in Hepatocellular Carcinoma

Victoria Chagoya de Sánchez, Enrique Chávez,
Gabriela Velasco-Loyden,
María Guadalupe Lozano-Rosas and
Alejandro Rusbel Aparicio-Cadena

Abstract

Hepatocellular carcinoma (HCC) is a pathology preceded mainly by cirrhosis of diverse etiology and is associated with uncontrolled dedifferentiation and cell proliferation processes. Many cellular functions are dependent on mitochondrial function, among which we can mention the enzymatic activity of PARP-1 and sirtuin 1, epigenetic regulation of gene expression, apoptosis, and so on. Mitochondrial dysfunction is related to liver diseases including cirrhosis and HCC; the energetic demand is not properly supplied and mitochondrial morphologic changes have been observed, resulting in an altered metabolism. There is a strong relationship between epigenetics and mitochondrion since the first one is dependent on the correct function of the last one. There is an interest to improve or to maintain mitochondrial integrity in order to prevent or reverse HCC; such is the case of IFC-305 that has a beneficial effect on mitochondrial function in a sequential model of cirrhosis-HCC. In this model, IFC-305 downregulates the expression of PCNA, thymidylate synthase, HGF and its receptor c-Met and upregulates the cell cycle inhibitor p27, thereby decreasing cell proliferation. Both effects, improvement of mitochondria function and reduction of tumor proliferation, suggest its use as HCC chemoprevention or as an adjuvant in chemotherapy.

Keywords: hepatocellular carcinoma, cell cycle, cell proliferation, mitochondria, epigenetics, IFC-305

1. Introduction

Hepatocellular carcinoma (HCC) represents 80% of the primary liver cancer and, in minor proportion, bile duct cancer and angiosarcoma of the blood vessels in the liver, but all of them have a poor prognosis. HCC is a major cause of cancer-related deaths globally. The incidence of HCC is increasing and has been rising in the last few decades [1]. The HCC is a complex pathology associated in 80–90% with chronic liver diseases like cirrhosis of diverse etiologies. Cirrhosis is a chronic degenerative disease of the hepatic parenchyma characterized by an inflammation process that leads to liver fibrogenesis. This process induces the loss of liver architecture and a diminution of functional parenchyma, which over time changes the environment of the cells resulting in chromosomal instability. The cause of cirrhosis transformation into HCC is not well known, but chromosomal instability could be an important factor for HCC generation in cirrhotic patients. The main problem of this pathology is the lack of early detection, recurrence of tumors following resection [2], and there are no effective therapies. To understand this complex pathology, it is convenient to have some knowledge of the structure and functions of the liver. Therapeutic options for HCC are very limited, and the incidence is very similar to the death rate per year. Only in the early stage of the disease, there are some approved therapies such as tumor ablation, surgical resection, and liver transplantation, but in advanced stages, when most patients are diagnosed, these treatments are not recommended. There is an average of 5-year survival below 20% with these therapies [3]. In intermediate and advanced stage-HCC, the approved options are transcatheter arterial chemoembolization (TACE) and the multi-kinase inhibitor, sorafenib. TACE therapy could extend survival to 2 years [3]. Sorafenib extends survival of patients with advanced stage disease for only 3 months, and this medication causes considerable adverse effects and offers no symptom palliation [4]. There are other several clinical trial efforts focused on therapies involving multiple signaling pathways, most commonly related to tyrosine-kinase growth factor receptors, but they have inferior survival benefits and several adverse effects. Immunotherapy has demonstrated some efficacy, but, in general, molecular characterization to find effective treatments of HCC is needed.

The liver is the largest internal and heterogeneous organ in the body constituted by different kinds of cells like hepatocytes, endothelial cells, cells of the bile duct, Kupffer cells, hepatic stellate cells (HSC), oval cells and pit cells [5]. The liver is an organ highly irrigated by the portal venous system and blood is distributed by the hepatic sinusoids and the hepatic artery [6]. About 80% of the liver cells are hepatocytes, and are epithelial cells that form cords with high metabolic activity and contain a complete set of organelles: mitochondria, peroxisomes, lysosomes, Golgi complex and a well-organized cytoskeleton [7]. The space between cords of hepatocytes and the endothelium is called the space of Disse. Endothelial cells constitute the wall of the hepatic sinusoids and are separated from the parenchymal cells by the space of Disse. They possess pores or fenestrae that permit the exchange of fluids [8]. These cells show endocytic activity and secrete several mediators such as interleukin-1 (IL-1), interleukin-6 (IL-6), interferon, and nitric oxide as paracrine modulators. Kupffer cells are the fixed macrophages of the liver that can migrate along sinusoids. Their main function is an immunomodulatory one [9]. Pit cells are intrahepatic leucocytes with natural killer cell activity [10] and exert a cytotoxic activity toward tumor and virus-infected cells [11]. HSC, also known as lipocytes, fat storing cells, perisinusoidal cells, and vitamin A storing cells, are quiescent in normal conditions.

When they are activated, they play an essential role in the synthesis and degradation of the extracellular matrix (ECM) proteins and fibrogenic cytokines, like hepatocyte growth factor (HGF), insulin growth factor (IGR), transforming growth factor-β (TGF-β), and, consequently, induce cirrhosis. Biliary epithelial cells participate in the formation of bile; they are transported to the bile ducts or Canals of Hering. These cells have the potential to become oval cells [7]. The cell-free hepatic tissue represents 20% of the liver volume and constitutes the ECM located in the Disse space. The ECM contains structural proteins like collagen of different types, glycoproteins, fibronectin, tenascin, laminin, entactin, and perlecan. Their function is to maintain the hepatic architecture and the organization of the entire organ. Hepatocytes contribute with 80–90% of the synthesis of liver collagen, which is degraded by metalloproteinases (MMPs) [12]. The liver has multiple functions needed for its own metabolism and for other organs; it participates intensely in the intermediary metabolism that occurs mainly in hepatocytes and is connected with the nutrients of the diet, reaching from the portal circulation, that is, in carbohydrates, proteins, and lipid metabolism. The liver also generates purines and pyrimidines for its own use and their distribution to other tissues in the form of adenosine, inosine, and hypoxanthine [13]. It also synthetizes and secretes plasma proteins and participates in the biotransformation of endogenous and exogenous compounds.

Previously, we have demonstrated that adenosine is a metabolic modulator of glucose and lipids in the liver and adipose tissue [14]. This molecule also modulates in vivo the energy charge in the liver [15]. The nucleoside adenosine is a substance with multiphysiological effects in different tissues, the central nervous system, and cardiovascular system; it is responsible for the modulation of the immune response and acts as metabolic regulator. Its action could be autocrine, paracrine, and endocrine; its metabolism is very active with a high turnover and a very short half-live. Adenosine presents circadian variations in the rat, which correlated with energetic homeostasis of the cell, modulation of membrane structure and function, cell proliferation, and genetic expression by regulating physiological methylation [16]. Exogenous adenosine administration to normal rats showed some pharmacological effects, like increased ATP levels simultaneous to a decrease in ADP and AMP, resulting in an increase of the energy charge of the liver [14]. Also, in the liver of fasted rats, adenosine induces an enhancement of glycogen synthesis [16] and an inhibition of fatty acid oxidation by inhibiting the extramitochondrial acyl CoA synthase and decreasing the plasma ketone bodies [17] These findings allowed us to demonstrate in vivo the Atkinson hypothesis of metabolism regulation by energy charge [18].

The redox state of the cell in different compartments, calculated by the NAD^+/NADH (NAD^+ and NADH nicotinamide adenine dinucleotide, oxidized and reduced) system, has been shown to be a key point in the control of metabolism [19]. Adenosine administration induces mitochondrial oxidation and promotes the oxidized state in the cytosol and mitochondria in the presence of fatty acid oxidation inhibition, which is induced by the nucleoside. It has been reported that adenosine modulates vasodilatation and vasoconstriction in the hepatic vessels controlling blood flow from the hepatic artery [20]. All these results observed in normal animals led us to test the effects of the nucleoside in several models of acute hepatotoxicity: one induced with ethanol [21], the second with cycloheximide, and the third with carbon tetrachloride (CCl_4). Although the toxic mechanism of each one is different, they yielded a similar response generating a fatty liver that was prevented by adenosine [21–23]. In this way, the nucleoside, through different mechanisms, protects the liver against acute toxicity.

Continuous acute hepatotoxicity results in chronic liver injury with subsequent cirrhosis, with accumulation of ECM proteins, mainly collagen type I [24], accompanied by a deficient degradation of deposited collagen [25]. These conditions will induce a change in liver architecture with loss of its function. This is a complex process, for which no effective treatment has been developed yet. To study the effects of adenosine in this process, a model of cirrhosis induced in rats with CCl_4 was developed, in which two conditions were tested: prevention during cirrhosis development and reversion once it is already established [26, 27]. The simultaneous administration of adenosine partially blocked the stimulated collagen synthesis induced by the hepatotoxin, maintained high levels of hepatic collagenase activity, resulting in 50% diminution of fibrosis [26]. The effect of the nucleoside was clearly observed also in the reversion model; it was tested in well-established cirrhosis after 10 weeks of CCl_4 administration. Five weeks after suspension of the toxin, animals were treated with saline or adenosine, the saline group increased the cirrhotic characteristics but the group of animals treated with the nucleoside revealed blocked fibrogenesis, increased collagen degradation and normalized collagen types ratio, promoted hepatocyte proliferation, accelerated normalization of liver function, and decreased oxidative stress. These results suggest adenosine as a potential therapeutic agent in the treatment of chronic hepatic disease.

The transfer of an interesting research finding to a clinical setting is complicated, but in collaboration with Dr. Francisco Hernández Luis from the National Autonomous University of Mexico's School of Chemistry, we prepared several adenosine derivatives that were tested in the CCl_4 induced cirrhosis. The aspartate of adenosine, named IFC-305, showed interesting results [28]; beneficial effects in structure and functional recovery were obtained with a fourfold lower dose of this adenosine derivative because it has a longer half-life. The hepatoprotective mechanism of IFC-305 on fibrogenesis was investigated by means of DNA microarrays analysis [29], showing that the expression of 413 differential genes deregulated in cirrhosis tended to be normalized by IFC-305 treatment. Fibrogenic genes, such as TGF-β, collagen type I, fibronectin I, increased their expression in cirrhotic groups, and IFC-305 diminished their expression supporting the antifibrogenic action of the compound. These results highly suggest a diminution of chromosomal instability. With the increased understanding in chromatin organization of the eukaryote genome at genetic and epigenetic levels and remembering the previously commented role of adenosine on physiological methylations, a possible epigenetic mechanism of the IFC-305 could participate in the obtained results. Global changes in DNA methylation, 5-hydroxymethylation and histone H4 acetylation were decreased in cirrhosis and after the IFC-305 treatment the normal values were recuperated. In contrast, the promoter of *Col1a1* gene is hypomethylated in cirrhosis but gains DNA methylation upon treatment with IFC-305, correlating with a decrease of Col1a1 transcript and protein level, showing that the treatment restores globally and specifically epigenetic modifications [30]. The microarray analysis also showed modification of immunity genes which where explored in the CCl_4 model; it was found that the IFC-305 compound reduced inflammatory cytokines and increased the anti-inflammatory ones like IL-10, supporting the modulation of the macrophage phenotypes M1 and M2 [31].

2. Hepatocytes proliferation in cirrhosis and cancer, modulation by IFC-305

The liver is an organ with regenerative capacity. Partial hepatectomy or diverse stimuli promote proliferation of parenchymal and non-parenchymal cells in order to recover the liver mass and architecture. This process is regulated by cell cycle proteins, cytokines, growth factors, and matrix remodeling [32].

In acute liver injury, there is a classic wound healing process in which inflammation triggers scar formation that is subsequently resolved to enable regeneration of the damaged hepatic parenchyma. However, when there is a chronic liver injury, the normal regenerative process is impaired, and instead a net deposition of fibrillar collagen is predominant [33].

Cirrhosis is characterized by a decrease in hepatocyte proliferation, in part, because liver cells have a limited regenerative capacity restricted by telomere length. After several rounds of replication, telomeres reach a critically short length that induces cell cycle arrest, senescence, and apoptosis of hepatocytes. Telomere shortening also activates DNA repair pathways leading to chromosomal fusions and instability [34]. During cirrhosis-activated HSC, inflammatory cells secrete proliferative and angiogenic cytokines that contribute to a proliferative condition milieu, including: HGF, vascular endothelial growth factor (VEGF), and IL-6 [33]. This proliferative milieu could stimulate the proliferation of altered hepatocytes carrying mutations of cell cycle checkpoint genes or could select genetically altered clones, promoting HCC [34].

Among the principal cell cycle checkpoints that are generally altered in HCC are the tumor suppressor p53 and Rb proteins. p53 is implicated in cell cycle control, DNA repair, apoptosis, and regulates different metabolic pathways [35, 36]. p53 is frequently mutated in HCC (28–50%) and core proteins from hepatitis B and C viruses can repress p53 activity [36]. The pRB protein is implicated in the progression from G1 into S phase. The Rb pathway is disrupted in more than 80% of human HCC [34]. Gankyrin binds Mdm2 promoting proteasomal degradation of p53 and pRb. Both gankyrin and Mdm2 proteins are frequently overexpressed in human HCC [34, 35]. p53 is also implicated in the stimulation of ATP production by oxidative phosphorylation (OXPHOS). p53 also decreases glycolysis and cellular reactive oxygen species (ROS) production by inducing a protein called TP53-induced glycolysis and apoptosis regulator (TIGAR). TIGAR blocks glycolysis by degrading fructose-2,6-bisphosphate. This inhibition redirects glucose-6-phosphate into the pentose phosphate pathway, which increases NADPH production increasing the antioxidant defenses. The inactivation of p53 should decrease OXPHOS and increase glycolysis and ROS production in cancer cells [37].

It has been demonstrated that IFC-305 is able to stimulate hepatocytes proliferation in CCl_4-induced cirrhotic liver through the upregulation of proliferating cell nuclear antigen (PCNA), HGF, and p53, with an increase in energy and preservation of mitochondrial function [38].

On the other hand, in a sequential model of cirrhosis-HCC induced by diethylnirosamine (DEN), IFC-305 caused a tumor reduction, and this protective effect was associated with decreased cell proliferation in the HCC stage. This effect was associated with a decreased expression of PCNA, thymidylate synthase, HGF and its receptor c-Met, and the induction of the cell cycle inhibitor p27. IFC-305 also induced a diminution of gankyrin expression contributing to restoring p53 protein expression to control levels [39].

How could the same compound IFC-305 have opposing effects on proliferation in normal versus transformed hepatocytes? These could be mediated partly by a differential expression of the HGF-c-Met pathway driven by IFC-305 treatment, and the dual role of HGF/c-Met in cirrhosis and liver tumorigenesis. HGF expression is restricted to cells of mesenchymal origin, whereas the receptor c-Met is expressed in epithelial and endothelial cells. HGF is implicated in cell proliferation, survival, morphogenesis, cell motility, and metastasis. This pathway plays a critical role in tissue protection and regeneration. It has been used as a therapeutic agent in fibrosis of different organs. The protective actions of HGF are associated with promotion of cell proliferation, migration, and morphogenesis that would help tissues reorganization [40]. Its protective role is also related to its anti-inflammatory action and its regulation of the cellular redox state, driven by upregulation of the antioxidant enzymes and glutathione reduced (GSH), as well as by repression of two major pro-oxidant systems: NADPH oxidase and/or Cyp2E1 [41]. Nevertheless, the HGF/c-Met pathway in HCC contributes to tumor development by stimulating cell proliferation, invasion, and metastasis [40]. We observed that, in the cirrhotic liver induced by CCl_4, the hepatoprotector IFC-305 incremented HGF expression [38], which could have a protective role in the regenerative capacity of the liver. On the other hand, in DEN-induced HCC, the IFC305 treatment downregulated HGF and c-Met expression, which contribute to liver tumorigenesis reduction [39]. HGF and c-Met can be potentiated by ROS in hepatoma cells [41, 42]. It was described that, in the sequential model of cirrhosis-HCC with DEN, there are dysfunctional mitochondria and the administration of IFC-305 restored the mitochondrial function and regulated parameters implicated in metabolism, as well as the mitochondrial dynamics modified by DEN intoxication [43]. Therefore, the IFC-305 could be suppressing expression of HGF via the improvement of mitochondrial redox in DEN carcinogenesis. On the other hand, the restoration by IFC-305 treatment of the p53 protein expression in CCl_4-induced cirrhosis and in DEN-induced carcinogenesis, among other effects, could contribute to the restoration of ATP production by OXPHOS and to the decrease of ROS production. However, the exact molecular mechanism by which IFC-305 causes different effects on hepatocytes proliferation in cirrhosis and HCC requires further clarification.

3. Mitochondrial alterations in the HCC: the effect of the IFC-305 compound

Mitochondria are responsible for energy metabolism in eukaryotic cells; they generate ATP through oxidative phosphorylation. In addition, an important part of the ATP synthesis is the donation of electrons by the tricarboxylic acids chain (TCA) to the electron transport chain (ETC), constituted by five complexes (I-V), NADH enters complex I and generates NAD^+, and complex V forms ATP. Mitochondria regulate the energetic state, the redox state, and the metabolism of the cells, being able to generate the epigenetic intermediaries becoming the main therapeutic target of many kinds of cancer [44].

As a response to stress, the cells acquire a metabolic adaptation, which is an important area of research due to its relationship with different illnesses [45]. In chronic liver diseases like cirrhosis, energetic deficiency and alterations in energy parameters have been demonstrated independently of their etiology [46]. Otto Warburg suggested that mitochondria from tumor cells supply energy through glycolytic flow due to lack of oxygen or genetic-epigenetic alterations that affect oxidative metabolism [47]. Mitochondrial dysfunction is implicated in metabolic reprogramming in HCC. The increased ROS production and the reduced ATP generation may contribute to the HCC malignancy [48]. Metabolic alterations may decrease the levels of acetyl CoA, which also plays an important role as modulator of gene expression [49]. In experimental models, including the CCl_4-induced cirrhosis, mitochondrial dysfunction has been demonstrated because impaired mitochondrial respiration and ATP decreased levels have been observed [50, 51]. A metabolic adaptation in response to the ATP diminished levels is increased glycolysis [51]. A consequence of oxidative stress in chronic liver diseases is the decrease in metabolic flux, which includes alterations in the TCA enzymes, such as isocitrate dehydrogenase (IDH), which can produce oncometabolites when it undergoes mutations [52].

The redox state can be represented by the NAD^+/NADH ratio, which is regulated by the ETC. Several enzymes depend on NAD^+ like sirtuin-1 (Sirt-1), a member of deacetylases, and poly (ADP-ribose) polymerase-1 (PARP-1). A Sirt-1 substrate is the peroxisome proliferator-activated receptor gamma co-activator 1-alpha (PGC-1α), which is upregulated in HCC and is responsible for orchestrating mitochondrial biogenesis, favoring accumulation of defective mitochondria [44]. On the other hand, PARP-1 modulates the transcription and DNA repair; however, in HCC, it is upregulated and is considered a hallmark of cancer [53]. The over-regulation of both enzymes in HCC may deplete the NAD^+ that can be related to loss of mitochondrial membrane potential (ψm) and mitochondrial dysfunction [54]. Alterations in ψm induce the process of mitochondrial dynamics as a repair response to possible damage to this organelle. Mitochondrial dynamics depends on two mechanisms: fission and fusion; the first one is caused by various types of stress and requires protein activity such as Drp-1, on the other hand, fusion requires the recovery of ψm and proteins such as mitofusin 1 and 2 (MFN 1 and 2) [44]. Mitochondrial fusion promotes cristae formation and normal mitochondria phenotype [55]. Morphological alterations in mitochondria determined through electronic microscopy in various models of hepatic fibrosis have been described a long time ago [56, 57].

Previously, it has been discussed some of the effects of adenosine (base molecule of IFC-305), which include increase in energy parameters and regulation of the redox state. Considering this background and what has been described regarding the metabolic and mitochondrial changes in chronic liver damage, such as cirrhosis and HCC, it was decided to evaluate whether IFC-305 had any mitochondrial effect in the sequential model of cirrhosis-HCC.

In the sequential model of cirrhosis-HCC, decreased mitochondrial respiration, determined through oxygen consumption, and a decreased ψm were found, which reflected in a diminished ATP synthesis. In fact, the dimeric form (active form) of the F1F0 complex of ATPase is lost [43].

On the other hand, alterations in the mitochondrial redox state were observed, determined through the ratio of the levels of β-hydroxybutyrate/acetoacetate (NAD^+/NADH). The activity of NAD-dependent enzymes was also affected, such is the case of IDH and PARP-1; this alteration induced a metabolic adaptation because increased levels of lactate were observed suggesting an increase in aerobic glycolysis [43].

It is known that the mitochondrion is capable of responding to several insults of stress through the activity of various nuclear-encoded proteins like PGC-1α and Sirt-1. However, the over-regulation of these proteins has been associated with the accumulation of dysfunctional mitochondria, as described above. In the model previously described, these proteins were found increased. Dysfunctional mitochondria have been related to their morphology, and we know that morphology is closely linked to dynamism. The ratio of Drp-1/MFN-2, proteins that regulate the mitochondrial dynamics, was increased favoring the fragmented form of mitochondria as verified through electron microscopy [43].

Important findings were observed with the IFC-305 treatment as described in **Table 1** [43].

Uncoupled mitochondria depicted lower ATP synthesis due to the altered ψm and complex I activity. Previously, it has been demonstrated that complex I is sensitive to DEN toxicity, as NAD^+ linked respiration is inhibited [58]. Recovery of these parameters with IFC-305 treatment was observed, including the activity of NAD^+-dependent IDH. The PARP-1 activity inhibition probably favored the NAD^+ availability and contributed to the maintenance of the redox state. Mitochondrial function preservation and restoration allowed the normalization of the metabolism observed by lactate levels diminution.

On the other hand, the decreased Sirt-1 and PGC-1α in the groups treated with IFC-305 suggested that abnormal mitochondrial accumulation was inhibited. In fact, mitochondrial dynamics regulation was induced by IFC-305. These results demonstrated mitochondrial impairment through functional, metabolic, and dynamic alterations in HCC, and the hepatoprotector IFC-305 helps to repair them, being a tumor suppressive mechanism.

These findings support the mitochondrial role in the establishment of HCC and the interplay with the nuclear genome as targets in the design of new therapeutic strategies for the HCC treatment. In this regard, the IFC-305 supports that idea and emerges as a new possible HCC therapy through mitochondrial regulation.

According to the above, there is a growing interest to find pharmacological strategies to block the effects of mitochondrial dysfunction in HCC. Regarding this, in the model of HCC induced with DEN, a study was conducted to determine the mitochondrial effects of ginkgolide B in

Mitochondrial parameter	Effect
Function	Maintained and recovered: • mitochondrial respiration • ATP synthesis • mitochondrial membrane potential • dimeric form of the F1F0 ATPase subunit • normal cellular redox state
Metabolic	• Recovered the normal mitochondrial redox state • recovered the IDH activity • reduced lactate production • diminished increased PARP-1 activity
Dynamics	Avoided the accumulation of dysfunctional mitochondria through: • down-regulation of PGC-1α and Sirt-1 • diminution of DRP-1/MFN-2 ratio • Sirt-3 increment

Table 1. Effects of IFC-305 administration in mitochondria in the sequential model of cirrhosis-HCC.

two different pharmaceutical formulations, finding a decrease in the mitochondrial generation of ROS and a decrease in the dissipation of the mitochondrial membrane potential [59]. Moreover, two of the most studied hepatoprotective compounds until now are resveratrol and N-acetylcysteine (NAC) [60]. On the one hand, resveratrol inhibits the formation of hepatocyte nodules in the DEN-induced HCC model plus phenobarbital administration; moreover, it is capable of modulating mitochondrial biogenesis [61]. On the other hand, NAC blocked phosphorylation of β-catenin, JNK, and c-jun activation, avoiding the development of liver damage in HCC transaldolase-deficient mice, a limiting enzyme for the non-oxidative branch of the pentose phosphate pathway, which is, at least in part, responsible for HCC generation [62]; furthermore, NAC stabilizes the mitochondrial membrane potential regulating mitochondrial dynamics [61].

4. Interaction of mitochondria and epigenetics in HCC: An overview

The epigenome can be altered not only by environmental factors, such as exposure to exogenous chemicals [63] but also by changes in the levels of endogenous cofactors and metabolites [64, 65]. The exact correlation between nucleus and mitochondrion allows for the maintenance of mitochondrial structure and function. On the one hand, the nuclear gene expression is regulated by mitochondrial intermediates, like acetyl-CoA, ATP, NAD^+, and s-adenosylmethionine, which are the link between the epigenome and calorie availability [47, 66]. In addition to the production of epigenetic substrates, mitochondria may be modified in their DNA (mtDNA). Some mitochondrial genes have been reported as hypermethylated in HCC; for example, mitochondrial ribosomal protein S12 (*Mrps12*), mitochondria-localized glutamic acid-rich protein (*Mgrap*), and transmembrane protein 70 (*Tmem70*) genes [67, 68]. On the other hand, the disruption of the step in the methylation of 5-mC to 5-hmC in the mitochondrial genome leads to the alteration of several OXPHOS genes, such as: NADH dehydrogenase (ubiquinone) 1 subunit C2 (NDUFC2), NADH dehydrogenase (ubiquinone) flavoprotein 1 (NDUFV1), NADH: ubiquinone oxidoreductase subunit S6 (NDUFS6) from complex 1. These modifications, added to the mitochondrial damage by oxidative stress, can favor the loss of ETC function. In addition to that, it has been reported that the mitochondrial genome damage can affect the expression of nuclear genes [69–71]. Moreover, there is a deregulation of hepatic one carbon, and TCA cycle, therefore it driving the aberrant epigenetics changes [72–74]. The main consequence of depressing the TCA cycle is the reduced availability of α-ketoglutarate, leading to a decrease in the activity of α-ketoglutarate-dependent proteins, which are responsible for the hydroxylation of many substrates in the cell that are important in epigenomic control [74].

Tumor cell metabolism can be linked to epigenetic changes during carcinogenesis; recent research has focused on epigenetic studies in relation to metabolic pathways [75, 76]. HCC is a heterogeneous disease affected by various lifestyles and environmental factors. Epigenetic alterations are frequently caused by these factors and contribute to hepatocarcinogenesis. During HCC development, different alterations in global DNA methylation have been described; for example, global hypomethylation leads to aberrant overexpression of oncogenes and large chromosomal instability [77, 78].

In cirrhosis and HCC, distinct patterns of aberrant DNA methylation associated with cirrhosis and HCC have been confirmed [79, 80].

5. Conclusion

The pathophysiology of HCC is multifactorial and involves mitochondrial dysfunction. Mitochondria usually generate relevant modulators of gene expression controlled by epigenetic mechanisms. These alterations induce chromosomic instability that could give advantages to subclones of cells to their outgrowth (**Figure 1**). Further studies are needed to find

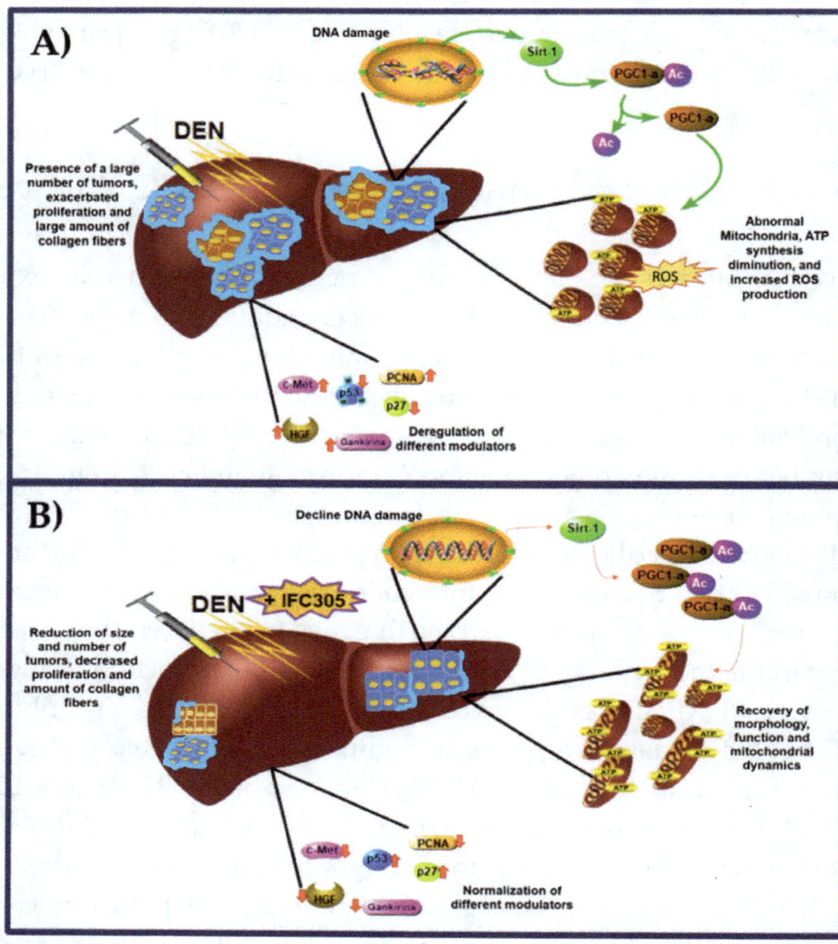

Figure 1. **(A)** In the model of liver injury induced by diethylnitrosamine (DEN), the architecture of the liver parenchyma is altered causing an exacerbated proliferation of various transformed clones, where the presence of a large number of tumors randomly distributed in each one is observed in the hepatic lobules. The preneoplastic nodules that form are surrounded by septa of collagen fibers; thus, favoring the evasion of the immune system and an ideal hypoxic microenvironment for the tumor cells. The genomic instability caused by the toxic as well as favoring mutations, for example in p53, and various alterations in different cellular modulators, among them HGF, c-Met, PCNA, gankyrin and p27. It also causes an increase of proteins, deacetylating PGC1-α, and, thus, modifies various nuclear genes exported to the mitochondria, causing accumulation of abnormal and dysfunctional mitochondria. **(B)** In the model of hepatocarcinoma induced by DEN, the administration of the adenosine derivative, IFC-305, has been shown to have various regulatory effects. The excessive accumulation of collagen fibers in preneoplastic nodules as well as the number and size of tumors are reduced. Also, cell morphology and DNA recover significantly. A decrease in the deacetylase Sirt-1, whose target is PCG1-α, has been observed, which allows the latter to remain acetylated and can be internalized to mitochondria, where it will promote its adequate morphology, dynamics and function. It has also been found that the compound IFC-305 acts on the levels of some important modulators in cancer (p53, HGF, C-Met…), maintaining or returning them to their concentrations under normal conditions. Overall, the aforementioned effects make this compound a possible therapeutic alternative.

therapeutic strategies capable of maintaining and improving the mitochondrial integrity to avoid alterations in the epigenetic regulation of nuclear- and mitochondrial-encoded genes. These effects could suppress failures in cell cycle checkpoints and the uncontrolled proliferation to prevent or reverse HCC as demonstrated for IFC-305.

Acknowledgements

This work was supported by Consejo Nacional de Ciencia y Tecnología (240315) and DGAPA-UNAM, grant numbers IN208915 VCS.

Abbreviations

HCC	hepatocellular carcinoma
PARP-1	poly (ADP-ribose) polymerase-1
TACE	transcatheter arterial chemoembolization
HSC	hepatic stellate cells
IL-1	interleukin-1
IL-6	interleukin-6
ECM	extracellular matrix
HGF	hepatocyte growth factor
IGR	insulin growth factor
TGF-β	transforming growth factor-β
MMPs	metalloproteinases
NAD+	nicotinamide adenine dinucleotide oxidized
NADH	nicotinamide adenine dinucleotide reduced
CCl4	carbon tetrachloride
IFC-305	aspartate of adenosine

VEGF	Vascular Endothelial Growth Factor
OXPHOS	oxidative phosphorylation
SCO2	chaperone protein "synthesis of cytochrome c oxidase 2"
ROS	reactive oxygen species
TIGAR	TP53-induced glycolysis and apoptosis regulator
PCNA	proliferating cell nuclear antigen
DEN	diethylnitrosamine
GSH	glutathione reduced
TCA	tricarboxylic acids chain
ETC	electron transport chain
IDH	isocitrate dehydrogenase
Sirt-1	sirtuin-1
PGC-1α	peroxisome proliferator-activated receptor gamma coactivator 1-alpha
ψm	mitochondrial membrane potential
MFN 1	mitofusin 1
MFN 2	mitofusin 2
NAC	N-acetylcysteine
mtDNA	mitochondrial DNA
Mrps12	mitochondrial ribosomal protein S12 gene
Mgrap	mitochondria-localized glutamic acid-rich protein gene
Tmem70	transmembrane protein 70 gene
NDUFC2	NADH dehydrogenase (ubiquinone) 1 subunit C2
NDUFV1	NADH dehydrogenase (ubiquinone) flavoprotein 1
NDUFS6	NADH: ubiquinone oxidoreductase subunit S6

Author details

Victoria Chagoya de Sánchez*, Enrique Chávez, Gabriela Velasco-Loyden, María Guadalupe Lozano-Rosas and Alejandro Rusbel Aparicio-Cadena

*Address all correspondence to: vchagoya@correo.ifc.unam.mx

Department of Cellular Biology and Development, Institute of Cellular Physiology, National Autonomous University of Mexico, Mexico City, Mexico

References

[1] Sanyal AJ, Yoon SK, Lencioni R. The etiology of hepatocellular carcinoma and consequences for treatment. The Oncologist. 2010;**15**(Suppl 4):14-22. DOI: 10.1634/theoncologist.2010-S4-14

[2] Cucchetti A, Piscaglia F, Cescon M, Ercolani G, Terzi E, Bolondi L, Zanello M, Pinna AD. Conditional survival after hepatic resection for hepatocellular carcinoma in cirrhotic patients. Clinical Cancer Research. 2012;**18**(16):4397-4405. DOI: 10.1158/1078-0432.CCR-11-2663

[3] Erstad DJ, Fuchs BC, Tanabe KK. Molecular signatures in hepatocellular carcinoma: A step toward rationally designed cancer therapy. Cancer. 2018. DOI: 10.1002/cncr.31257

[4] Sanoff HK, Chang Y, Lund JL, O'Neil BH, Dusetzina SB. Sorafenib effectiveness in advanced hepatocellular carcinoma. The Oncologist. 2016;**21**(9):1113-1120. DOI: 10.1634/theoncologist.2015-0478

[5] Rappaport A. Physioanatomic considerations. In: Schiff L, Schiff ER, editors. Diseases of the Liver. Philadelphia: Lippincott Company; 1987. pp. 1-46

[6] Tygstrup N, Winkler K, Mellemgaard K, Andreassen M. Determination of the hepatic arterial blood flow and oxygen supply in man by clamping the hepatic artery during surgery. The Journal of Clinical Investigation. 1962;**41**:447-454. DOI: 10.1172/JCI104497

[7] Jones AL, Hradek GT, Renston RH, Wong KY, Karlaganis G, Paumgartner G. Autoradiographic evidence for hepatic lobular concentration gradient of bile acid derivative. The American Journal of Physiology. 1980;**238**(3):G233-G237. DOI: 10.1152/ajpgi.1980.238.3.G233

[8] Zucker SG, Brown JL. Physiology of the liver. In: Fenton Schaffner HB, Edward Berk J, editors. Bockus Gastroenterology. Philadelphia, Pennsylvania: Saunders Company; 1995. pp. 1858-1905

[9] Laskin DL. Nonparenchymal cells and hepatotoxicity. Seminars in Liver Disease. 1990;**10**(4):293-304. DOI: 10.1055/s-2008-1040485

[10] Kaneda K, Wake K. Distribution and morphological characteristics of the pit cells in the liver of the rat. Cell and Tissue Research. 1983;**233**(3):485-505

[11] Ramadori G, Rieder H, Knittel T. Hepatic transport and bile secretion: Physiology and pathophysiology. In: Tavolini N, Berk PD, editors. Biology and Pathobiology of Sinusoidal Liver Cells. New York: Raven Press; 1993. pp. 83-102

[12] Chojkier M, Lyche KD, Filip M. Increased production of collagen in vivo by hepatocytes and nonparenchymal cells in rats with carbon tetrachloride-induced hepatic fibrosis. Hepatology. 1988;**8**(4):808-814

[13] Chagoya V. Interrelaciones metabolicas entre tejidos. Adaptación metabólica al ayuno y al ejercicio. In: Castillón E, editor. Bioquímica. España: EMALSA, S.A; 1986. pp. 1183-1194

[14] Chagoya de Sanchez V, Brunner A, Pina E. In vivo modification of the energy charge in the liver cell. Biochemical and Biophysical Research Communications. 1972;**46**(3):1441-1445

[15] De Sanchez VC, Pina E. Adenosine, a glucogenic and lipogenic compound. FEBS Letters. 1972;**19**(4):331-334

[16] Chagoya de Sanchez V, Hernandez-Munoz R, Sanchez L, Vidrio S, Yanez L, Suarez J. Twenty-four-hour changes of S-adenosylmethionine, S-adenosylhomocysteine adenosine and their metabolizing enzymes in rat liver; possible physiological significance in phospholipid methylation. The International Journal of Biochemistry. 1991;**23**(12):1439-1443

[17] De Sanchez VC, Piña E. The redox state of NAD+/NADH systems in rat liver during in vivo inhibition of fatty acid oxidation by adenosine. FEBS Letters. 1977;**83**(2):321-324

[18] Chagoya de Sánchez V, Piña E. Support for energy-charge model. Trends in Biochemical Sciences. 1978;**3**:N14-N15

[19] Hohorst HJ, Kreutz FH, Reim M, Huebener HJ. The oxidation/reduction state of the extramitochondrial DPN/DPNH system in rat liver and the hormonal control of substrate levels in vivo. Biochemical and Biophysical Research Communications. 1961;**4**:163-168

[20] Lautt WW. Mechanism and role of intrinsic regulation of hepatic arterial blood flow: Hepatic arterial buffer response. The American Journal of Physiology. 1985;**249**(5 Pt 1): G549-G556

[21] Hernandez-Munoz R, Santamaria A, Garcia-Sainz JA, Pina E, Chagoya de Sanchez V. On the mechanism of ethanol-induced fatty liver and its reversibility by adenosine. Archives of Biochemistry and Biophysics. 1978;**190**(1):155-162

[22] Garcia-Sainz JA, Hernandez-Munoz R, Santamaria A, de Sanchez VC. Mechanism of the fatty liver induced by cycloheximide and its reversibility by adenosine. Biochemical Pharmacology. 1979;**28**(8):1409-1413

[23] Hernandez-Munoz R, Glender W, Diaz Munoz M, Adolfo J, Garcia-Sainz JA, Chagoya de Sanchez V. Effects of adenosine on liver cell damage induced by carbon tetrachloride. Biochemical Pharmacology. 1984;**33**(16):2599-2604

[24] Friedman SL. Mechanisms of hepatic fibrogenesis. Gastroenterology. 2008;**134**(6):1655-1669. DOI: 10.1053/j.gastro.2008.03.003

[25] Perez Tamayo R. Is cirrhosis of the liver experimentally produced by CCl4 and adequate model of human cirrhosis? Hepatology. 1983;**3**(1):112-120

[26] Hernandez-Munoz R, Diaz-Munoz M, Suarez J, Chagoya de Sanchez V. Adenosine partially prevents cirrhosis induced by carbon tetrachloride in rats. Hepatology. 1990;**12**(2): 242-248

[27] Hernandez-Munoz R, Diaz-Munoz M, Suarez-Cuenca JA, Trejo-Solis C, Lopez V, Sanchez-Sevilla L, Yanez L, De Sanchez VC. Adenosine reverses a preestablished CCl4-induced micronodular cirrhosis through enhancing collagenolytic activity and stimulating hepatocyte cell proliferation in rats. Hepatology. 2001;**34**(4 Pt 1):677-687. DOI: 10.1053/jhep.2001.27949

[28] Chagoya de Sánchez V, Hernandez-Luis F, Díaz-Muñoz M, Hernández-Muñoz R. Role of the energy state of liver cells in cirrhosis development and treatment. In: Michelli ML, editor. Liver Cirrhosis: Causes, Diagnosisand Treatment. Nova Science Publisher; 2011. pp. 31-59

[29] Perez-Carreon JI, Martinez-Perez L, Loredo ML, Yanez-Maldonado L, Velasco-Loyden G, Vidrio-Gomez S, Ramirez-Salcedo J, Hernandez-Luis F, Velazquez-Martinez I, Suarez-Cuenca JA, Hernandez-Munoz R, de Sanchez VC. An adenosine derivative compound, IFC305, reverses fibrosis and alters gene expression in a pre-established CCl(4)-induced rat cirrhosis. The International Journal of Biochemistry & Cell Biology. 2010;**42**(2):287-296. DOI: 10.1016/j.biocel.2009.11.005

[30] Rodriguez-Aguilera JR, Guerrero-Hernandez C, Perez-Molina R, Cadena-Del-Castillo CE, de Vaca RP, Guerrero-Celis N, Dominguez-Lopez M, Murillo-de-Ozores AR, Arzate-Mejia R, Recillas-Targa F, de Sanchez VC. Epigenetic effects of an adenosine derivative in a Wistar rat model of liver cirrhosis. Journal of Cellular Biochemistry. 2018. DOI: 10.1002/jcb.26192

[31] Pérez-Cabeza de Vaca R, Domínguez-López M, Guerrero-Celis N, Rodríguez-Aguilera JR, Chagoya de Sánchez V. Inflammation is regulated by the adenosine derivative molecule IFC-305, during reversion of cirrhosis in a CCl4 rat model. International Immunopharmacology. 2018;**54**:12-23

[32] Delgado-Coello B, Briones-Orta MA, Macias-Silva M, Mas-Oliva J. Cholesterol: Recapitulation of its active role during liver regeneration. Liver International. 2011;**31**(9): 1271-1284. DOI: 10.1111/j.1478-3231.2011.02542.x

[33] Wallace MC, Friedman SL. Hepatic fibrosis and the microenvironment: Fertile soil for hepatocellular carcinoma development. Gene Expression. 2014;**16**(2):77-84. DOI: 10.3727/105221614X13919976902057

[34] El-Serag HB, Rudolph KL. Hepatocellular carcinoma: epidemiology and molecular carcinogenesis. Gastroenterology. 2007;**132**(7):2557-2576. DOI: 10.1053/j.gastro.2007.04.061

[35] Jin Y, Ding K, Wang D, Shen M, Pan J. Novel thiazole amine class tyrosine kinase inhibitors induce apoptosis in human mast cells expressing D816V KIT mutation. Cancer Letters. 2014;**353**(1):115-123. DOI: 10.1016/j.canlet.2014.07.017

[36] Shiraha H, Yamamoto K, Namba M. Human hepatocyte carcinogenesis (review). International Journal of Oncology. 2013;**42**(4):1133-1138. DOI: 10.3892/ijo.2013.1829

[37] Wallace DC. Mitochondria and cancer. Nature Reviews. Cancer. 2012;**12**(10):685-698. DOI: 10.1038/nrc3365

[38] Chagoya de Sanchez V, Martinez-Perez L, Hernandez-Munoz R, Velasco-Loyden G. Recovery of the cell cycle inhibition in CCl(4)-induced cirrhosis by the adenosine derivative IFC-305. International Journal of Hepatology. 2012;**2012**:212530. DOI: 10.1155/2012/212530

[39] Velasco-Loyden G, Perez-Martinez L, Vidrio-Gomez S, Perez-Carreon JI, Chagoya de Sanchez V. Cancer chemoprevention by an adenosine derivative in a model of

cirrhosis-hepatocellular carcinoma induced by diethylnitrosamine in rats. Tumour Biology. 2017;**39**(2):1010428317691190. DOI: 10.1177/1010428317691190

[40] Nakamura T, Sakai K, Matsumoto K. Hepatocyte growth factor twenty years on: Much more than a growth factor. Journal of Gastroenterology and Hepatology. 2011;**26** (Suppl 1):188-202. DOI: 10.1111/j.1440-1746.2010.06549.x

[41] Gómez-Quiroz LE, Gutiérrez-Ruiz MC, Marquardt JU, Factor VM, Thorgeirsson SS. Redox regulation by HGF/c-Met in liver disease. In: Muriel P, editor. Liver Pathophysiology: Therapies and Antioxidants. 2017. pp. 375-387

[42] Miura D, Miura Y, Yagasaki K. Resveratrol inhibits hepatoma cell invasion by suppressing gene expression of hepatocyte growth factor via its reactive oxygen species-scavenging property. Clinical & Experimental Metastasis. 2004;**21**(5):445-451

[43] Chavez E, Lozano-Rosas MG, Dominguez-Lopez M, Velasco-Loyden G, Rodriguez-Aguilera JR, Jose-Nunez C, Tuena de Gomez-Puyou M, Chagoya de Sanchez V. Functional, metabolic, and dynamic mitochondrial changes in the rat cirrhosis-hepatocellular carcinoma model and the protective effect of IFC-305. The Journal of Pharmacology and Experimental Therapeutics. 2017;**361**(2):292-302. DOI: 10.1124/jpet.116.239301

[44] Boland ML, Chourasia AH, Macleod KF. Mitochondrial dysfunction in cancer. Frontiers in Oncology. 2013;(3). DOI: 292. 10.3389/fonc.2013.00292

[45] Eltzschig HK, Carmeliet P. Hypoxia and inflammation. The New England Journal of Medicine. 2011;**364**(7):656-665. DOI: 10.1056/NEJMra0910283

[46] Hernandez-Munoz R, Glender W, Diaz-Munoz M, Suarez J, Lozano J, Chagoya de Sanchez V. Alterations of ATP levels and of energy parameters in the blood of alcoholic and nonalcoholic patients with liver damage. Alcoholism, Clinical and Experimental Research. 1991;**15**(3):500-503

[47] Wallace DC, Fan W. Energetics, epigenetics, mitochondrial genetics. Mitochondrion. 2010;**10**(1):12-31. DOI: 10.1016/j.mito.2009.09.006

[48] Hsu CC, Lee HC, Wei YH. Mitochondrial DNA alterations and mitochondrial dysfunction in the progression of hepatocellular carcinoma. World Journal of Gastroenterology. 2013;**19**(47):8880-8886. DOI: 10.3748/wjg.v19.i47.8880

[49] Pietrocola F, Galluzzi L, Bravo-San Pedro JM, Madeo F, Kroemer G. Acetyl coenzyme a: A central metabolite and second messenger. Cell Metabolism. 2015;**21**(6):805-821. DOI: 10.1016/j.cmet.2015.05.014

[50] Hernandez-Munoz R, Diaz-Munoz M, Chagoya de Sanchez V. Effects of adenosine administration on the function and membrane composition of liver mitochondria in carbon tetrachloride-induced cirrhosis. Archives of Biochemistry and Biophysics. 1992;**294**(1):160-167

[51] Nishikawa T, Bellance N, Damm A, Bing H, Zhu Z, Handa K, Yovchev MI, Sehgal V, Moss TJ, Oertel M, Ram PT, Pipinos II, Soto-Gutierrez A, Fox IJ, Nagrath D. A switch in

the source of ATP production and a loss in capacity to perform glycolysis are hallmarks of hepatocyte failure in advance liver disease. Journal of Hepatology. 2014;**60**(6):1203-1211. DOI: 10.1016/j.jhep.2014.02.014

[52] Dang L, Yen K, Attar EC. IDH mutations in cancer and progress toward development of targeted therapeutics. Annals of Oncology. 2016;**27**(4):599-608. DOI: 10.1093/annonc/mdw013

[53] Hanahan D, Weinberg RA. Hallmarks of cancer: The next generation. Cell. 2011;**144**(5):646-674. DOI: 10.1016/j.cell.2011.02.013

[54] Morales J, Li L, Fattah FJ, Dong Y, Bey EA, Patel M, Gao J, Boothman DA. Review of poly (ADP-ribose) polymerase (PARP) mechanisms of action and rationale for targeting in cancer and other diseases. Critical Reviews in Eukaryotic Gene Expression. 2014;**24**(1):15-28

[55] Liesa M, Borda-d'Agua B, Medina-Gomez G, Lelliott CJ, Paz JC, Rojo M, Palacin M, Vidal-Puig A, Zorzano A. Mitochondrial fusion is increased by the nuclear coactivator PGC-1beta. PLoS One. 2008;**3**(10):e3613. DOI: 10.1371/journal.pone.0003613

[56] Moller B, Dargel R. Structural and functional impairment of mitochondria from rat livers chronically injured by thioacetamide. Acta Pharmacologica et Toxicologica (Copenh). 1984;**55**(2):126-132

[57] Jezequel AM, Mancini R, Rinaldesi ML, Macarri G, Venturini C, Orlandi F. A morphological study of the early stages of hepatic fibrosis induced by low doses of dimethylnitrosamine in the rat. Journal of Hepatology. 1987;**5**(2):174-181

[58] Boitier E, Merad-Boudia M, Guguen-Guillouzo C, Defer N, Ceballos-Picot I, Leroux JP, Marsac C. Impairment of the mitochondrial respiratory chain activity in diethylnitrosamine-induced rat hepatomas: Possible involvement of oxygen free radicals. Cancer Research. 1995;**55**(14):3028-3035

[59] Ghosh S, Dungdung SR, Choudhury ST, Chakraborty S, Das N. Mitochondria protection with ginkgolide B-loaded polymeric nanocapsules prevents diethylnitrosamine-induced hepatocarcinoma in rats. Nanomedicine (London, England). 2014;**9**(3):441-456. DOI: 10.2217/nnm.13.56

[60] Chavez E, Reyes-Gordillo K, Segovia J, Shibayama M, Tsutsumi V, Vergara P, Moreno MG, Muriel P. Resveratrol prevents fibrosis, NF-kappaB activation and TGF-beta increases induced by chronic CCl4 treatment in rats. Journal of Applied Toxicology. 2008;**28**(1):35-43. DOI: 10.1002/jat.1249

[61] Chávez E, Galicia M, Muriel P. Are N-acetylcysteine and resveratrol effective treatments for liver disease? In: Muriel P, editor. Liver Pathophysiology: Therapies and Antioxidants. London, United Kingdom: Academic Press, Elsevier; 2017. pp. 729-742

[62] Perl A, Hanczko R, Telarico T, Oaks Z, Landas S. Oxidative stress, inflammation and carcinogenesis are controlled through the pentose phosphate pathway by transaldolase. Trends in Molecular Medicine. 2011;**17**(7):395-403. DOI: 10.1016/j.molmed.2011.01.014

[63] Baccarelli A, Bollati V. Epigenetics and environmental chemicals. Current Opinion in Pediatrics. 2009;**21**(2):243-251

[64] Herceg Z, Vaissiere T. Epigenetic mechanisms and cancer: An interface between the environment and the genome. Epigenetics. 2011;**6**(7):804-819. DOI: 10.4161/epi.6.7.16262

[65] Turner BM. Epigenetic responses to environmental change and their evolutionary implications. Philosophical Transactions of the Royal Society of London. Series B, Biological Sciences. 2009;**364**(1534):3403-3418. DOI: 10.1098/rstb.2009.0125

[66] Lozano-Rosas MG, Chávez E, Aparicio-Cadena AR, Velasco-Loyden G, Chagoya de Sánchez V. Mitoepigenetics and hepatocellular carcinoma. Hepatoma Research. 2018;**4**: 1-14. DOI: 10.20517/2394-5079.2018.48

[67] Shock LS, Thakkar PV, Peterson EJ, Moran RG, Taylor SM. DNA methyltransferase 1, cytosine methylation, and cytosine hydroxymethylation in mammalian mitochondria. Proceedings of the National Academy of Sciences of the United States of America. 2011;**108**(9):3630-3635. DOI: 10.1073/pnas.1012311108

[68] Mizukami S, Yafune A, Watanabe Y, Nakajima K, Jin M, Yoshida T, Shibutani M. Identification of epigenetically downregulated Tmem70 and Ube2e2 in rat liver after 28-day treatment with hepatocarcinogenic thioacetamide showing gene product downregulation in hepatocellular preneoplastic and neoplastic lesions produced by tumor promotion. Toxicology Letters. 2017;**266**:13-22. DOI: 10.1016/j.toxlet.2016.11.022

[69] Malik AN, Czajka A. Is mitochondrial DNA content a potential biomarker of mitochondrial dysfunction? Mitochondrion. 2013;**13**(5):481-492. DOI: 10.1016/j.mito.2012.10.011

[70] Singh KK, Kulawiec M, Still I, Desouki MM, Geradts J, Matsui S. Inter-genomic cross talk between mitochondria and the nucleus plays an important role in tumorigenesis. Gene. 2005;**354**:140-146. DOI: 10.1016/j.gene.2005.03.027

[71] Ye C, Tao R, Cao Q, Zhu D, Wang Y, Wang J, Lu J, Chen E, Li L. Whole-genome DNA methylation and hydroxymethylation profiling for HBV-related hepatocellular carcinoma. International Journal of Oncology. 2016;**49**(2):589-602. DOI: 10.3892/ijo.2016.3535

[72] Maier K, Hofmann U, Reuss M, Mauch K. Dynamics and control of the central carbon metabolism in hepatoma cells. BMC Systems Biology. 2010;**4**:54. DOI: 10.1186/1752-0509-4-54

[73] Stubbs M, Griffiths JR. The altered metabolism of tumors: HIF-1 and its role in the Warburg effect. Advances in Enzyme Regulation. 2010;**50**(1):44-55. DOI: 10.1016/j.advenzreg.2009.10.027

[74] Puszyk WM, Trinh TL, Chapple SJ, Liu C. Linking metabolism and epigenetic regulation in development of hepatocellular carcinoma. Laboratory Investigation. 2013;**93**(9):983-990. DOI: 10.1038/labinvest.2013.94

[75] Cyr AR, Domann FE. The redox basis of epigenetic modifications: From mechanisms to functional consequences. Antioxidants & Redox Signaling. 2011;**15**(2):551-589. DOI: 10.1089/ars.2010.3492

[76] Shyh-Chang N, Locasale JW, Lyssiotis CA, Zheng Y, Teo RY, Ratanasirintrawoot S, Zhang J, Onder T, Unternaehrer JJ, Zhu H, Asara JM, Daley GQ, Cantley LC. Influence of threonine metabolism on S-adenosylmethionine and histone methylation. Science. 2013;**339**(6116):222-226. DOI: 10.1126/science.1226603

[77] Herath NI, Leggett BA, MacDonald GA. Review of genetic and epigenetic alterations in hepatocarcinogenesis. Journal of Gastroenterology and Hepatology. 2006;**21**(1 Pt 1):15-21. DOI: 10.1111/j.1440-1746.2005.04043.x

[78] Calvisi DF, Ladu S, Gorden A, Farina M, Lee JS, Conner EA, Schroeder I, Factor VM, Thorgeirsson SS. Mechanistic and prognostic significance of aberrant methylation in the molecular pathogenesis of human hepatocellular carcinoma. The Journal of Clinical Investigation. 2007;**117**(9):2713-2722. DOI: 10.1172/JCI31457

[79] Shen J, Wang S, Zhang YJ, Kappil M, Wu HC, Kibriya MG, Wang Q, Jasmine F, Ahsan H, Lee PH, Yu MW, Chen CJ, Santella RM. Genome-wide DNA methylation profiles in hepatocellular carcinoma. Hepatology. 2012;**55**(6):1799-1808. DOI: 10.1002/hep.25569

[80] Nishida N, Kudo M, Nagasaka T, Ikai I, Goel A. Characteristic patterns of altered DNA methylation predict emergence of human hepatocellular carcinoma. Hepatology. 2012; **56**(3):994-1003. DOI: 10.1002/hep.25706

11

Liver Cancer Treatment by Chinese Medicines and their Active Compounds

Ming Hong, Ning Wang and Yibin Feng

Abstract

Recent studies have indicated that traditional Chinese medicines (CMs) and their active compounds play an important role in liver cancer treatment by preventing tumor formation, inhibiting tumor growth, metastasis and recurrence as well as improving the quality of life and reducing side effects of radiotherapy and chemotherapy. Mechanism studies have proved the advantage of multicomponent, multitarget and multipathway combinational regulation by CMs in liver cancer treatment. This chapter emphatically introduces the molecular mechanisms underlying liver cancer treatment by CMs. In addition, we also put forward discussion on existing obstacles and prospect of the future development on liver cancer treatment using CMs, in terms of providing a comprehensive understanding of action of CMs in liver cancer treatment.

Keywords: TCM, Chinese medicines, Chinese herbal medicines, Anticancer, Antimetastasis, Antiangiogenesis, adjuvant therapy, complementary, alternative treatment

1. Introduction

Primary liver cancer is a serious disease threatening human health. It was the sixth most frequent cancer, and the second leading cause of cancer death worldwide according to the reports from the International Liver Cancer Association in 2014 [1]. The most common type of liver cancer is hepatocellular carcinoma (HCC), which is originated from hepatocyte. Other types of liver cancer, such as hepatoblastoma and intrahepatic cholangiocarcinoma, are relatively uncommon. Recognized risk factors for liver cancer include viral hepatitis B or C infection, obesity and alcohol abuse. In developing countries such as African countries and China, Hepatitis B or C is the major cause of liver cancer, whereas in developed countries such as the European Union and United States, the predominant cause of liver cancer is cirrhosis caused by alcohol abuse or obesity [2]. In addition, inherited factor may also increase the risk of liver cancer. Recent studies have found that some patients developed liver cancer with inherited susceptible genes from their parents [3]. Usually, liver cancer has no symptoms at the early stages; with the tumor progression, symptoms such as yellow skin, abdominal pain, abdominal mass, nausea or liver dysfunction appear and rapidly deteriorate. Generally, the prognosis of liver cancer is poor, because only 10–20% patients with early detection can receive curative resection surgery. In addition, surgical resection is unavailable for cirrhotic patients as increased risk of fatal complications may occur during resection on cirrhotic livers [4]. Other conventional cancer treatment options such as radiation and chemotherapy are not routinely used for liver cancer as the liver is chemotherapy-refractory and not tolerant to radiation [5, 6]. In recent decades, several novel targeted therapies have been developed for liver cancer treatment. The National Comprehensive Cancer Network (NCCN) guidelines recommend sorafenib as the standard frontline therapy for patients with unresectable HCC but with well-preserved liver function [7, 8]. Other locoregional or adjuvant therapies such as the percutaneous ablation (ethanol injection and radiofrequency ablation), intra-arterial radiolabeled lipiodol, intra-arterial chemotherapy, transarterial chemoembolization (TACE), interferon, adoptive immunotherapy and complementary and alternative medicine are recommended for providing opportunity for liver transplantation or extending disease-free survival and improving survival quality. For patients who are diagnosed with early stage liver cancer, the 5-year survival rate is about 31%. If the tumor has invaded to the surrounding organs or lymph nodes, the 5-year survival rate will decrease to 11%. If the cancer has metastasized to distant organs, the 5-year survival rate is only 3% [9].

Traditional Chinese medicine (TCM) is one of the most popular complementary and alternative medicine in cancer patients worldwide. In China, TCM is based on the foundation of about 2500 years of folk medical practice, which have been covered by the National Health Insurance Program and supported by the government in both Mainland of China and Taiwan. Different from the western medicines that are based on modern human anatomy and pathology, TCM is mainly focused on the identification of functional entities. In the view of TCM, health is based on the harmonious interaction of the internal functional entities and the external environment. The primary functional entities used by TCM include gas (Qi), blood (Xie), internal organs (Zang-fu) and the meridians (Jing-luo) that are main channels of communication of Qi and Xie in the body and link Zang-Fu with the superficial areas of the body [10, 11]. There are various forms of TCM, which have been used for cancer patients, such as the herbal remedies, acupuncture, moxibustion, breathing exercise and dietary therapy. These therapies may have potential in improving the overall survival in cancer patients and the survival quality.

2. The understanding of liver cancer in traditional Chinese medicine

In TCM, liver cancer is associated with the presence of an "abdominal mass" called "zheng jia" (癥瘕). "Zheng" (癥) means fixed mass in the abdomen with fixed pain, while "Jia" (瘕)

refers to abdominal mass occurs intermittently with no fixed pain. According to TCM literature, the symptoms of liver cancer include abdominal distention, jaundice, abdominal fullness and oppression. Those symptoms can be concluded as "Jiju" (积聚), which means syndromes caused by abdominal lump with pain or swelling. In TCM, the causes of liver cancer can be divided into internal factors and external factors. The internal factors include individual congenital constitution and emotional conditions. The emotions are considered as the major internal causes of liver cancer in TCM. Emotions are regarded as internal, normal, physiological response to stimulus from the external factors. The negative emotions with high intensity and prolonged duration may cause serious damage to the internal organs and influence the healthy condition of the whole body. External factors include unhealthy dietary habits and lifestyle such as alcohol beverage and contaminated food or over exhaustion. These factors can lead to spleen and body disharmony. Other external factors such as the environment also play an important role in the process of tumorigenesis. For example, the wet climate is considered as an induction factor for liver cancer in TCM. Both internal and external factors may cause stagnation of qi, spleen deficiency and the accumulation of dampness, which can eventually lead to liver cancer.

3. The role of Chinese medicines and their active compounds in liver cancer treatment

3.1. Chinese medicines and their active compounds for preventing liver cancer

From a TCM point of view, a good doctor should prevent and cure potential disease in the initiating stage. "Treating before getting illness" is one of the preponderant thoughts of TCM in dealing with disease and health. It is important to prevent the occurrence of liver cancer by keeping healthy diet and lifestyle according to the TCM theories. As we have discussed earlier, spleen deficiency may cause the occurrence of liver cancer. Symptoms such as ascites and abdominal distention are all related to spleen deficiency. According to the relationship among the TCM five internal organs (heart, liver, spleen, lungs and kidneys), the spleen and the liver can influence on each other. Therefore, spleen deficiency can also restrict the liver function. In order to strengthen spleen health and protect liver function, people should avoid taking too much spicy and "cold" food such as pepper, green beans and cold water. Alcohol beverage can also induce spleen deficiency by aggravating the dampness in the body. But moderate drinking are beneficial for preventing liver diseases such as liver cancer according to TCM theories [12].

Many Chinese medicines (CMs) and its active compounds are effective in reducing inflammation as confirmed by modern science [13, 14]. Recent studies have demonstrated that inflammation is a major stimulus for hepatic carcinogenesis and some CMs may prevent liver cancer by inhibiting inflammation in liver. Xiao Chai Hu Tang (XCHT) is an herbal medicine formula used in some Asian countries for treating chronic viral liver diseases. According to the TCM theories, XCHT can modulate Qi activity and balance between Yin and Yang. Recent studies found that XCHT can prevent chronic hepatitis C-related liver cancer by suppressing inflammation and inhibiting fibrosis in the liver [15]. Shi Quan Da Bu Tang (SQDBT) is a classic TCM herbal diet formula that was documented in the "Tai Ping Imperial Grace Formulary" in Song dynasty. In TCM, SQDBT were used to regulate Qi and treat Yang deficiency. Modern scientific research show that SQDBT can relieve chronic viral liver diseases by reducing inflammatory processes and controlling serum alanine transaminase (ALT) levels, thus it may prevent liver cancer development [16]. Other TCM herbal extracts or isolates such as the Salvia Miltiorrhiza extracts, Schisandra chinensis extracts, silymarin, glycyrrhizin, baicalein and baicalin may prevent liver cancer by relieving chronic liver diseases associated hepatic steatosis and fibrosis [17–21].

3.2. Chinese medicines and their active compounds for inhibiting liver cancer development

Invigorating Qi and strengthening the spleen; relieving Qi stagnancy in liver, clearing heat and detoxifying, activating blood circulation to dissipate blood stasis, supplementing Qi and nourishing yin are the main principles in treating primary liver cancer with TCM. Inhibiting tumor growth, suppressing metastasis and preventing recurrence with TCM is the key to restrain liver cancer development. According to a large-scale cohort study in Taiwan, Jia Wei Xiao Yao San (JWXYS) and Chai Hu Shu Gan Tang (CHSGT) are the most common TCM prescriptions for liver cancer treatment. These TCM formulae can significantly inhibit tumor development and improve survival in patients with primary liver cancer [22]. JWXYS are used for invigorating the spleen and nourishing blood, it is effective for relieving Qi stagnancy in liver. Besides its antihepatoma effects, JWXYS can also inhibit colon cancer and breast cancer [23, 24]. CHSGT are also used for dispersing the Qi stagnancy in liver. Different from the JWXYS that focuses on invigorating the spleen, CHSGT is mainly applied for activating Qi movement and relieving pain. Both of these formulae have been safely used in liver cancer treatment for patients in China, Taiwan and Hong Kong, with few side effects being reported. Some pharmacological studies also revealed that a lot of CMs extracts or isolates could inhibit liver cancer growth or metastasis both *in vitro* and *in vivo*. This includes but not limited to Coptidis Rhizome extracts, Radix Bupleuri extracts, Radix Salvia Miltiorrhiza extracts, silymarin, berberine, Wogonin, bufalin and curcumin [25–28].

3.3. Chinese medicines and their active compounds for improving the quality of life and reducing the side effects of conventional therapy in liver cancer patients

As most of the liver cancer patients are diagnosed with late-stage cancer, only 20% patients may have the chance to receive curative treatment. In this case, improving the quality of life and reducing the side effects of conventional therapy are very important for liver cancer patients. The common side-effects of conventional therapies, such as nausea, vomiting, fever, abdominal pain, loss of appetite, alopecia and myelosuppression may lead to noncompliance of treatment and thus affect treatment outcomes and reduce the quality of life. According to a series of randomized clinical trials, CMs are effective in extending survival time, improving quality of life, and reducing side effects of conventional therapies for liver cancer patients [29]. For example, Ophiopogonis Radix and Galli Gigerii Endothelium Corneum (Ji Nei Jing) are most commonly used CMs for appetite improvement; Astragali Radix is widely used for alleviating fatigue; Artemisiae Scopariae Herba is recommended for abating jaundice; Toosendan Fructus and Corydalis Rhizoma are effective in relieving abdominal pain; Pericarpium Arecae, Polyporus, Poria can be used to treat ascites [26].

4. The molecular mechanism on liver cancer treatment by Chinese medicines and their active compounds

4.1. Traditional Chinese medicines and its active compounds for inhibiting the proliferation and inducing cell death in liver cancer cells

Jie Du Xiao Zheng Yin (JDXZY) is a typical TCM formula for liver cancer treatment. Recent studies have found that JDXZY can suppress the proliferation of liver cancer cells in a dose- and time-dependent manner [30]. *In vivo* studies also confirmed that JDXZY could increase the tumor apoptotic index and reduce tumor size in nude mice. Mechanism studies showed that JDXZY may induce human hepatoma HepG2 cell apoptosis by mitochondrial-related pathway. Treatment with JDXZY can activate caspase-9 and caspase-3 as well as up-regulate the ratio of Bax/Bcl-2, which may partially demonstrate its antihepatoma effects. In addition, another study also found that JDXZY could inhibit the proliferation of HepG2 cells by arresting the cell cycle at the G0/G1 phase [31].

Bufalin is a digoxin-like agent isolated from Chansu which is a precious CMs extracted from parotoid glands of toads. Previous studies found that bufalin exhibited significant anticancer activities in many cancer cell lines *in vitro* and *in vivo*. A recent research showed that bufalin can suppress AKT-related signaling pathway in HepG2 and HCCLM3 cell lines. After bufalin treatment, the proliferation-related proteins in AKT/GSK3beta/beta-catenin/E-cadherin-signaling pathway were significantly inhibited [32]. Thus, bufalin may be a potential anti-hepatoma agent by inhibiting the proliferation of cancer cell.

Gekko swinhonis Guenther also called ShouGong in TCM; it was a widely used anticancer drug in China for hundreds of years. Modern science has demonstrated that one of the major active components in *Gekko swinhonis* Guenther is sulfated polysaccharide–protein complex (GSPP). Previous studies showed that GSPP can suppress the proliferation of liver cancer cells and arrest the cell cycle in SMMC-7721 cells with little direct toxicity [33]. In addition, Gepsin, the monomeric protein in GSPP also showed strong inhibition on the proliferation of hepatocarcinoma Bel-7402 cells [34].

Many researches have revealed the strong anticancer activity of berberine. The protective effects of berberine on liver diseases including liver cancer have been widely studied by our groups. The quaternary ammonium salt derived from Coptidis Rhizome (Huanglian in TCM) can induce both autophagy and apoptosis in hepatocellular carcinoma cells (HCC). Further mechanisms studies demonstrated that berberine could induce mitochondrial apoptotic signaling pathway in MHCC97-L and HepG2 cells via upregulating Bax expression. Furthermore, berberine could also induce autophagic cell death in HCC cells through inhibiting the activity of Akt and activating the p38 MAPK-signaling pathway [35].

4.2. Chinese medicines and their active compounds for inducing liver cancer cells differentiation

Panaxydol is one of the bioactive components in Panax Notoginseng (Sanqi in TCM). Panax Notoginseng is a famous hemostatic in TCM and it can also relieve other blood disorders, such as blood stasis or blood deficiency. Recent studies have shown that the panaxydol could induce cell differentiation in human HCC cell lines SMMC-7721 [36]. Ultrastructure morphology observation confirmed that there have obvious cell morphologic changes after panaxydol treatment. The activity of several differentiation related proteins such as alkaline phosphatase and albumin were increased, while AFP activity was significantly decreased after panaxydol treatment. These results showed that panaxydol may be a potential antihepatoma agent by inducing tumor cell differentiation.

Gepsin can also inhibit liver cancer development by inducing cancer cells differentiation. Studies showed that after gepsin treatment, the HCC cell line Bel-7402 presents ultrastructural morphology of differentiation. Western blot results revealed that the differentiation related proteins such as the AFP protein secretion significantly decreased, while ALB protein expression was obviously up-regulated on gepsin-treated cancer cells [34].

Ginseng is one of the most widely used herbs in TCM for thousands of years. Ginsenosides are the main bio-active components in Ginseng. There are many reports verified the anticancer effect of ginsenosides *in vitro* and *in vivo*. For example, ginsenosides-Rh2 (G-Rh2) can inhibit the proliferation of SMMC-7721 cells as well as induce the mature and normality of cell ultrastructure morphology. The expression of AFP, gamma-GT and heat-resistant ALP were also significantly decreased after 10 mg/ml G-Rh2 treatment [37].

4.3. Chinese medicines and their active compounds for averting the invasion and metastasis of liver cancer cells

Ardipusilloside I is a triterpene-saponin separated from the TCM herbs *Ardisia pusilla* A. DC. Recent studies have revealed its anticancer effects through inhibition invasion and metastasis of HCC cells [38]. Both *in vitro* and *in vivo* studies demonstrated that Ardipusilloside I may suppress migration of HCC cells partially by decreasing the expression of the metalloproteinase (MMP)-2 and MMP-9 proteins. In addition, Ardipusilloside I can activate Rac1 protein and further induce E-cadherin which may result in inhibition of cancer cells migration.

As we have discussed earlier, GSPP and its monomeric protein gepsin are effective in inhibiting the proliferation of HCC cells. Recent studies found that GSPP was also effective in suppressing the migration of HCC cells [33]. GSPP treatment remarkably decreased the concentration of intracellular calcium. Many studies have demonstrated that low intracellular calcium concentration is associated with reduced cancer migration. GSPP treatment could remarkably decrease the concentration of intracellular calcium. Thus, the antimigration effect by GSPP may be partially a consequence of downregulation of intracellular calcium concentration together with an upregulation of actin filaments polymerization in HCC cells.

The hepatic protective effects of Radix Salviae have been verified through its extensive use in TCM. Recent studies also found that aqueous extracts of Radix Salviae can inhibit the development of liver cancer by suppressing the metastasis and recurrence in animal models [21]. *In vitro* study showed that Radix Salviae treatment significantly decreased the expression of Intercellular Adhesion Molecule 1(ICAM-1) in SMMC-7721 cells. In addition, it could suppress the invasion of SMMC-7721 cell and make the fibronectin-attached cells exfoliated. The cell adhesion ability of HCC-HCC, HCC-lymphocyte and HCC-endothelial cell also decreased after Radix Salviae treatment. The tumor xenograft mice model also confirmed the antimetastasis effects of Radix Salviae on posthepatectomy liver cancer *in vivo*.

Curcumin, a polyphenol isolated from the rhizome of Curcuma longa (Jiang in TCM) has potential anti-cancer effects in many types of cancers. However, due to its poor aqueous solubility, the clinical application of curcumin has been limited. A recent study has used the polymeric nanoparticle formulation of curcumin to improve its solubility as well as anticancer activity [39]. The results showed that when used as a combination with sorafenib, the modified curcumin can suppress the proliferation and invasion of HCC cells *in vitro*. Furthermore, *in vivo* study also found curcumin could inhibit liver cancer growth and lung metastases. Mechanisms study found curcumin and sorafenib synergistically inhibited the expression of MMP9 by down-regulating NF-kappaB/p65-signaling pathway. Taken together, the polymeric nanoparticle formulation of curcumin may exhibit antitumor activity by inhibiting liver cancer metastasis.

4.4. Chinese medicines and their active compounds for inhibiting angiogenesis in liver cancer treatment

Angiogenesis is a physiological process during which new blood vessels are produced and developed based on the original vessels. As angiogenesis plays a crucial role in tumor growth and metastasis, the novel antitumor therapies targeting angiogenesis may provide new hopes for cancer treatment. Livistona Chinensis seeds (EELC) have been used for centuries in TCM for cancer treatment. HCC xenograft mice model confirmed that EELC can inhibit tumor angiogenesis through the Notch-signaling pathway [40]. After EELC treatment, *in vivo* results showed remarkable decrease in intratumoral microvessel density (MVD) in the HCC xenograft mice tumors. In addition, the angiogenesis-related proteins such as the VEGF-A and VEGFR-2 were significantly decreased after EELC treatment. The mechanism study demonstrated that the antiangiogenesis effect was related with the inhibition of the Notch pathway as the expression of Notch, Dll4 and Jagged1 were down regulated according to the real-time polymerase chain reaction (RT-PCR) results.

Yang Zheng Xiao Ji (YZXJ) is a commercial TCM product for supplementary treatment of advanced liver cancer. Some clinical trials indicated that YZXJ may improve the curative effect of interventional chemotherapy for advanced liver cancer patients. *In vitro* studies showed that YZXJ can inhibit the matrigel-based sandwich tubule formation and cell migration. Western blot results confirmed that inhibition of the activation of focal adhesion kinase may at least in part confer the YZXJ-induced inhibition of cell migration and tube formation [41]. These results indicated that YZXJ could be a potential antihepatoma TCM product via suppressing tumor angiogenesis.

Asparagus polysaccharide, the bioactive derivate from Asparagus, is a common TCM herbal diet that may exhibit anticancer activity according to previous researches. One study has explored the adjunctive effects of asparagus polysaccharide in liver cancer chemotherapy [42]. Their results showed that asparagus polysaccharide significantly suppressed liver cancer growth in combination with transcatheter arterial chemoembolization (TACE) therapy in orthotopic HCC rat model. Tumor angiogenesis may be the major target for asparagine gelatinous in liver cancer treatment. Several angiogenesis markers such as CD34 and VEGF significantly decreased after asparagine gelatinous treatment. The expression of MVD markers also remarkably reduced in asparagus polysaccharide treated liver tumors. These results suggested that asparagus polysaccharide with TACE could apparently inhibit the tumor angiogenesis *in vivo*; asparagus polysaccharide might be a potential adjunvant therapy for TACE in treating liver cancer.

4.5. Chinese medicines and their active compounds for enhancing immunological function in liver cancer patient

The TCM formula Songyou Yin (SYY) was developed by Professor Zhao-You Tang for liver cancer treatment. Recent studies have found that the antimetastasis and anti-recurrence effects by SYY may be correlated with its immunomodulation activity. SYY can significantly extend survival and inhibit the tumor growth and metastasis in tumor-burdened mice. SYY remarkably increased the ratio of CD4/CD8 in peripheral blood and decreased the serum TGF-beta1 activity as well as the percentage of Treg cells both in spleen and peripheral blood. Thus, the TCM product SYY may strengthen the immunity of liver cancer patient and prevent tumor recurrence [43].

Mylabris mixture is a popular anticancer TCM formula which mainly consists of the Mylabris extracts, Tangerine Peel and Millet Sprout. Recent studies found that Mylabris mixture could obviously suppress the growth of liver cancer H22 cells by improving the immunological function in mice model [44]. After Mylabris mixture treatment, the stimulation index of T-lymphocyte transformation and proportion of NK cells were apparently increased. The subpopulation percentage of T lymphocytes also significantly increased after Mylabris mixture treatment. Up-regulation on the secretion of interferon-gamma and interleukin-4 by T lymphocytes also confirmed the immunoloregulation effects by Mylabris mixture.

A recent study has explored the immunoloregulation effects of ultrasound-guided intratumoral injection of TCM formula "Star-99" in HCC in mice model. Star-99 can improve the cellular immunity and induce HCC cell apoptosis by increasing the level of plasma IL-2 and TNF-alpha. The cytokines IL-2 can be considered as an immunological response modifier. It can improve the activity of lymphocyte and the anti-tumor effects of NK, CTL and LAK cells as well as cytokine secretion. In addition, another experiment also found that many lymphocytes can be observed in the tumor tissues after the Star-99 treatment [45]. The electron microscope results observed that the microvilli on the surface of the lymphocytes attacked the cancer cells. The membrane of tumor cell in contact with the sensitized T lymphocyte became broken with the organelle and the nucleus dissolved and the vacuolation of the cytoplasm as well. This phenomenon further illustrate that the Star-99 could stimulate and induce the cellular immunity function of the organism.

Previous studies revealed the TCM herbal product Kanglaite (KLT) which mainly consists of Jobstears Seed oil exhibits anticancer and immunoregulation activities. According to a clinical study, KLT treatment can improve the immunological function via increasing the proportion of T cells and NK cells in the blood of HCC patients [46]. *In vivo* study in tumor-bearing mice showed that KLT enhanced the immune system by increasing the secretion of several cytokines such as the IFN-gamma and IL-2, and up-regulate the proportion of CD4+ T cells in mice. These events further improved the killing activity of NK cells and CD8+ T cells against the HepG2 cells. KLT treatment also up-regulate the mRNA level of some NF-kappaB responsive genes in CD4+ cells. In conclusion, KLT may have immunomodulatory activity at least partially through the activating of NF-kappaB mediated gene transcription in CD4+ T cells.

4.6. Chinese medicines and their active compounds for reversing drug resistance in liver cancer treatment

Astragaloside is a saponin isolated from Radix Astragali, one of the popular TCM herbs. Astragaloside has been reported to be an effective agent in reversing multidrug resistance (MDR) of cancer treatment. A recent study found that astragaloside can modulate the expression of P-glycoprotein in human hepatic cancer cells Bel-7402 and reverse 5-fluorouracil resistance in chemotherapy. As P-glycoprotein majorly is responsible for the drug efflux in cancer treatment, the down-regulation of P-glycoprotein will inhibit P-glycoprotein-mediated drug efflux and improve the efficacy of chemotherapies [47]. Thus, astragaloside may be a potential anticancer drug for reversing drug resistance in liver cancer treatment.

Polyphyllin D is a saponin derived from a TCM herb Paris Polyphylla. The herb of Paris Polyphylla has been used for liver cancer treatment in China for thousands years. Previous study showed that polyphyllin D can induce apoptosis in multi-drug resistant HepG2 cells [48]. Further mechanism study demonstrated that polyphyllin D may elicit mitochondrial fragmentation in HCC cells. When treating polyphyllin D directly to the isolated mitochondria, the mitochondria exhibited strong swelling with deep transmembrane depolarization. In addition, significant apoptosis-inducing factor release could be observed from the multidrug-resistant HepG2 cells. These results suggest that polyphyllin D may be a potential anti-cancer agent targeting drug resistance in HCC cells by inducing mitochondrial damage.

Piper betel leaves (PBL) are enriched with medication properties in TCM for many centuries. Modern researches have proven that PBL has antioxidation activity and may inhibit gene mutation. Recent study has found that PBL extract can inhibit total Glutathione S-transferase (GST) and alpha class of GST (GSTA) in HepG2 cells [49]. Further study showed PBL could enhance the sensitivity of HCC cells to chemotherapy. The results revealed that the cytotoxicity of cisplatin was apparently increased in cell with PBL treatment, with the mechanism related to the inhibition of multidrug resistance protein 2. These results indicated that PBL extract may reduce drug resistance and improve the efficacy of chemotherapy in liver cancer treatment.

5. Future prospect of liver cancer treatment by Chinese medicines and their active compounds

CMs and its active compounds have a long history for anticancer treatment in China. In recent decades, many TCM formulae, herbal extracts or isolates have been developed to treat liver cancer, especially for patients with advanced-stage liver cancer. According to both clinical studies and basic researches, CMs have less toxicity and exhibit multitarget anticancer activity. In China, the antihepatoma effects of several TCM products have been verified by clinical trials, such as the Songyou Yin and Kanglaite injection. Many studies have proven that CMs had beneficial effects in relieving fatigue and pain, preventing respiratory tract infections and alleviating gastrointestinal symptoms in liver cancer patients.

However, there are also some problems with CMs in current cancer treatment that should be considered seriously. First of all, most of the CMs are extracted from plants or animals, their pharmacological active components are still unknown CMs. Second, the adverse effects, contraindications and corresponding clinical data of CMs are rarely indicated by TCM doctors or CMs manufacturers. Third, the frequent occurrence of fatal accidents such as allergy and phlebitis has been observed during TCM treatment especially in TCM injection treatment. Finally, although there are many clinical trials on CMs for liver cancer treatment, none of them were large multicenter trials with strict and standard criteria CMs. In this case, it is difficult to give an accurate conclusion about the effects of CMs for liver cancer treatment when conducting a meta-analysis. Therefore, large-scale multicenter clinical trials with strict and standard criteria are urgently needed for the development of TCM in liver cancer treatment. According to the previous studies, combination of CMs and its active compounds with surgery, TACE or chemotherapy may protect liver function, enhance the patients' immune response, and reduce the side effects and complications of conventional therapy as well as prolong lifespan. With the rapid development of modern scientific research, the combination therapy with TCM will be definitely promising for future liver cancer treatment.

Acknowledgements

This research was partially supported by the research council of the University of Hong Kong 8 (Project Code: 104001764 & 104002320) and donations of Modern oncology of Chinese Medicine (Project code: 20006276) and the Gaia Family Trust, New Zealand (Project code: 20007008).

Author details

Ming Hong, Ning Wang and Yibin Feng*

*Address all correspondence to: yfeng@hku.hk

School of Chinese Medicine, Li Ka Shing Faculty of Medicine, The University of Hong Kong, Pok Fu Lam, Hong Kong, China

References

[1] Nault, J.C. Reports from the international liver cancer association (ilca) congress 2014. *Journal of Hepatology* 2015, *62*, 477-482.

[2] MacLachlan, J.H., Cowie, B.C. Liver cancer is the fastest increasing cause of cancer death in Australians. *The Medical Journal of Australia* 2012, *197*, 492-493.

[3] Zhang, X.F., Bian, J.C., Zhang, X.Y., Zhang, Z.M., Jiang, F., Wang, Q.M., Wang, Q.J., Cao, Y.Y., Tang, B.M. Are polymorphisms of n-acetyltransferase genes susceptible to primary liver cancer in Luoyang, China? *World Journal of Gastroenterology: WJG* 2005, *11*, 1457-1462.

[4] Wang, J.H., Kuo, Y.H., Wang, C.C., Chen, C.L., Cheng, Y.F., Hsu, H.C., Lu, S.N. Surgical resection improves the survival of selected hepatocellular carcinoma patients in Barcelona clinic liver cancer stage c. *Digestive and Liver Disease : Official Journal of the Italian Society of Gastroenterology and the Italian Association for the Study of the Liver* 2013, *45*, 510-515.

[5] Kudo, M. Surveillance, diagnosis, treatment, and outcome of liver cancer in Japan. *Liver Cancer* 2015, *4*, 39-50.

[6] Benckert, C., Bruns, C. The role of liver resection in the treatment of hepatocellular cancer. *Der Chirurg; Zeitschrift fur alle Gebiete der operativen Medizen* 2015, *86*, 803.

[7] Kelley, R.K. Adjuvant sorafenib for liver cancer: wrong stage, wrong dose. *The Lancet. Oncology* 2015, *16*, 1279-1281.

[8] Woo, H.Y., Heo, J. Sorafenib in liver cancer. *Expert Opinion on Pharmacotherapy* 2012, *13*, 1059-1067.

[9] Kudo, M., Izumi, N., Ichida, T., Ku, Y., Kokudo, N., Sakamoto, M., Takayama, T., Nakashima, O., Matsui, O., Matsuyama, Y. Report of the 19th follow-up survey of primary liver cancer in Japan. *Hepatology Research: The Official Journal of the Japan Society of Hepatology* 2016, *46*, 372-390.

[10] Wang, A., Lin, L., Wang, Y. Traditional Chinese herbal medicine penthorum chinense pursh: A phytochemical and pharmacological review. *The American Journal of Chinese Medicine* 2015, *43*, 601-620.

[11] Zhang, W.B., Wang, G.J., Fuxe, K. Classic and modern meridian studies: A review of low hydraulic resistance channels along meridians and their relevance for therapeutic effects in traditional Chinese medicine. *Evidence-based Complementary and Alternative Medicine: eCAM* 2015, *2015*, 410979.

[12] Ji, G., Wang, L., Zhang, S.H., Liu, J.W., Zheng, P.Y., Liu, T. Effect of Chinese medicine qinggan huoxuefang on inducing hsc apoptosis in alcoholic liver fibrosis rats. *World Journal of Gastroenterology : WJG* 2006, *12*, 2047-2052.

[13] Wen, Y., Zhan, Y., Liu, H., Zhao, T., Yang, L., Zhang, H., Dong, X., Li, P. Yi qi qing re gao formula ameliorates puromycin aminonucleoside-induced nephrosis by suppressing inflammation and apoptosis. *BMC Complementary and Alternative Medicine* 2015, *15*, 155.

[14] Wei, Y., Luo, Q.L., Sun, J., Chen, M.X., Liu, F., Dong, J.C. Bu-shen-yi-qi formulae suppress chronic airway inflammation and regulate th17/treg imbalance in the murine ovalbumin asthma model. *Journal of Ethnopharmacology* 2015, *164*, 368-377.

[15] Miyanishi, K., Hoki, T., Tanaka, S., Kato, J. Prevention of hepatocellular carcinoma: Focusing on antioxidant therapy. *World Journal of Hepatology* 2015, *7*, 593-599.

[16] Rino, Y., Tarao, K. Anti-inflammatory drugs reduce the risk of hepatocellular carcinoma development. *ISRN Oncology* 2011, *2011*, 390676.

[17] Zhu, S.Y., Dong, Y., Tu, J., Zhou, Y., Zhou, X.H., Xu, B. Silybum marianum oil attenuates oxidative stress and ameliorates mitochondrial dysfunction in mice treated with d-galactose. *Pharmacognosy Magazine* 2014, *10*, S92-99.

[18] Park, H.J., Lee, S.J., Song, Y., Jang, S.H., Ko, Y.G., Kang, S.N., Chung, B.Y., Kim, H.D., Kim, G.S., Cho, J.H. Schisandra chinensis prevents alcohol-induced fatty liver disease in rats. *Journal of Medicinal Food* 2014, *17*, 103-110.

[19] Wang, E., Bussom, S., Chen, J., Quinn, C., Bedognetti, D., Lam, W., Guan, F., Jiang, Z., Mark, Y., Zhao, Y., *et al.* Interaction of a traditional chinese medicine (phy906) and cpt-11 on the inflammatory process in the tumor microenvironment. *BMC Med Genomics* 2011, *4*, 38.

[20] Dhiman, R.K., Chawla, Y.K. Herbal medicines for liver diseases. *Digestive Diseases and Sciences* 2005, *50*, 1807-1812.

[21] Sun, J., Zhou, X., Liu, Y. Study on preventive and therapeutic effect of radix salviae miltiorrhizae on recurrence and metastasis of liver cancer. *Zhongguo Zhong xi yi jie he za zhi Zhongguo Zhongxiyi jiehe zazhi = Chinese Journal of Integrated Traditional and Western Medicine/Zhongguo Zhong xi yi jie he xue hui, Zhongguo Zhong yi yan jiu yuan zhu ban* 1999, *19*, 292-295.

[22] Liao, Y.H., Lin, C.C., Lai, H.C., Chiang, J.H., Lin, J.G., Li, T.C. Adjunctive traditional Chinese medicine therapy improves survival of liver cancer patients. *Liver International: Official Journal of the International Association for the Study of the Liver* 2015, *35*, 2595-2602.

[23] Lai, J.N., Wu, C.T., Wang, J.D. Prescription pattern of Chinese herbal products for breast cancer in Taiwan: A population-based study. *Evidence-Based Complementary and Alternative Medicine: eCAM* 2012, *2012*, 891893.

[24] Chao, T.H., Fu, P.K., Chang, C.H., Chang, S.N., Chiahung Mao, F., Lin, C.H. Evidence-based Chinese medicine research, G. Prescription patterns of Chinese herbal products for post-surgery colon cancer patients in Taiwan. *Journal of Ethnopharmacology* 2014, *155*, 702-708.

[25] Zhai, X.F., Qiao, C.X., Liu, Q., Chen, Z., Ling, C.Q. Quality assessment of clinical research on liver cancer treated by intra-arterial infusion of Chinese medicine. *Chinese Journal of Integrative Medicine* 2014, *20*, 870-875.

[26] Liu, X., Li, N. Regularity analysis on clinical treatment in primary liver cancer by traditional Chinese medicine. *Zhongguo Zhong yao za zhi = Zhongguo zhongyao zazhi = China Journal of Chinese Materia Medica* 2012, *37*, 1327-1331.

[27] Li, M., Qiao, C., Qin, L., Zhang, J., Ling, C. Application of traditional Chinese medicine injection in treatment of primary liver cancer: A review. *Journal of Traditional Chinese Medicine = Chung i tsa chih ying wen pan/sponsored by All-China Association of Traditional Chinese Medicine, Academy of Traditional Chinese Medicine* 2012, *32*, 299-307.

[28] Wu, M.C. Traditional Chinese medicine in prevention and treatment of liver cancer: Function, status and existed problems. *Zhong xi yi jie he xue bao = Journal of Chinese Integrative Medicine* 2003, *1*, 163-164.

[29] Li, X.Q., Ling, C.Q. Chinese herbal medicine for side effects of transarterial chemoembolization in liver cancer patients: A systematic review and meta-analysis. *Zhong xi yi jie he xue bao = Journal of Chinese Integrative Medicine* 2012, *10*, 1341-1362.

[30] Cao, Z., Chen, X., Lin, W., Zhao, J., Zheng, L., Ye, H., Liao, L., Du, J. Jiedu xiaozheng yin decoction inhibits hepatoma cell proliferation by inducing apoptosis via the mitochondrial-mediated pathway. *Molecular Medicine Reports* 2015, *12*, 2800-2806.

[31] Cao, Z., Lin, W., Huang, Z., Chen, X., Zhao, J., Zheng, L., Ye, H., Liu, Z., Liao, L., Du, J. Ethyl acetate extraction from a Chinese herbal formula, jiedu xiaozheng yin, inhibits the proliferation of hepatocellular carcinoma cells via induction of g0/g1 phase arrest in vivo and in vitro. *International Journal of Oncology* 2013, *42*, 202-210.

[32] Qiu, D.Z., Zhang, Z.J., Wu, W.Z., Yang, Y.K. Bufalin, a component in chansu, inhibits proliferation and invasion of hepatocellular carcinoma cells. *BMC Complementary and Alternative Medicine* 2013, *13*, 185.

[33] Chen, D., Yao, W.J., Zhang, X.L., Han, X.Q., Qu, X.Y., Ka, W.B., Sun, D.G., Wu, X.Z., Wen, Z.Y. Effects of gekko sulfated polysaccharide-protein complex on human hepa-

toma smmc-7721 cells: Inhibition of proliferation and migration. *Journal of Ethnopharmacology* 2010, *127*, 702-708.

[34] Wu, X., Chen, D., Xie, G.R. Effects of gekko sulfated polysaccharide on the proliferation and differentiation of hepatic cancer cell line. *Cell Biology International* 2006, *30*, 659-664.

[35] Wang, N., Feng, Y., Zhu, M., Tsang, C.M., Man, K., Tong, Y., Tsao, S.W. Berberine induces autophagic cell death and mitochondrial apoptosis in liver cancer cells: The cellular mechanism. *Journal of Cellular Biochemistry* 2010, *111*, 1426-1436.

[36] Wang, Z.J., Song, L., Guo, L.C., Yin, M., Sun, Y.N. Induction of differentiation by panaxydol in human hepatocarcinoma smmc-7721 cells via camp and map kinase dependent mechanism. *Yakugaku zasshi: Journal of the Pharmaceutical Society of Japan* 2011, *131*, 993-1000.

[37] Zeng, X.L., Tu, Z.G. Induction of differentiation by ginsenoside rh2 in hepatocarcinoma cell smmc-7721. *Ai zheng = Aizheng = Chinese Journal of Cancer* 2004, *23*, 879-884.

[38] Lou, L., Ye, W., Chen, Y., Wu, S., Jin, L., He, J., Tao, X., Zhu, J., Chen, X., Deng, A., *et al.* Ardipusilloside inhibits survival, invasion and metastasis of human hepatocellular carcinoma cells. *Phytomedicine: International Journal of Phytotherapy and Phytopharmacology* 2012, *19*, 603-608.

[39] Hu, B., Sun, D., Sun, C., Sun, Y.F., Sun, H.X., Zhu, Q.F., Yang, X.R., Gao, Y.B., Tang, W.G., Fan, J., *et al.* A polymeric nanoparticle formulation of curcumin in combination with sorafenib synergistically inhibits tumor growth and metastasis in an orthotopic model of human hepatocellular carcinoma. *Biochemical and Biophysical Research Communications* 2015, *468*, 525-532.

[40] Lin, W., Zhao, J., Cao, Z., Zhuang, Q., Zheng, L., Zeng, J., Hong, Z., Peng, J. Livistona chinensis seeds inhibit hepatocellular carcinoma angiogenesis in vivo via suppression of the notch pathway. *Oncology Reports* 2014, *31*, 1723-1728.

[41] Jiang, W.G., Ye, L., Ji, K., Frewer, N., Ji, J., Mason, M.D. Inhibitory effects of yangzheng xiaoji on angiogenesis and the role of the focal adhesion kinase pathway. *International Journal of Oncology* 2012, *41*, 1635-1642.

[42] Weng, L.L., Xiang, J.F., Lin, J.B., Yi, S.H., Yang, L.T., Li, Y.S., Zeng, H.T., Lin, S.M., Xin, D.W., Zhao, H.L., *et al.* Asparagus polysaccharide and gum with hepatic artery embolization induces tumor growth and inhibits angiogenesis in an orthotopic hepatocellular carcinoma model. *Asian Pacific Journal of Cancer Prevention : APJCP* 2014, *15*, 10949-10955.

[43] Zhang, Q.B., Meng, X.T., Jia, Q.A., Bu, Y., Ren, Z.G., Zhang, B.H., Tang, Z.Y. Herbal compound songyou yin and moderate swimming suppress growth and metastasis of liver cancer by enhancing immune function. *Integrative Cancer Therapies* 2016 Sep;15(3): 368–75.

[44] Zhou, A.G., Zhang, Y., Kong, D.Y., Wang, Y., Zhang, H.Z., Wang, S.J., Kui, G., Hong, S., Ge, H.L., Ren, Q.H., *et al.* Tumor inhibiting and immunoloregulation effects of mylabris

mixture on h22 cancer-bearing mice. *Zhong xi yi jie he xue bao = Journal of Chinese Integrative Medicine* 2006, *4*, 504-508.

[45] Lin, L.W., Sun, Y., He, Y.M., Gao, S.D., Xue, E.S., Lin, X.D., Yu, L.Y., Lin, X.F., Yang, Y.H. Percutaneous intratumoral injection of traditional Chinese herbal compound medicine star-99 in treatment of hepatocellular carcinoma of mice. *Hepatobiliary & Pancreatic Diseases International: HBPD INT* 2004, *3*, 49-54.

[46] Huang, X., Qin, J., Lu, S. Kanglaite stimulates anticancer immune responses and inhibits hepg2 cell transplantation induced tumor growth. *Molecular Medicine Reports* 2014, *10*, 2153-2159.

[47] Wang, P.P., Xu, D.J., Huang, C., Wang, W.P., Xu, W.K. Astragaloside reduces the expression level of p-glycoprotein in multidrug-resistant human hepatic cancer cell lines. *Molecular Medicine Reports* 2014, *9*, 2131-2137.

[48] Ong, R.C., Lei, J., Lee, R.K., Cheung, J.Y., Fung, K.P., Lin, C., Ho, H.P., Yu, B., Li, M., Kong, S.K. Polyphyllin d induces mitochondrial fragmentation and acts directly on the mitochondria to induce apoptosis in drug-resistant hepg2 cells. *Cancer Letters* 2008, *261*, 158-164.

[49] Young, S.C., Wang, C.J., Hsu, J.D., Hsu, J.L., Chou, F.P. Increased sensitivity of hep g2 cells toward the cytotoxicity of cisplatin by the treatment of piper betel leaf extract. *Archives of Toxicology* 2006, *80*, 319-327.

12

HCC in Elderly Patients: Curative Intraoperative Strategies and Management in Recurrences

Stefania Brozzetti, Simone Bini, Leonardo Luca Chiarella, Katia Fazzi, Michele Di Martino and Mario Bezzi

Abstract

Hepatocellular carcinoma (HCC) incidence is growing among general population and especially in elderly patients. Recent development in surgical technique, surgical equipment, interventional radiology, and radiotherapy (hadrontherapy) allows us to use different techniques and approaches in order to treat this cancer. Patients are conventionally considered disease-free after a 10-year recurrence-free period. Commonly, patients remain into a lifelong follow-up and recurrences are treated as they show. In this chapter, we will give description and indications of different curative techniques, especially hepatic resections and Radio-frequency thermal ablation (RFTA). We will also describe and give indications to palliative care techniques such as transarterial chemoembolization (TACE), Selective Internal Radio-Therapy (SIRT), hadrontherapy, and supportive care. The aim of this chapter is to give information to clinicians and specialists dealing with the disease about the most effective approach to treat HCC, taking into account not only biological age, but also "physiological age," performance status, comorbidities, and number of liver operative treatments. This chapter highlights that patients advanced in age are in particular need of a tailored medicine, where benefits are well weighted against invasivity of treatment and its side effects, in spite of assuring the best QoL and survival.

Keywords: HCC elderly, HCC metastases, HCC intervention radiology, HCC surgery, HCC patient management, HCC hadrontherapy, HCC liver resection, HCC cryoablation, HCC laser ablation, RFTA, TACE

1. Introduction

Hepatocellular carcinoma (HCC) is characterized by high clinical and biological variability [1]. Diagnosis and treatment of HCC always require multidisciplinary approaches.

Treatment requires commonly to make a decision between several specific interventions and to choose the one that allows the best risk-benefit ratio for a chosen patient.

Therapeutical approach shall take into account acute cirrhotic impairment risk and patient management experience, thus to avoid iatrogenic prognosis worsening.

Nowadays, patients older than 75 years account for 22% of HCC patients [2]. That is due to treatment and technological advancements which allow to reach an overall survival of decades, if therapy is well pondered; patients are kept in lifelong follow-up and intervention is timed well.

Therapeutical approaches to treat HCC can be divided into surgical approaches, such as major hepatic resection, minor hepatic resection, and wedge resection. Nonsurgical approaches are interventional radiology, chemotherapy, and most recently hadrontherapy. Since people older in age frequently have several comorbidities, often a specific less invasive therapeutical approach is needed.

Age is not a good outcome predictor: fit elderly patients may tolerate radical and invasive approaches, while unfit patients may not [3]. Treatment of older adults must take into account multiple issues related to the condition of aging itself. First of all, patient's frailty, thus invasive approaches are commonly excluded in patients advanced in age; on the other hand, noninvasive treatments are often palliative and do not achieve a satisfactory disease-free survival (DFS) or long-term survival (LTS) [3, 4]. Into this complex scenario, treatment strategies should also consider obstacles to cure the patients either physical or psychological, illness awareness, linguistic or cultural barriers, poverty, depression, and family environment.

Giving indication for or against invasive treatments is arduous in elderly. A decision for intervention shall consider either oncological principles and radical excision on one side or performance status, tolerability of treatment, and actual life expectancy on the other. HCC patients are not only in need for specific treatments, they must also be guided through routine activities in order to ameliorate their own hepatopathic condition, such as lifestyle correction (diet, water and salt assumption, physical activity, and smoking); instructions to the patient himself and to his family for therapeutical adhesion and instruction for early recognition of cirrhotic impairment or therapeutical side effects.

Physiological age is a new fundamental concept which is crucial in evaluating an advance in aged patient's performance status beyond his chronological age, which is still today too often used as a threshold to exclude or include a patient into specific treatment protocols [4].

The aim of this chapter is to give guidelines about management of elderly patients suffering from HCC and to give indications to treat those suffering from HCC as primary malignancy, recurrent illness, or metastatic disease either.

2. Patient management

2.1. Epidemiology and risk factors

Hepatocellular carcinoma (HCC) is the fifth most common cancer worldwide and the third most common cause of cancer mortality. In almost all populations, males have higher liver cancer rates than females, with male/female ratios usually averaging between 2:1 and 4:1 [1, 2].

HCC global distribution varies by region, incidence rate, sex, and also, by etiology. Normally, HCC incidence in female peaks 5 years later than males. Age-specific onset patterns are likely related to differences in the dominant hepatitis virus in population, age at viral infection, and the existence of other risk factors. As for average age at infection, normally, HCV carriers became infected in adulthood, while HBV carriers tend to become infected in childhood [2].

Recently, a significant increase in HCC incidence in hepatitis-free patients was noted; this index had a boost and went from 22% in 2000–2004 to 31% in 2010–2014 (database ITALICA) [5]. Among nonvirus-related hepatopathy, incidence of HCC in Alcoholic fatty liver disease patients (AFLD-patients) remains stable (17 vs. 19%), while a significant incidence increase was seen in Non Alcoholic fatty liver disease Patients (NAFLD-Patients) or in patients suffering from cryptogenic cirrhosis (0.5 vs. 9%) [5].

Often NAFLD-patients are demanding to treat; patients in this group have commonly several comorbidities such as metabolic syndrome; therefore, they need a more accurate and multidimensional clinical evaluation in order to choose the best treatment and achieve the best outcome from their condition.

HCV interferon-mediated clearance, associated with mild to severe fibrosis reduces hepatopathy progression and cirrhosis incidence, thus HCC's incidence reduction in SVR patients is expectable.

HCC hazard in HBV replication-controlled infection is reduced but not abolished, although effective antiviral therapy reduces HCC incidence in HBV- or HCV-positive patients [6].

Sudden HCC recurrence was reported by several papers after Direct Acting Antiretrovirals (DAA) mediated HCV clearance [7]. Other papers have found similar incidence of HCC after DAA-mediated HCV clearance when compared to IFN-mediated SVR but considering an overall 24-month follow-up [7]. HCC incidence after HCV clearance is still not sufficiently evaluated.

2.2. Elderly management and evaluation

More than two-third of patients newly diagnosed with HCC are aged >65 years [8], and this number is expected to increase as the world population ages. Furthermore, there is heterogeneity in the aging process, which further contributes to the complexity of treatment decisions. These factors contribute to age-related variations in treatment patterns and outcomes, potentially resulting in increased likelihood of under- or overtreatment, which can influence both risk of treatment toxicity and survival [9].

Geriatric patients may be extremely complex to treat due to comorbidities that may affect them. Therefore, a clinical evaluation is fundamental to assess the best treatment for each patient.

Aspects that must be considered comprehend not only biological age, HCC stage, and liver status, but also general patient conditions, performance status, and, in particular, individual and familial psychological frame, will to fight against the disease, and treatment tolerability. All these parameters are included into the concept of physiological age which goes far beyond chronological age and considers many crucial aspects of aging which is an extremely individual process.

Since chronologic age alone is a poor descriptor of heterogeneity in the aging process, a systematic and evidence-based way to assess physiological age is needed to guide treatment decisions.

Comprehensive geriatric assessment (CGA) is defined as a multidimensional, interdisciplinary diagnostic process focusing on determining an older person's medical, psychosocial, and functional capabilities to develop a coordinated and integrated plan for treatment and long-term follow-up [10] (**Table 1**).

Important reasons to perform GA in older patients with cancer are detection of unidentified problems and risks for which targeted interventions can be applied and prediction of adverse outcomes (e.g., toxicity, other relevant items such as functional or cognitive decline, postoperative complications); and better estimation of residual life expectancy and lethality of the malignancy in the context of competing comorbidities and general health problems. There is

COMPREHENSIVE GERIATRIC ASSESSMENT
• Medical history and tumor staging; • Physical examination and physical performance test; • Karnofsky Performance Status; • Activities of daily living (ADL); • Instrumental activities of daily living (IADL); • Charlson comorbidity score and review of medication; • Geriatric depression scale; • Mini mental state; • Nutritional status (BMI, albumin, haemoglobin, transferrin); • Social and economic conditions; • Geriatric Syndromes (Dementia/ Depression/Delirium, Neglect or Abuse, Failure to thrive, Osteoporosis, Falls, Incontinence)

Table 1. Considered parameters in Comprehensive geriatric Assessment.

clear evidence that GA items independently predict OS in a variety of oncology diseases and treatment settings. Poorer OS in older patients with cancer and deficits identified in geriatric domains might potentially be explained by several factors (e.g., increased risk of death resulting from causes other than cancer, increased death resulting from cancer because of less aggressive treatment, or death resulting from complications of cancer treatment) [9].

Patients with risk factors, in particular if older in age, must be lifelong under clinical surveillance for HCC onset. Principal conditions that require normally a twice per year follow-up are advanced cirrhosis, active HCV infection or cleared HCV infection, and HBV-controlled infection. Surveillance is made by liver-US and serum α-fetoprotein assessment. Oncological-marker-only surveillance is not recommendable and since cirrhotic parenchyma is on average poorly explorable, imaging shall be performed by a hepatobiliary dedicated team. Suspect nodules shall be further investigated by CT scan or hepatospecific MRI, which allows to make in the same session either a noninvasive diagnosis or staging when nodule is >10 mm in diameter [11]. Noninvasive diagnosis is cost-effective and a big advantage especially for elderly in poor performance status.

Patients older in age are the cohort that receives the highest benefit in early cancer detection since lower stage HCCs are associated with less invasive interventions, faster recovery, lower mortality rate, and better QoL [4].

Therefore, geriatric patients shall be educated to strictly comply to follow-up timing and to change their lifestyle in order to ameliorate liver function and reduce liver damage.

HCC shall never be considered as a single-cell malignancy: it is a whole organ malignancy; cell transformation is due to liver damage from hepatotropic viruses, toxins, and metabolic syndrome [2, 4]. Even a radical liver resection that cures the single malignancy does not exclude the onset of further lesions and rarely metastases after radical resection is possible [12].

The aim of HCC treatment is to freeze the disease into a chronic stage and to treat lesions as they show. There are several possible treatments that allow in some cases extremely long survival, even in metastatic patients [12].

Management of HCC patients can be extremely complex, so only dedicated multidisciplinary teams shall treat these patients who are regularly discussed into liver units [4].

3. Surgical therapy

3.1. Hepatic resection

Hepatic resection is the gold standard in noncirrhotic liver. In western countries, HCC incidence is raising, mostly due to NAFLD and metabolic syndrome [13].

Patients with these pathologic conditions can develop HCC in the absence of cirrhosis or severe fibrosis [14], although hepatic parenchyma shall not be considered healthy since steatosis is determinable in 50% of patients and steatohepatitis (NASH) in 25% [15, 16]. A multicentric study confirmed that HCC patients suffering from metabolic syndrome have higher postoperative hepatic failure, mortality, and morbidity rates [15, 16].

Nevertheless, hepatic resection on metabolic syndrome-liver has excellent oncologic effectiveness and leads to long-time survival [16].

In cirrhotic patients, hepatic resection is the first-line treatment for single HCC nodule and preserved hepatic function, strict indications for hepatic resection are serum-bilirubin <1.5 mg/dl and Hepatic Portal-Venous Gradient (HPVG) ≤10 mmHg or platelets ≥100,000 [17].

Resection in patients with light portal hypertension and nonenrollable for liver transplant shall be well weighted against locoregional treatments [17].

Cirrhotic liver resection can be a safe practice in well-selected patients with low morbidity and mortality rates [18]. Selection shall be lead through a global, multiparametric evaluation of the patient and shall pass beyond a dogmatic data interpretation.

All guidelines agree that is needed to select cirrhotic patients for hepatic resection thus to achieve the best outcome, but selection criteria are not universally accepted, the ones suggested from several surgical groups are not based on strong evidence. Therefore, it is necessary to develop a multiparametric evidence-based prognostic score to allow to evaluate a "tailored" operative risk and expected survival.

Tailored-risk evaluation is even more important in elderly patients since aging is a strict-individual process, multidimensional evaluation, and CGA score, in particular, are crucial to assess whether advanced in aged patients can be either enrolled or not for surgery with a deep gap in quality of life and overall survival [4].

Child-Pugh class B patients are routinely excluded from surgery; however, in some cases, satisfying outcome was achieved by performing limited hepatic resections in strictly selected patients, with mild serum bilirubin raise (≤2 mg/dl) and without portal hypertension [19] (**Table 2**).

Laparoscopic or robotic approaches could widen indications to Child-Pugh class B patients due to their little invasivity.

In elderly patients, these approaches are extremely interesting.

HEPATIC RESECTION FOR HCC- INDICATION
• Non-cirrhotic liver (HBV/HCV related liver disease, AFLD, NAFLD); • Cirrhotic liver: Child Pugh A-B (5-7), MELD <10 Serum bilirubin <1,5 mg/dL HPVG ≤ 10 Platelets ≥ 100.000; • Tumor staging/ chance of radical resection; • No severe comorbidities/ ASA I-III;

Table 2. Indications to liver resection in HCC patient.

Hepatic surgery obtains excellent results in elderly patients, even if cirrhotic. Advance age alone is no more a contraindication to surgery.

However, elderly patients, cirrhotic or not, are often excluded from surgery due to comorbidities that rise ASA score and operative risk. Mini-invasive procedures on the one hand make operative time longer and worsen blood-gases control; on the other hand, they allow to spare hepatic parenchyma and shorten hospitalization and recovery [20]. Therefore, patients treated with mini-invasive surgery vs. open achieve a better outcome, especially if elderly, who often suffer longer hospitalizations either physically (reduced physical activity and nosocomial infection risk) and psychologically (depression, confusion, and dizziness) [20].

As reported by a recent meta-analysis, even better outcome is achieved with surgery (open or mini-invasive) vs. transarterial chemoembolization (TACE), which is the most used palliative care technique for HCC, whose advantage remains consistent even in advance HCC, even if vascular invasion is present, so up to stage Barcelona Clinic Liver Cancer (BCLC) stageC [17, 21].

Portal hypertension is often associated with hepatic damage. However, several studies proved that hepatic residual functionality and not portal hypertension affects short- and long-time outcome of hepatic resections [22, 23].

Patients with mild portal hypertension and preserved hepatic functionality can receive limited resections with morbidity, mortality, and OS similar to patients without portal hypertension [19].

HCC frequently develops and spreads through the portal system and that is why several authors recommend performing anatomical resections; these studies prove a better OS and local disease control for anatomic resection vs. wedge resection [24, 25].

More recently, a large Japanese retrospective study (more than 72,000 patients) proved superiority of anatomical resection only for HCC diameter >2 and <5 cm. Superiority is not proven if HCC diameter is <2 cm since portal diffusion risk is very low or >5 cm because other factors influence prognosis [26].

It is also possible to match a parenchyma-sparing surgery with anatomical resection, thanks to subsegmental US-guided resections [27]. This technique with laparoscopic subglissonian or extraglissionan approach is not of common use, due to its technical difficulty and exclusion criteria, that are ascites and moderate to severe portal hypertension. The approach remains interesting and future technical development is possible, especially thanks to robotic surgery. Subsegmental resection shall not be performed for advanced HCC (diameter >2 cm) in order to respect oncologic principles of a radical resection [27]. The procedure allows to spare liver parenchyma, and it may be really interesting for elderly even if cirrhotics with an early-HCC diagnosis.

3.2. Liver transplantation

Liver transplantation (LT) is considered the first-line treatment for cirrhotic patients. LT indications are given following the Milan criteria: single HCC nodules (diameter <5 cm) or less than 3 HCC nodules all <3 cm and in any case nonresectable [17].

A modest expansion to Milan criteria was given by "up to seven criteria," which had achieved satisfactory results in patients without extrahepatic metastases and/or macrovascular invasion. A prospective validation is needed [28].

An increasing number of older patients with end-stage liver disease (ESLD) are evaluated for liver transplantation (LT). In fact, patients aged ≥65 years represent one of the fastest-growing patient populations in LT [29]. The most extreme of these patients, those aged ≥70 years, are associated with several difficult clinical dilemmas. Firstly, advanced patient age is associated with higher risk and poorer outcomes after complex surgical procedures [30]. LT in advanced age patients is associated with increased risk for infection and cardiovascular impairment, increased resource utilization, and lower patient survival [31]. Since the number of adult candidates on the waiting list continues to rise and organ availability remains unable to fully meet this demand, proper organ allocation and utilization are critically important.

Equivalent outcomes can be achieved in elderly recipients and age alone should not be used as a barrier to LT.

Recent data for waitlist registrants on the SRTR registry suggest that <12% of waitlisted patients are aged ≥65 years, but this proportion has steadily increased over the past decade. Continued improvements in care in pre- and posttransplant medicine and surgery suggest that this age group will continue to grow on the waiting list. With this demographic shift in the ESLD, more elderly patients will be considered for LT, and the use of scarce donor livers will need to be addressed because these recipients have a shorter life expectancy compared with younger patients. Despite the shortened lifespan, single-centered reports have shown equivalent posttransplant survival in super-selected patients [32, 33].

Due to physical and psychological impairment, elderly patients are often considered unfit for liver transplantation, since in super-selected groups only satisfying result in LT is achieved, surgical resection remains, for elderly, the first-line approach when performable.

4. Nonsurgical therapies

4.1. Intervention radiology

4.1.1. Radiofrequency thermoablation and microwave thermoablation

Percutaneous radiofrequency thermoablation (RFTA) and microwave thermoablation (MWA) are considered the standard care for patients with BCLC 0-A HCC, who are not eligible for surgical treatment.

Percutaneous ablation techniques are indicated for HCC nodules <2 cm, while nodules with diameter between 2 and 3 cm need to be discussed in a multidisciplinary unit in order to determine an appropriate management plan (**Table 3**). In patients with a single HCC nodule less than 2 cm in diameter, a complete necrosis ratio of 97% is expected [34].

RADIOFREQUENCY THERMO-ABLATION (RTA)- INDICATIONS
• HCC nodules diameter < 2 cm / 2-3 cm in selected cases • Contraindication for Subglissonian localization, near to vessels or biliary branches due to heat-sink effect • Contraindication in advanced cirrhosis Child-Pugh > B7 or important ascites

Table 3. Indications to Radio-Frequency Thermal Ablation.

Several randomized studies have documented the superiority of surgical resection over percutaneous ablation techniques in terms of efficacy, while thermoablation has shown lower morbidity, mortality, hospitalization rates, and costs [35].

MWA and RFTA have shown comparable safety and effective results, although MWA seems to have certain theoretical advantages compared to RFTA: shorter procedure, higher ablation temperature, larger area of necrosis, lower probability of biliary duct injury, and reduction in the heat-sink effect through a more uniform heating in the volume of ablation. However, these advantages have not been confirmed in clinical practice. Although EASL guidelines recommend the use of MWA for nodules up to 4 cm, a recent phase II trial, comparing the two techniques in patients with similar mean lesion volumes, showed no significant difference between them in terms of outcome and recurrence ratio [36].

RFTA and MWA can also be safely and effectively performed via a video laparoscopic (VL) approach [37]. VL allows the operator to treat nodules that would normally not be eligible for a percutaneous approach due to nonaccessible locations and allows for hybrid management of patients with multiple nodules (e.g., surgical resection and RFTA on additional nonresectable nodules).

Percutaneous ablation techniques are a precious tool in management of elderly patients with multiple comorbidities.

HCC is often methacronous and new nodules are expected to develop during follow-up after the first tumor. Therefore, it is crucial to perform an appropriate follow-up in patients who have been treated for HCC, in order to detect new nodules at an early stage, so that the least invasive treatment available can be delivered. This is particularly relevant in elderly patients, or those who have already undergone extensive hepatic resection, who might not be eligible for surgery.

Percutaneous ablation is a recommended treatment modality, when indicated, due to its mini-invasive nature, high effectiveness, low rates of adverse events, short hospitalization times, and its relatively few contraindications.

4.1.2. Transarterial chemoembolization

Transarterial chemoembolization (TACE) is a palliative treatment that is routinely used in patients with HCC that are neither eligible for surgery nor for percutaneous ablation, and in stage BCLC B HCC. TACE is indicated for asymptomatic patients in Child-Pugh class up to B7 and PS ≤ 1 [17] (**Table 4**).

A study found no significant difference in survival following TACE in patients with Child-Pugh Class 8–9 compared to class 7; however, patients with Child-Pugh 8–9 had a significant worse prognosis and more dangerous side effects [38].

TACE is not indicated for patients with signs of HCC vascular invasion, metastases, untreatable ascites, jaundice, thrombosis of a major portal vessel, and HCC nodules >10 cm. In these cases, due to an already compromised liver function, there is a high risk of liver failure and eventually death.

Drug-eluting beads TACE (DEB-TACE) is a more recent variation of conventional TACE (cTACE) that uses embolizing beads eluted with doxorubicin as a chemotherapeutic agent. It has shown overall similar effectiveness, but less systemic side effects compared to cTACE.

Randomized trials have found superior outcomes with DEB-TACE compared to cTACE in patients with Child-Pugh class B and/or PS ≥ 1 [39, 40].

Although contrast-enhanced CT (CECT) or MRI with hepatospecific contrast agent is recommended for TACE outcome evaluation, contrast-enhanced US (CEUS) could be an appropriate alternative in patients with less than four nodules [41].

If imaging follow-up detects residual or recurrent HCC nodules, TACE can be repeated up to three times per nodule. Treatment failure is considered when there are no signs of lesion response, as assessed using the mRECIST criteria, after two treatments or if there is no complete response after three treatments [42]; in eastern countries, different staging criteria, RECICIL, are actually in use [43].

TACE has been proved safe and effective in elderly as well as in younger patients. In particular, a prospective study found that elderly patients suffered from the same complication rates as nonelderly, while effectiveness rates were similar [44].

More important than age is the liver functional status, and the patient's performance status that mostly affects the safety profile of TACE. Therefore, TACE can be an effective palliative treatment able to give benefits in terms of disease control and improved quality of life in elderly patients with HCC.

TRANS-ARTERIAL CHEMO-EMBOLIZATION (TACE)	
Indications	**Controindications**
• Patients not elegible for surgery nor percutaneous ablation; • Child Pugh 8-9; • Performance Status ≤1	• Nodules >10 cm; • Vascular invasion/ Thrombosis of major portal vessels; • Metastases; • Untreatable ascites; • Jaundice

Table 4. Indications to Trans Arterial Chemo-Embolization.

TACE can also be combined with percutaneous ablation, particularly in patients with tumor recurrence within 1 year since the initial treatment, those with tumor diameters of 3.1–5.0 cm, and those with tumor recurrences after initial treatment with thermoablation, where sequential TACE-thermoablation might be the best treatment option [45].

The benefit of this sequential approach is due to the occlusion of hepatic arterial flow by means of embolization before ablation. Furthermore, lipiodol and gelatine sponge particles used in TACE reduce the portal flow around the tumor by filling the peripheral portal vein via multiple arterioportal communications. Therefore, the reduced cooling effect of the hepatic blood flow on ablation-induced thermal coagulation allows the achievement of an enlarged ablation zone which might reduce recurrence rates.

4.1.3. Transarterial radioembolization

Transarterial radioembolization (TARE) is a palliative brachytherapy for HCC. Radioactive substances (I131-lipidol or Y90-beads) are delivered into the tumor by injecting them selectively into its feeding arteries.

This is a complex technique that requires a high-level specialization and has potentially severe side effects such as hepatic, intestinal, and lung toxicity [17]. Therefore, it should only be performed in specialized centers, with high volume activity and experience with this procedure.

Given the fact that TARE has minimal embolizing effects, it can be safely performed even in patients with thrombosis of the portal vein or its branches.

It can be used as a first-line treatment when TACE is not recommended, such as in the case of large or multifocal HCC or if there are signs of portal thrombosis. However, liver function must be conserved (Child-Pugh ≤7, bilirubin ≤2.0 mg/dl, no ascites) [17].

TARE has also been shown to be an appropriate bridge or downstaging treatment in order to meet liver transplantation criteria [17, 46].

Furthermore, TARE can be used as a second-line treatment in patients who did not respond to TACE or who are intolerant to chemotherapy [17, 47].

Mean survival for Child-Pugh class A or B patients who underwent TARE is, respectively, 17.2 and 7.7 months [48, 49]. Mean survival for patients with portal vein thrombosis is 9 months, while for those with intrahepatic portal thrombosis is 17 months [50].

A study has revealed similar results in terms of overall survival (OS) and toxicity between cTACE and TARE in patients with nonresectable HCC [51]; another study has shown a better time-to-progression (TTP) and lower toxicity following TARE compared to TACE [52].

TARE cannot be performed in patients with a pulmonary shunt >20% or if other vascular anomalies may cause irradiation of visceral organs (stomach and intestine) [17].

Indications for this treatment are often controversial and should only be discussed in dedicated multidisciplinary teams. The difficulty in determining the precise indications of TARE is in part due to the lack of cost-effectiveness studies and the fact that its therapeutical equivalence to TACE has only been proved in selected patients. TARE is usually indicated in patients with stage BCLC C HCC, especially those with portal vein thrombosis and preserved liver function.

TARE is usually not indicated in elderly patients, who often have a compromised liver function, and therefore, risks of liver failure and death are high. TARE can be performed in elderly with good performance status and liver functionality as a second-line treatment in patients with treatment failure following TACE.

TARE has not been shown superior to sorafenib in treating advanced HCC; therefore, sorafenib could be a safer treatment in elderly patients who can tolerate chemotherapy [53].

4.1.4. Other

4.1.4.1. Percutaneous ethanol injection (PEI)

PEI induces cell necrosis through dehydration, protein denaturation, and small vessel disruption. It is not often used since it can only be performed in lesions <2 cm and it has a higher recurrence ratio than percutaneous ablation. It has indication only in lesions that are not considered safe for ablation due to their localization [54].

Compared to PEI, RF has shown better outcomes in terms of overall survival, survival at 1, 2, and 3 years, and cancer-free survival at 1, 2, and 3 years. This is probably due to the better performance of RF in terms of complete necrosis of the lesion and the low percentage of local recurrence [54].

RF requires fewer treatment sessions and shorter hospitalization than ethanol injection: although the quality of life of these patients was not evaluated, there was a decrease in hospitalization rates [54].

4.1.4.2. Cryoablation

Cell death with cryoablation is different than that with thermal ablation. The freezing process results in both intracellular and extracellular ice formation, both of which can result in cellular death, but by different mechanisms. Since the ablation zone is reperfused after the ice ball melts, the result is a rapid release of cellular debris into the systemic circulation. This probably explains the systemic complications of cryoablation (i.e., cryoshock) that are rare with heat-based ablation. Thermoablation is the preferred ablation method for treating HCC in patients with cirrhosis because of the increased risk of bleeding and of disseminated intravascular coagulation-like reaction (called cryoshock) associated with cryoablation [55, 56]. Therefore, although many studies have shown that small-volume cryoablation is feasible in patients with cirrhosis and HCC, it is difficult to justify the additional risk of cryoablation in these patients when viable heat-based alternatives are available [55].

4.1.4.3. Laser ablation (LA)

The term laser ablation refers to the thermal tissue destruction by conversion of absorbed light (usually infrared) into heat. Infrared energy penetrates tissue for 12–15 mm in depth; heat is conducted beyond this range thereby creating a larger ablation area. Optical penetration has been shown to be increased in malignant tissue compared to normal parenchyma [57].

Local tissue properties, in particular perfusion, have a significant impact on the size of the ablation zone. Highly perfused tissue and large blood vessels act as a heat sink, since infrared energy is absorbed by erythrocytic heme and transported away from the target area. This phenomenon makes normal liver parenchyma relatively more resistant to LA than tumor tissue and this is the rationale for using hepatic inflow occlusion techniques such as arterial embolization (TACE) in conjunction with laser therapy [57].

Light transmission into tissues and the size of the ablation zone increase with higher laser power, as does the local tissue temperature reached during ablation, with consequent higher risk of overheating and carbonization of the adjacent normal tissue.

The use of water-cooled laser application sheaths allows the use of a higher laser power output while preventing carbonization [58]. When using multiple water-cooled higher power fibers, ablation zones of up to 80 mm diameter can be obtained.

Major complications of LA are liver failure, segmental infarction, hepatic abscess, cholangitis, bile duct injury, and hemorrhage. The technique is considered safe by rates of 1.8% for major complications and a mortality rate of 0.1% [59] and can also be used safely in elderly patients with advanced liver disease up to Child–Pugh class B [57]. Tumor seeding after percutaneous biopsy and ablative therapies is a well-known phenomenon, but it has rarely been reported following laser ablation [57].

A recent study compared LA and TACE in patients with a single large HCC and found a significant superiority in multifiber-LA vs. TACE in terms of recurrence rates, especially in nodules >4 cm, while OS was similar between both groups [60].

Ablation size is critical to predict outcome; patients with lesions >6 cm or with multifocal disease (more than five nodules) are usually managed with other treatment modalities.

LA can be used with a curative intent only in patients with early-stage HCC. In this setting, it has shown similar outcomes compared to RFTA when treating nodules <3 cm [57, 60].

In patients with advanced local HCC, LA should only be used as a palliative treatment. The use of laser ablation is not currently extensively adopted for the treatment of HCC, but given the promising outcomes shown in recent studies and the expected technical advancements, it could become an increasingly more important treatment modality for HCC in the near future.

4.2. Chemotherapy

Systemic therapy is recommended for HCC patients in stage BCLC-C with conserved liver functionality (Child-Pugh A), good performance status, advanced disease, and/or extrahepatic diffusion. Systemic therapy is also recommended for patients with progressive HCC after locoregional treatments or HCC with vascular invasion not enrollable for other local treatments [17].

Target therapy with sorafenib proved to give survival benefits versus either placebo or cytotoxic and hormonal therapy [61].

Observational studies suggest that sorafenib administration in Child-Pugh B patients is as safe as administration in class A patients [62].

Recently, RESORCE trial showed survival benefit in regorafenib administration vs. placebo for HCC patients that went to tumor progression after sorafenib administration; all patients had tyrosine kinases-associated adverse effects [63].

Cytotoxic chemotherapy, such as doxorubicin or FOLFOX4 scheme, can be considered in patients with conserved liver functionality and after that sorafenib therapy has suspended for adverse effects [17] (**Table 5**).

Adverse effects of sorafenib especially dermatological, hypertension, or diarrhea in the first month of treatment are a frequent cause of treatment failure; it was proved that half-dose administration after adverse effects is associated with survival benefits [64].

In some cases, for fit and super-selected patients, intolerant to sorafenib, in case of oligometa-static disease, a different disease management can be done. Mini-invasive surgical therapy along with intervention radiology may be able to remove several metastases and treat them as they show; once the primitive tumor is surgically resected, a chronic metastatic disease can be surgically controlled with survival benefits [12]. Only case reports on this field have been published, but these authors believe that more research shall be done with multicentric clinical trials to prove what has been shown only in case reports.

Elderly can hardly ever be treated with surgical therapy due to their frailty and low PS even if in many cases, biological age does not correspond to chronological age. Sorafenib showed similar results in terms of safety and effectiveness in elderly and younger HCC populations. When administering systemic therapy, careful baseline evaluation is needed for patient's selection in elderly population, including discussion about antiplatelet therapy discontinuation, and caution in PS ≥ 1 patients, as well as active management of toxicity.

Asthenia and bleeding are more frequent in the elderly. The higher frequency of bleeding is explained by concomitant antiplatelet treatments, and major asthenia is frequent in PS ≥ 1 elderly patients [65].

A multidimensional evaluation is crucial for elderly patients and also in advanced HCC, and decision to start systemic therapy shall be made by experienced and dedicated units.

Adverse Effects of Sorafenib
• Dermatological toxicity; • Hypertension; • Diarrhea; • Nausea and vomiting; • Haematological toxicity

Table 5. Most common adverse effects of Sorafenib.

4.3. Best supportive care

Palliative treatments and supportive care aim at ameliorating patients QoL and at giving relief by symptoms. Terminal-stage HCC may have several symptoms associated with liver dysfunction due to cirrhosis, such as ascites, esophageal hemorrhage, and hepatic encephalopathy. Abdominal pain and asthenia are common.

Paracetamol and opioids are the safest drugs for pain control in hepatopathics; Non Steroideal Antinflammatory Drugs (NSAIDs) shall be avoided due to hemorrhage risk, kidney dysfunction risk, and resistant ascites development.

Radiotherapy is effective in pain control due to bone metastases; control results complete in 50% of patients and partial in 80–90% [66].

Percutaneous cementoplasty is effective in controlling HCC vertebral metastases' pain [67]. Brain metastases are rare and selected cases can be treated with stereotaxic radiotherapy [68].

Malnutrition and cachectic-state is common in end-stage oncological patients, in particular if affected by noncontrolled cirrhosis which enhances weight loss and muscular tissue loss.

Nutritional state assessment is important in HCC patients and was observed that prognostic nutritional index can predict survival expectancy in HCC patients [69].

4.4. Frontiers in palliative treatment of HCC: hadrontherapy

Hadrontherapy or heavy charged particle therapy (CPT) is one of the newest palliative treatments available against HCC.

Hadrontherapy technology is based on charged particles (carbon ions), which accelerated by cyclotrons or synchrotrons are conveyed into a beam to irradiate the tumor. Different from X-rays, charged particles have a sharp Bragg's peak which is even sharper than the one of protons; therefore, they release a great part of their energy at a specific level of tissue penetration which is proportional to their kinetic energy.

This technology allows to concentrate cellular damage into a very small area; therefore, CPT has higher tumor control probability (TCP) and relative biological effectiveness (RBE) than other radiotherapy techniques, it can also reduce organs at risk (OAR) and nonmalignant tissue complications probability (NTCP) [70].

Due to the physical properties of charged particles and, in particular, the possibility to generate a heavy concentrated damage, hypofractioning is possible with good results in terms of adverse effects.

Clinical trials on CPT are still running; first data are hopeful; in a Japanese study that used CPT in nontreatable HCC, a 5-year local control rate was 81% and survival was 33%; results are similar to those for proton therapy with 20 fractions, but by using a total of 4 fractions in 2 days [71]. Good results are also obtained with difficult to treat porta-hepatis HCC [69]. As for HCC metastases, they can be treated with a 50.4 Gy irradiation in 12 fractions [12, 71].

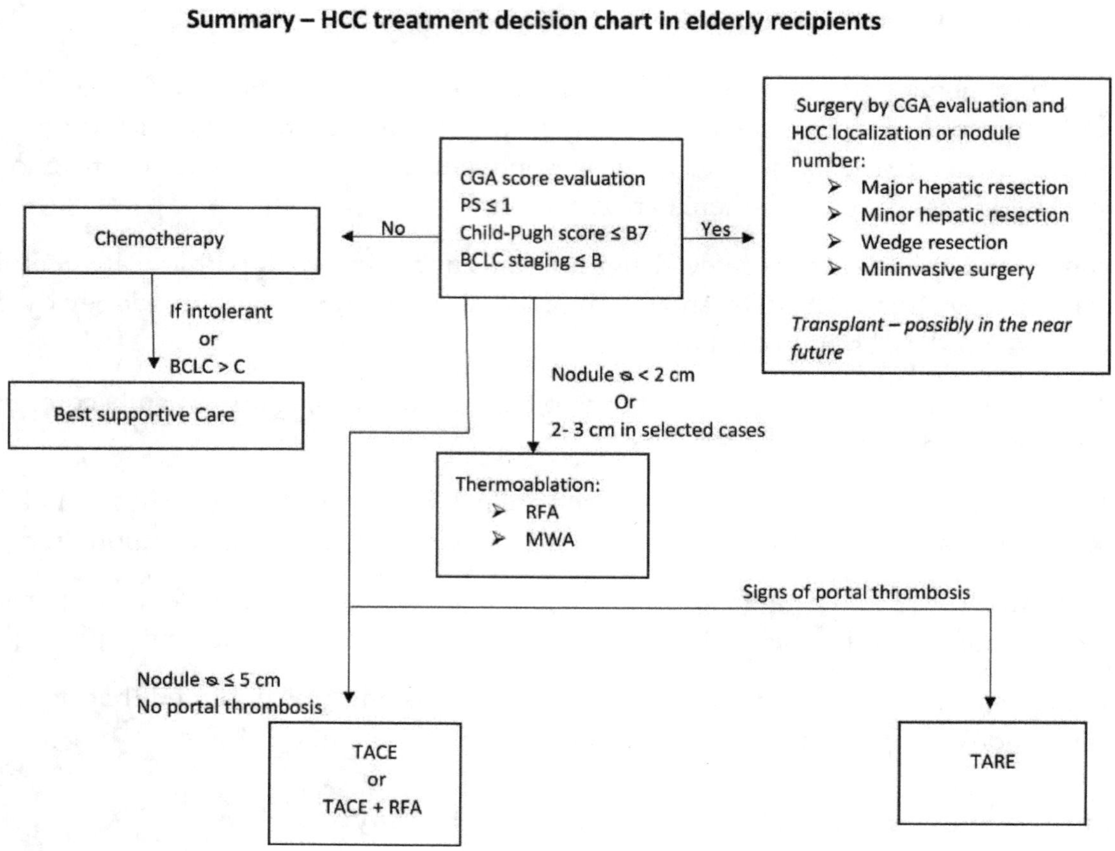

Figure 1. Summary—HCC treatment decision chart in elderly recipients.

These treatments are still experimental but results of trials until now are encouraging, in the next future hadrontherapy may be one of the pillaRs of advance HCC treatment.

Hadrontherapy may be extremely interesting as a treatment also for elderlies, since it has little adverse effect and thanks to hypofractioning and noninvasivity; in the future, it may become a treatment of choice for difficult-to-treat HCC in elderly and for metastatic disease. It may ensure long-time tumor control and good QoL even in people advanced in age; the only issue of this treatment is its high cost-effectiveness ratio, even though cost-effectiveness trials for CPT are not still published a CPT apparatus costs around US$ 200 million; only three carbon ion centers are available in Western Europe, seven in Asia (Japan and China), and none in US [65] (**Figure 1**).

5. Conclusion

The aim of this chapter is to give information and indications about the most recent operative and nonoperative existing techniques to treat HCC. Focus on older adults' case evaluation is of extreme importance; because lifespan enlargement will produce, in next decades, a sharp rise in HCC incidence among elderlies [2].

It is strongly believed, by this multidisciplinary team, that early diagnosis is the key for HCC eradication in general population and in particular in elderly: dealing with a lower-staged cancer allows to use both less invasive and more radical treatments. Patients would then suffer less hospitalization time; would have faster recovery and lower infection risk [4]. Hospitalization time and subsequent infections are the most common cause of death for hospitalized elderly patients. Early-HCCs grow slowly when they develop in elderlies and when removed surgically or with interventional radiology mean (RFTA or MWA) recurrences appear after a sufficient time latency thus to make it possible to chronicize the disease and allow to reach survival rates not different from general population [4].

The elderlies are a very heterogenic population; therefore, this kind of patients cannot be treated with a standardized protocol, but a tailored approach is needed. Each patient has its own comorbidities that must be taken into account; moreover, aging itself is an extremely individual process and different patients may have wide differences in performance status and therefore different treatment indications. Life expectancy, comorbidities, liver functionality, cancer progression, patient's therapy compliance, psychological status, and performance status shall be all taken into account when cases are discussed into multidisciplinary teams in order to assure the best treatment, and therefore, the best OS and QoL.

Author details

Stefania Brozzetti[1*], Simone Bini[1], Leonardo Luca Chiarella[1], Katia Fazzi[1], Michele Di Martino[2] and Mario Bezzi[2]

*Address all correspondence to: stefania.brozzetti@uniroma1.it

1 Department of Surgery "Pietro Valdoni", University of Rome La Sapienza, Policlinico Umberto I, Rome, Italy

2 Department of Radiological Sciences, University of Rome La Sapienza, Policlinico Umberto I, Rome, Italy

References

[1] Cabibbo G, Enea M, Attanasio M, Bruix J, Craxí A, Cammà, C. A meta-analysis of survival rates of untreated patients in randomized clinical trials of hepatocellular carcinoma. Hepatology. 2010;**51**(4):1274-1283. DOI: 10.1002/hep.23485

[2] El-Serag HB, Rudolph KL. Hepatocellular carcinoma: Epidemiology and molecular carcinogenesis. Gastroenterology. 2007;**132**(7):2557-2576. DOI: 10.1053/j.gastro.2007.04.061

[3] Basso U, Monfardini S. Multidimensional geriatric evaluation in elderly cancer patients: A practical approach. European Journal of Cancer Care. 2004;**13**(5):424-433. DOI: 10.1111/j.1365-2354.2004.00551

[4] Brozzetti S, Bezzi M, de Sanctis GM, Andreoli GM, de Angelis M, Miccini M, Tocchi A, et al. Elderly and very elderly patients with hepatocellular carcinoma: Strategy for a first line treatment. Annali Italiani di Chirurgia. 2014;**85**(2):1-10

[5] Leoni S, Piscaglia F, Serio I, Terzi E, Pettinari I, Croci L, Bolondi L, et al. Adherence to AASLD guidelines for the treatment of hepatocellular carcinoma in clinical practice: Experience of the Bologna Liver Oncology Group. Digestive and Liver Disease. 2014;**46**(6):549-555. DOI: 10.1016/j.dld.2014.02.012

[6] Van der Meer AJ, Veldt BJ, Feld JJ, Wedemeyer H, Dufour JF, Lammert F, Duarte-Rojo A, et al. Association between sustained virological response and all-cause mortality among patients with chronic hepatitis C and advanced hepatic fibrosis. JAMA. 2012;**308**:2584-2593

[7] Schietroma I, Scheri GC, Pinacchio C, Statzu M, Pascale FG. Hepatitis C virus and hepatocellular carcinoma—Pathogenetic mechanisms and impact of direct-acting antivirals. Open Virology Journal. 2018;**12**:16-25. DOI: 10.2174/1874357901812010016

[8] Liu P, Xie S, Hu S, Cheng X, Gao T, Zhang C. Age-specific sex difference in the incidence of hepatocellular carcinoma in the United States. Oncotarget. 2017;**8**(40):68131-68137

[9] Wildiers H, Heeren P, Puts M, Topinkova E, Janssen-Heijnen MLG, Extermann M, Hurria A, et al. International society of geriatric oncology consensus on geriatric assessment in older patients with cancer. Journal of Clinical Oncology. 2014;**32**(24):2595-2603. DOI: 10.1200/JCO.2013.54.8347

[10] Extermann M, Hurria A. Comprehensive geriatric assessment for older patients with cancer. Journal of Clinical Oncology. 2007;**25**:1824-1831

[11] Ayuso C, Rimola J, Vilana R, Burrel M, Darnell A, García-Criado Á, Brú C, et al. Diagnosis and staging of hepatocellular carcinoma (HCC): Current guidelines. European Journal of Radiology. 2018;**101**:72-81. DOI: 10.1016/j.ejrad.2018.01.025

[12] Brozzetti S, Bini S, Fazzi K, Chiarella LL, Ceccarossi V, Lucia, De C, Toma, De G. Case report—Metastases in a low-stage middle-graded HCC in cleared HCV infection, non-cirrhotic liver: Surgical therapy. International Journal of Surgery Case Reports. 2018;**47**:19-21. DOI: 10.1016/j.ijscr.2018.04.013

[13] Siegel AB, Zhu AX. Metabolic syndrome and hepatocellular carcinoma: Two growing epidemics with a potential link. Cancer. 2009;**115**:5651-5661

[14] Piscaglia F, Svegliati-Baroni G, Barchetti A, Pecorelli A, Marinelli S, Tiribelli C, Bellentani S, et al. Clinical patterns of hepatocellular carcinoma in nonalcoholic fatty liver disease: A multicenter prospective study. Hepatology. 2016;**63**:827-838

[15] Vigano L, Conci S, Cescon M, Fava C, Capelli P, D'Errico A, Torzilli G, et al. Liver resection for hepatocellular carcinoma in patients with metabolic syndrome: A multicenter matched analysis with HCV-related HCC. Journal of Hepatology. 2015;**63**:93-101

[16] Cauchy F, Zalinski S, Dokmak S, Fuks D, Farges O, Castera L, Paradis V, et al. Surgical treatment of hepatocellular carcinoma associated with the metabolic syndrome. The British Journal of Surgery. 2013;**100**:113-121

[17] Dufour JF, Greten TF, Raymond E, Roskams T, De T, Ducreux M, Governing E, European Organisation for Research and Treatment of Cancer, et al. EASL—EORTC clinical practice guidelines: Management of hepatocellular carcinoma. Journal of Hepatology. 2012;**56**(4):908-943. DOI: 10.1016/j.jhep.2011.12.001

[18] Krenzien F, Strucker B, Raschzok N, Ollinger R, Pascher A, Bahra M, Sauer I, Schmelzle M, Pratschke J, Andreou A. Liver transplantation and liver resection for cirrhotic patients with hepatocellular carcinoma: Comparison of long-term survivals. Transplant International. 2017;**30**:28-46. DOI: 10.1111/tri.13065

[19] Roayaie S, Jibara G, Tabrizian P, Park JW, Yang J, Yan L, Schwartz M, et al. The role of hepatic resection in the treatment of hepatocellular cancer. Hepatology. 2015;**62**:440-451

[20] Gerges FJ, Kanazi GE, Jabbour-Khoury SI. Anesthesia for laparoscopy: A review. Journal of Clinical Anesthesia. 2006;**18**(1):67-78. DOI: 10.1016/j.jclinane.2005.01.013

[21] Hyun MH, Lee Y, Kim JH, Lee CU, Jung YK, Seo YS, Byun KS, et al. Hepatic resection compared to chemoembolization in intermediate to advanced stage hepatocellular carcinoma: A meta-analysis of high-quality studies. Hepatology. 2018;**15**. DOI: 10.1002/hep

[22] Ishizawa T, Hasegawa K, Aoki T, Takahashi M, Inoue Y, Sano K, Imamura H, et al. Neither multiple tumors nor portal hypertension are surgical contraindications for hepatocellular carcinoma. Gastroenterology. 2008;**134**:1908-1916

[23] Giannini EG, Savarino V, Farinati F, Ciccarese F, Rapaccini G, Marco MD, Benvegnu L, et al. Influence of clinically significant portal hypertension on survival after hepatic resection for hepatocellular carcinoma in cirrhotic patients. Liver International. 2013;**33**: 1594-1600

[24] Cucchetti A, Qiao GL, Cescon M, Li J, Xia Y, Ercolani G, Shen F, et al. Anatomic versus nonanatomic resection in cirrhotic patients with early hepatocellular carcinoma. Surgery. 2014;**155**:512-521

[25] Agrawal S, Belghiti J. Oncologic resection for malignant tumors of the liver. Annals of Surgery. 2011;**253**(4):656-665. DOI: 10.1097/SLA.0b013e3181fc08ca

[26] Eguchi S, Kanematsu T, Arii S, Okazaki M, Okita K, Omata M, Takayasu K, et al. Comparison of the outcomes between an anatomical subsegmentectomy and a non-anatomical minor hepatectomy for single hepatocellular carcinomas based on a Japanese nationwide survey. Surgery. 2008;**143**(4):469-475. DOI: 10.1016/j.surg.2007.12.003

[27] Torzilli G, Procopio F, Cimino M, Del Fabbro D, Palmisano A, Donadon M, Montorsi M. Anatomical segmental and subsegmental resection of the liver for hepatocellular carcinoma: A new approach by means of ultrasound-guided vessel compression. Annals of Surgery. 2010;**251**:229-235

[28] Cascales-Campos P, Martinez-Insfran L a, Ramirez P, Ferreras D, Gonzalez-Sanchez MR, Sanchez-Bueno F, Parrilla P, et al. Liver transplantation in patients with hepatocellular carcinoma outside the Milan criteria after downstaging: Is it worth it? Transplantation Proceedings. 2018;**50**(2):591-594. DOI: 10.1016/j.transproceed.2017.09.063

[29] Kim WR, Stock PG, Smith JM, Heimbach JK, Skeans MA, Edwards EB, et al. OPTN/SRTR 2011 annual data report: Liver. American Journal of Transplantation. 2013;**13**(Suppl. 1):73-102

[30] Finlayson E, Fan Z, Birkmeyer JD. Outcomes in octogenarians undergoing high-risk cancer operation: A national study. Journal of the American College of Surgeons. 2007;**205**:729-734

[31] Berg CL, Steffick DE, Edwards EB, Heimbach JK, Magee JC, Washburn WK, et al. Liver and intestine transplantation in the United States 1998-2007. American Journal of Transplantation. 2009;**9**(4 Pt 2):907-931

[32] Lipshutz GS, Hiatt J, Ghobrial RM, Farmer DG, Martinez MM, Yersiz H, et al. Outcome of liver transplantation in septuagenarians: A single-centre experience. Archives of Surgery. 2007;**142**:775-781

[33] Wilson GC, Quillin RC, Wima K, Sutton JM, Hoehn RS, Hanseman DJ, Shah SA, et al. Is liver transplantation safe and effective in elderly (≥70 years) recipients? A case-controlled analysis. HPB. 2014;**16**(12):1088-1094. DOI: 10.1111/hpb.12312

[34] Wang Y, Luo Q, Li Y, Deng S, Wei S, Li X. Radiofrequency ablation versus hepatic resection for small hepatocellular carcinomas: A meta-analysis of randomized and nonrandomized controlled trials. PLoS One. 2014;**9**:e84484

[35] Huang J, Yan L, Cheng Z, Wu H, Du L, Wang J, Xu Y, et al. A randomized trial comparing radiofrequency ablation and surgical resection for HCC conforming to the Milan criteria. Annals of Surgery. 2010;**252**:903-912

[36] Vietti Violi N, Duran R, Guiu B, Cercueil JP, Aubé C, Digklia A, Denys A, et al. Efficacy of microwave ablation versus radiofrequency ablation for the treatment of hepatocellular carcinoma in patients with chronic liver disease: A randomised controlled phase 2 trial. The Lancet Gastroenterology & Hepatology. 2018;**3**(5):317-325. DOI: 10.1016/S2468-1253(18)30029-3

[37] Herbold T, Wahba R, Bangard C, Demir M, Drebber U, Stippel DL. The laparoscopic approach for radiofrequency ablation of hepatocellular carcinoma—Indication, technique and results. Langenbeck's Archives of Surgery. 2013;**398**(1):47-53. DOI: 10.1007/s00423-012-1018-5

[38] Yamakado K, Miyayama S, Hirota S, Mizunuma K, Nakamura K, Inaba Y, Yamaguchi M, et al. Subgrouping of intermediate-stage (BCLC stage B) hepatocellular carcinoma based on tumor number and size and Child-Pugh grade correlated with prognosis after transarterial chemoembolization. Japanese Journal of Radiology. 2014;**32**(5):260-265. DOI: 10.1007/s11604-014-0298-9

[39] Golfieri R, Giampalma E, Renzulli M, Cioni R, Bargellini I, Bartolozzi C, Breatta AD, et al. Randomised controlled trial of doxorubicin-eluting beads vs conventional chemoembolisation for hepatocellular carcinoma. British Journal of Cancer. 2014;**111**:255-264

[40] Lammer J, Malagari K, Vogl T, Pilleul F, Denys A, Watkinson A, Pitton M, et al. Prospective randomized study of doxorubicin-eluting-bead embolization in the treatment of hepatocellular carcinoma: Results of the PRECISION V study. Cardiovascular and Interventional Radiology. 2009;**33**:41-52

[41] Moschouris H, Malagari K, Papadaki MG, Kornezos I, Gkoutzios P, Tepelenis N, Matsaidonis D. Short-term evaluation of liver tumors after transarterial chemoembolization: Limitations and feasibility of contrast-enhanced ultrasonography. Abdominal Imaging. 2011;**36**(6):718-728. DOI: 10.1007/s00261-011-9690-4

[42] Lencioni R, Llovet J. Modified RECIST (mRECIST) assessment for hepatocellular carcinoma. Seminars in Liver Disease. 2010;**30**(01):052-060. DOI: 10.1055/s-0030-1247132

[43] Kudo M, Trevisani F, Abou-Alfa GK, Rimassa L. Hepatocellular carcinoma: Therapeutic guidelines and medical treatment. Liver Cancer. 2017;**6**(1):16-26. DOI: 10.1159/000449343

[44] Cohen MJ, Bloom AI, Barak O, Klimov A, Nesher T, Shouval D, Shibolet O, et al. Transarterial chemo-embolization is safe and effective for very elderly patients with hepatocellular carcinoma. World Journal of Gastroenterology. 2013;**19**(16):2521-2528. DOI: 10.3748/wjg.v19.i16.2521

[45] Peng Z-W, Zhang Y-J, Liang H-H, Lin X-J, Guo R-P, Chen M-S. Recurrent hepatocellular carcinoma treated with sequential transcatheter arterial chemoembolization and RF ablation versus RF ablation alone: A prospective randomized trial. Radiology. 2012;**262**(2):689-700. DOI: 10.1148/radiol.11110637

[46] Kallini JR, Gabr A, Ali R, Abouchaleh N, Riaz A, Baker T, Lewandowski RJ, et al. Pretransplant intra-arterial liver-directed therapy does not increase the risk of hepatic arterial complications in liver transplantation: A single-center 10-year experience. Cardiovascular and Interventional Radiology. 2017;**41**(2):231-238. DOI: 10.1007/s00270-017-1793-z

[47] Moreno-Luna LE, Yang JD, Sanchez W, Paz-Fumagalli R, Harnois DM, Mettler TA, Roberts LR, et al. Efficacy and safety of transarterial radioembolization versus chemoembolization in patients with hepatocellular carcinoma. Cardiovascular and Interventional Radiology. 2013;**36**(3):714-723. DOI: 10.1007/s00270-012-0481-2

[48] Salem R, Lewandowski RJ, Mulcahy MF, Riaz A, Ryu RK, Ibrahim S, Atassi B, et al. Radioembolization for hepatocellular carcinoma using yttrium-90 microspheres: A comprehensive report of long-term outcomes. Gastroenterology. 2010;**138**:52-64

[49] Sangro B, Carpanese L, Cianni R, Golfieri R, Gasparini D, Ezziddin S, Paprottka PM, et al. Survival after yttrium-90 resin microsphere radioembolization of hepatocellular carcinoma across Barcelona clinic liver cancer stages: A European evaluation. Hepatology. 2011;**54**:868-878

[50] Mazzaferro V, Sposito C, Bhoori S, Romito R, Chiesa C, Morosi C, Maccauro M, et al. Yttrium-90 radioembolization for intermediate-advanced hepatocellular carcinoma: A phase 2 study. Hepatology. 2013;**57**:1826-1837

[51] Kooby DA, Egnatashvili V, Srinivasan S, Chamsuddin A, Delman KA, Kauh J, Staley CA 3rd, et al. Comparison of yttrium-90 radioembolization and transcatheter arterial chemoembolization for the treatment of unresectable hepatocellular carcinoma. Journal of Vascular and Interventional Radiology. 2010;**21**:224-230

[52] Salem R, Lewandowski RJ, Kulik L, Wang E, Riaz A, Ryu RK, Sato KT, et al. Radioembolization results in longer time-to-progression and reduced toxicity compared with chemoembolization in patients with hepatocellular carcinoma. Gastroenterology. 2011;**140**:497-507 e492

[53] Gramenzi A, Golfieri R, Mosconi C, Cappelli A, Granito A, Cucchetti A, Trevisani F, et al. Yttrium-90 radioembolization vs sorafenib for intermediate-locally advanced hepatocellular carcinoma: A cohort study with propensity score analysis. Liver International. 2015;**35**(3):1036-1047. DOI: 10.1111/liv.12574

[54] Orlando A, Leandro G, Olivo M, Andriulli A, Cottone M. Radiofrequency thermal ablation vs. percutaneous ethanol injection for small hepatocellular carcinoma in cirrhosis: Meta-analysis of randomized controlled trials. American Journal of Gastroenterology. 2009;**104**(2):514-524. DOI: 10.1038/ajg.2008.80

[55] Jansen MC, van Hillegersberg R, Schoots IG, et al. Cryoablation induces greater inflammatory and coagulative responses than radiofrequency ablation or laser induced thermotherapy in a rat liver model. Surgery. 2010;**147**(5):686-695

[56] Hinshaw JL, Lubner MG, Ziemlewicz TJ, Lee FT, Brace CL. Percutaneous tumor ablation tools: Microwave, radiofrequency, or cryoablation—What should you use and why? Radiographics. 2014;**34**(5):1344-1362. DOI: 10.1148/rg.345140054

[57] Gough-Palmer A-L. Laser ablation of hepatocellular carcinoma—A review. World Journal of Gastroenterology. 2008;**14**(47):7170. DOI: 10.3748/wjg.14.7170

[58] Vogl TJ, Straub R, Zangos S, Mack MG, Eichler K. MR-guided laser-induced thermotherapy (LITT) of liver tumours: Experimental and clinical data. International Journal of Hyperthermia. 2004;**20**:713-724

[59] Vogl TJ, Straub R, Eichler K, Woitaschek D, Mack MG. Malignant liver tumors treated with MR imaging guided laser-induced thermotherapy: Experience with complications in 899 patients (2,520 lesions). Radiology. 2002;**225**:367-377

[60] Morisco F, Camera S, Guarino M, Tortora R, Cossiga V, Vitiello A, Ravaioli F, et al. Laser ablation is superior to TACE in large-sized hepatocellular carcinoma: A pilot case-control study. Oncotarget. 2018;**9**(25):17483-17490. DOI: 10.18632/oncotarget.24756

[61] Manuscript A, Review S. Sorafenib for treatment of hepatocellular carcinoma: A systematic review. Digestive Diseases and Sciences. 2013;**57**(5):1122-1129. DOI: 10.1007/s10620-012-2136-1

[62] Kudo M, Ikeda M, Takayama T, Numata K, Izumi N, Furuse J, Kokudo N, et al. Safety and efficacy of sorafenib in Japanese patients with hepatocellular carcinoma in clinical practice: A subgroup analysis of GIDEON. Journal of Gastroenterology. 2016;**51**(12):1150-1160. DOI: 10.1007/s00535-016-1204-2

[63] Tovoli F, Granito A, De Lorenzo S, Bolondi L. Regorafenib for the treatment of hepatocellular carcinoma. Drugs Today (Barc). 2018;**54**(1):5-13

[64] Reig M, Torres F, Rodriguez-Lope C, Forner A, LLarch N, Rimola J, Darnell A, et al. Early dermatologic adverse events predict better outcome in HCC patients treated with sorafenib. Journal of Hepatology. 2014;**61**:318-324

[65] Edeline J, Crouzet L, Le Sourd S, Larible C, Brunot A, Le Roy F, Boucher E, et al. Sorafenib use in elderly patients with hepatocellular carcinoma: Caution about use of platelet aggregation inhibitors. Cancer Chemotherapy and Pharmacology. 2015;**75**(1):215-219. DOI: 10.1007/s00280-014-2645-z

[66] He J, Zeng ZC, Tang ZY, Fan J, Zhou J, Zeng MS, Wang JH, et al. Clinical features and prognostic factors in patients with bone metastases from hepatocellular carcinoma receiving external beam radiotherapy. Cancer. 2009;**115**:2710-2720

[67] Kodama H, Aikata H, Uka K, Takaki S, Mori N, Waki K, Jeong SC, et al. Efficacy of percutaneous cementoplasty for bone metastasis from hepatocellular carcinoma. Oncology. 2007;**72**:285-292

[68] Choi HJ, Cho BC, Sohn JH, Shin SJ, Kim SH, Kim JH, Yoo NC. Brain metastases from hepatocellular carcinoma: Prognostic factors and outcome: Brain metastasis from HCC. Journal of Neuro-Oncology. 2009;**91**:307-313

[69] Pinato DJ, North BV, Sharma R. A novel, externally validated inflammation-based prognostic algorithm in hepatocellular carcinoma: The prognostic nutritional index (PNI). British Journal of Cancer. 2012;**106**:1439-1445

[70] Durante M, Orecchia R, Loeffler JS. Charged-particle therapy in cancer: Clinical uses and future perspectives. Nature Reviews. Clinical Oncology. 2017;**14**(8):483-495. DOI: 10.1038/nrclinonc.2017.30

[71] Kamada T, Tsujii H, Blakely EA, Debus J, De Neve W, Durante M, Chu WT, et al. Carbon ion radiotherapy in Japan: An assessment of 20 years of clinical experience. The Lancet Oncology. 2015;**16**(2):e93-e100. DOI: 10.1016/S1470-2045(14)70412-7

Permissions

All chapters in this book were first published in LC, by InTech Open; hereby published with permission under the Creative Commons Attribution License or equivalent. Every chapter published in this book has been scrutinized by our experts. Their significance has been extensively debated. The topics covered herein carry significant findings which will fuel the growth of the discipline. They may even be implemented as practical applications or may be referred to as a beginning point for another development.

The contributors of this book come from diverse backgrounds, making this book a truly international effort. This book will bring forth new frontiers with its revolutionizing research information and detailed analysis of the nascent developments around the world.

We would like to thank all the contributing authors for lending their expertise to make the book truly unique. They have played a crucial role in the development of this book. Without their invaluable contributions this book wouldn't have been possible. They have made vital efforts to compile up to date information on the varied aspects of this subject to make this book a valuable addition to the collection of many professionals and students.

This book was conceptualized with the vision of imparting up-to-date information and advanced data in this field. To ensure the same, a matchless editorial board was set up. Every individual on the board went through rigorous rounds of assessment to prove their worth. After which they invested a large part of their time researching and compiling the most relevant data for our readers.

The editorial board has been involved in producing this book since its inception. They have spent rigorous hours researching and exploring the diverse topics which have resulted in the successful publishing of this book. They have passed on their knowledge of decades through this book. To expedite this challenging task, the publisher supported the team at every step. A small team of assistant editors was also appointed to further simplify the editing procedure and attain best results for the readers.

Apart from the editorial board, the designing team has also invested a significant amount of their time in understanding the subject and creating the most relevant covers. They scrutinized every image to scout for the most suitable representation of the subject and create an appropriate cover for the book.

The publishing team has been an ardent support to the editorial, designing and production team. Their endless efforts to recruit the best for this project, has resulted in the accomplishment of this book. They are a veteran in the field of academics and their pool of knowledge is as vast as their experience in printing. Their expertise and guidance has proved useful at every step. Their uncompromising quality standards have made this book an exceptional effort. Their encouragement from time to time has been an inspiration for everyone.

The publisher and the editorial board hope that this book will prove to be a valuable piece of knowledge for researchers, students, practitioners and scholars across the globe.

List of Contributors

Xi-Dai Long
Department of Pathology, the Affiliated Hospital of Youjiang Medical University for Nationalities, Baise, China
Department of Liver Surgery, Ren Ji Hospital, School of Medicine, Shanghai Jiao Tong University, Shanghai, China
Guangxi Clinic Research Center of Hepatobiliary Diseases, Baise, China

Yan Deng
Department of Epidemiology, Youjiang Medical University for Nationalities, Baise, China

Xiao-Ying Huang, Jin-Guang Yao, Qun-Ying Su, Xue-Min Wu, Juan Wang and Bing-Chen Huang
Department of Pathology, the Affiliated Hospital of Youjiang Medical University for Nationalities, Baise, China

Qun-Qing Xu and Xiao-Ying Zhu
Guangxi Clinic Research Center of Hepatobiliary Diseases, Baise, China

Chao Wang
Department of Medicine, the Affiliated Hospital of Youjiang Medical University for Nationalities, Baise, China

Qiang Xia
Department of Liver Surgery, Ren Ji Hospital, School of Medicine, Shanghai Jiao Tong University, Shanghai, China

Mark A. Feitelson
College of Science and Technology, Temple University, Philadelphia, Pennsylvania, United States

Kevin Labadie, Kevin M. Sullivan and James O. Park
University of Washington, Seattle, WA, USA

Mohammad Telfah, Mohammed Al-Jumayli and Anwaar Saeed
Department of Medicine, Division of Medical Oncology, University of Kansas Medical Center Kansas City, Westwood, Kansas, USA

Vasileia Ntomi and Anna Paspala
Third Department of Surgery, National and Kapodistrian University of Athens, Attikon University Hospital, Athens, Greece

Dimitrios Schizas
First Department of Surgery, National and Kapodistrian University of Athens, Laikon General Hospital, Athens, Greece

Chih-Che Lin and Chao-Long Chen
Department of general surgery and liver transplant center, Chang Gung Memorial Hospital, Kaohsiung, Taiwan

Ahmed Mohammed Abdel Aziz Elsarawy
Liver transplant center, Chang Gung Memorial Hospital, Kaohsiung, Taiwan

Andra-Iulia Suceveanu
Faculty of Medicine, Department of Gastroenterology, Emergency Hospital of Constanta, Ovidius University, Constanta, Romania

Laura Mazilu and Andreea-Daniela Gheorghe
Faculty of Medicine, Department of Oncology, Emergency Hospital of Constanta, Ovidius University, Constanta, Romania

Anca Pantea Stoian
University of Medicine and Farmacy, Carol Davila, Department of Diabetes, Nutrition and Metabolic Disease, Bucharest, Romania

Felix Voinea
Faculty of Medicine, Department of Urology, Emergency Hospital of Constanta, Ovidius University, Constanta, Romania

Adrian-Paul Suceveanu
Faculty of Medicine, Department of Internal Medicine, Emergency Hospital of Constanta, Ovidius University, Constanta, Romania

Qun-Ying Su, Xiao-Ying Huang, Jin-Guang Yao, Xue-Min Wu and Bing-Chen Huang
Department of Pathology, The Affiliated Hospital of Youjiang Medical University for Nationalities, Baise, China

Jun Lu and Qiang Xia
Department of Liver Surgery, Renji Hospital, School of Medicine, Shanghai Jiao Tong University, Shanghai, China

Chao Wang
Department of Digestive Medicine, The Affiliated Hospital of Youjiang Medical University for Nationalities, Baise, China

Xi-Dai Long
Department of Pathology, The Affiliated Hospital of Youjiang Medical University for Nationalities, Baise, China
Department of Liver Surgery, Renji Hospital, School of Medicine, Shanghai Jiao Tong University, Shanghai, China
Guangxi Clinic Research Center of Hepatobiliary Diseases, Baise, China

Feiyu Chen, Ning Wang and Yibin Feng
School of Chinese Medicine, Li Ka Shing Faculty of Medicine, The University of Hong Kong, China

Victoria Chagoya de Sánchez, Enrique Chávez, Gabriela Velasco-Loyden, María Guadalupe Lozano-Rosas and Alejandro Rusbel Aparicio-Cadena
Department of Cellular Biology and Development, Institute of Cellular Physiology, National Autonomous University of Mexico, Mexico City, Mexico

Ming Hong, Ning Wang and Yibin Feng
School of Chinese Medicine, Li Ka Shing Faculty of Medicine, The University of Hong Kong, Pok Fu Lam, Hong Kong, China

Stefania Brozzetti, Simone Bini, Leonardo Luca Chiarella and Katia Fazzi
Department of Surgery "Pietro Valdoni", University of Rome La Sapienza, Policlinico Umberto I, Rome, Italy

Michele Di Martino and Mario Bezzi
Department of Radiological Sciences, University of Rome La Sapienza, Policlinico Umberto I, Rome, Italy

Index

www.ingramcontent.com/pod-product-compliance
Lightning Source LLC
LaVergne TN
LVHW081028210926
848485LV00004B/975